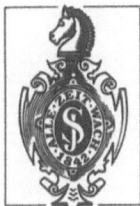

T. Omae, A. Zanchetti (Eds.)

How Should Elderly Hypertensive Patients Be Treated?

Proceedings of Satellite Symposium to the 12th Scientific Meeting of the International Society of Hypertension, May 1988, Kyoto, Japan

With 60 Figures

Springer Japan KK

Dr. TERUO OMAE
Director of Hospital
National Cardiovascular Center Hospital
Suita, Osaka, 565 Japan

Dr. ALBERTO ZANCHETTI
Professor
Centro di Fisiologia Clinica e Ipertensione
Ospedale Maggiore di Milano
Instituto di Clinica Medica IV
Università di Milano
20122 Milan, Italy

The publication of this volume was made possible by a grant from Bayer AG and
Bayer Yakuhin, Ltd.

ISBN 978-4-431-68342-1   ISBN 978-4-431-68340-7 (eBook)
DOI 10.1007/978-4-431-68340-7

Typesetting: Koford Prints (Pte) Ltd., Singapore

Preface

The percentage of the population which is elderly has been increasing steadily in many countries in the world; and as this tendency continues, the question of how to treat the elderly rises in importance. The problem of how to manage hypertension in the elderly has become one of the most important issues in the prevention and treatment of cardiovascular disease. However, not many of the clinical studies performed so far to evaluate the effects of antihypertensive drug treatment have included the elderly. Many important problems remain unsolved. How much beneficial effect can be expected from active antihypertensive drug treatment in the elderly? How can isolated systolic hypertension, which is frequently encountered in the elderly, have better prognosis when treated? When is drug treatment indicated, to what level should blood pressure be reduced and maintained in the elderly, and how should drugs be selected?

The elderly also frequently bear other medical problems, either recognized or unrecognized, such as mental depression, respiratory problems, infection, malignant neoplasms, and water and electrolyte imbalances. The body's ability to eliminate drugs also decreases with age and necessitates modified dosage.

The 12th Scientific Meeting of the International Society of Hypertension held in Kyoto, Japan on May 22–26, 1988 included the satellite symposium. "How Should Elderly Hypertensive Patients Be Treated?" which focused on the pathophysiology and outcome of elderly hypertensive patients. Data presented there on the comparison of morbidity and mortality results in various therapeutic trials involving the elderly have been compiled here to provide a comprehensive guide of elderly hypertensive studies up to date.

TERUO OMAE
ALBERTO ZANCHETTI

List of Contributors

Chairmen

W. BIRKENHÄGER   Department of Medicine, Zuiderziekenhuis
Groene Hilledijk 315, 3075 EA Rotterdam
The Netherlands

C. DOLLERY   Department of Medicine
Royal Postgraduate Medical School
Ducane Road, London W12 ONN, UK

T. OGIHARA   Department of Medicine and Geriatrics
Osaka University Medical School
1-1-50, Fukushima, Fukushima-ku, Osaka
553 Japan

T. OMAE   National Cardiovascular Center
5-7-1, Fujishirodai, Suita, Osaka, 565 Japan

T. OZAWA   Department of Geriatrics
School of Medicine, Kochi Medical School
Kohasu, Oko-cho, Nankoku, Kochi
781-51 Japan

A. ZANCHETTI   Centro di Fisiologia Clinica e Ipertensione
Ospedale Maggiore di Milano, Istituto
di Clinica Medica IV, Universitá di Milano
Via Sforza 35, 20122 Milan, Italy

Speakers

A. AMERY   Hypertension and Cardiovascular Rehabilitation
Unit, University of Leuven
Hérestraat 49, B-3000 Leuven, Belgium

W. BIRKENHÄGER   Department of Medicine, Zuiderziekenhuis
Groene Hilledijk 315, 3075 EA Rotterdam
The Netherlands

C. BULPITT   Division of Geriatric Medicine
                    Hammersmith Hospital
                    Ducane Road, London W12 OHS, UK

C. DOLLERY   Department of Clinical Pharmacology
                    Royal Postgraduate Medical School
                    Ducane Road, London W12 ONN, UK

K. KURAMOTO   Tokyo Metoropolitan Geriatric Hospital
                    35-2, Sakae-cho, Itabashi-ku, Tokyo, 173 Japan

Y. KURIYAMA   Department of Internal Medicine
                    National Cardiovascular Center
                    5-7-1, Fujishirodai, Suita, Osaka, 565 Japan

G. LEONETTI   Istituto Clinica Medica Generale e Terapia
                    Medica, Università di Milano
                    Centro Fisiologia Clinica e Ipertensione
                    Ospendale Maggiore, Via Sforza 35, 20122
                    Milan, Italy

P. LUND-JOHANSEN   Section of Cardiology, Medical Department
                    University of Bergen
                    Haukeland Hospital, N-5016, Bergen, Norway

K. UEDA   School of Health Science, Kyushu University
                    3-1-1, Maidashi, Higashi-ku, Fukuoka, 812 Japan

P. WEIDMANN   Medizinische Poliklinik, University of Berne
                    Freiburgstrasse 3, CH-3010 Berne, Switzerland

Poster Presentaters

R. CARRETTA   Instituto di Patologia Medica dell Universita
                    c/o Dspedale di Cattinara, 34149 Trieste, Italy

R. JANSEN   Division of General Internal Medicine
                    University Hospital Nijmegen
                    Geert Grooteplein Zuid 8, P.O. Box 9101, 6500
                    HB Nijmegen, The Netherlands

A. KAWAMOTO   Department of Medicine and Geriatrics
                    Kochi Medical School
                    Kohasu, Oko-cho, Nankoku, Kochi, 781–51 Japan

F. LATTANZI   Instituto di Fisiologia Clinica del C.N.R.
                    Universita di Pisa
                    Via P. Savi 8, 56100 Pisa, Italy

P. LIJNEN   Hypertension Unit, Campus Gasthuisberg
                    Herestraat 49, B-3000 Leuven, Belgium

H. MIKAMI   Department of Medicine and Geriatrics
                   Osaka University Medical School
                   1-1-50, Fukushima, Fukushima-ku, Osaka
                   533 Japan

M. NAKAMARU   Department of Medicine and Geriatrics
                   Osaka University Medical School
                   1-1-50, Fukushima, Fukushima-ku, Osaka
                   533 Japan

S. NOVO   Institute of Clinical Medicine
                   University of Palermo
                   Viale delle Alpi 86, 90144 Palermo, Italy

A. NOZAWA   The 2nd Department of Internal Medicine
                   Sapporo Medical College
                   S-1, W-16, Chuo-ku, Sapporo, 060 Japan

T. OSHIMA   First Department of Internal Medicine
                   Hiroshima University School of Medicine
                   1-2-3, Kasumi, Minami-ku, Hiroshima, 734 Japan

M. PETITTO   Section of Cardioangiology, II Medical School
                   Naples University
                   II Traversa T. De Amicis No. 51, 80145 Napoli
                   Italy

J. PROBSTFIELD   Clinical Trials Branch, DECA-NHLBI
                   Federal Bldg. 5C-10, 7550 Wisconsin Avenue
                   Bethesda, MD 20892, USA

J. ROSENFELD   Hypertension Clinic, Beilinson Medical Center
                   Petah Tikva 49100, Israel

T. ROSENTHAL   Hypertension Unit
                   Tel Aviv University Medical School
                   The Chaim Sheba Medical Center
                   Tel Hashomer, 52621 Israel

M. SAFAR   Centre de Diagnostic, Hopital Broussais
                   96 rue Didot, 75674 Paris Cedex 14, France

E. TAIOLI   Instituto di Ricerche Farmacologiche
                   "Mario Negri"
                   Via Eritrea 62, 20157 Milan, Italy

Table of Contents

Session 1

Morbidity and Mortality of Elderly Hypertensives: Results from the
Long-Term Prospective Study in Hisayama, a Japanese Community
K. UEDA, T. OMAE, Y. HASUO, M. FUJISHIMA 3

Discussion 15

Hypertension in the Elderly
A. AMERY, J. STAESSEN, R. FAGARD, R. VAN HOOF 17

Discussion 31

Clinical Pharmacological Considerations in the Treatment of
Hypertension in the Elderly
C.M. NEWMAN, C.T. DOLLERY 33

Discussion 47

Session 2

Hemodynamics in Treatment with Calcium Antagonists
P. LUND-JOHANSEN, P. OMVIK 53

Discussion 67

Antihypertensive Drugs and Cerebral Circulation
Y. KURIYAMA, T. SAWADA, T. OMAE 69

Discussion 83

Treatment of the Hypertensive Diabetic: Focus on Calcium
Channel Blockade
P. WEIDMANN, B.N. TROST, P. FERRARI 85

Discussion 101

Calcium Antagonists in Combination Therapy
G. LEONETTI, A ZANCHETTI 103

Discussion 111

Posters

Prevalence, Treatment, and Control of Hypertension in the
Elderly: Study on Blood Pressure in Elderly Outpatients (SPAA)
E. TAIOLI, C. ALLI, F. AVANZINI, G. BETTELLI, F. COLOMBO,
R. CORSO, M.A. DEVOTO, M. DI TULLIO, R. MARCHIOLI,
G. MARIOTTI, M. RADICE, G. TOGNONI, M. VILLELLA,
A. ZUSSINO 117

Comparison of Cardiovascular Regulatory Functions in Elderly
Hypertensive Patients and Normal Elderly Subjects
A. KAWAMOTO, K. SHIMADA, K. MATSUBAYASHI,
T. CHIKAMORI, O. KUZUME, H. ISHIDA, H. OGURA,
T. OZAWA 123

Role of Dipyridamole-Echocardiography Tests in the Diagnosis of
Coronary Artery Disease in Hypertensives
F. LATTANZI, A.R. LUCARINI, E. PICANO, S. SEVERI, E. ORSINI,
A. DISTANTE, A. SALVETTI, A. L'ABBATE 127

The Systolic Hypertension in the Elderly Program (SHEP):
Rationale, Design, Recruitment, and Baseline Data
J.L. PROBSTFIELD, W.B. APPLEGATE, J.D. CURB, N.O. BORHANI,
C.M. HAWKINS, J.A. CUTLER, B.R. DAVIS, C.D. FURBERG,
E. LAKATOS, L.B. PAGE, H.M. PERRY, JR., W. MCFATE SMITH 135

Antihypertensive Therapy with Uncontrolled Systolic Pressure
and Increased Aortic Rigidity
M.E. SAFAR, PH.L. SOUBIES, A.M. SAFAVIAN, R.G. ASMER,
ST. LAURENT 143

Role of Intracellular Free Calcium in the Hypotensive Response
to Nifedipine
T. OSHIMA, H. MATSUURA, K. MATSUMOTO, K. KIDO,
T. OTSUKI, T. SHINGU, I. INOUE, G. KAJIYAMA 151

Determinants of the Hypotensive Action of Nitrendipine and
Atenolol in African Black Patients
P. LIJNEN, J.R. M'BUYAMBA-KABANGU, B. LEPIRA,
R. FAGARD, A. AMERY 157

The Role of Renal Calcium Handling in the Hypotensive
Response to Long-Term Nifedipine Administration in Essential
Hypertensives
A. NOZAWA, K. KIKUCHI, T. HASEGAWA, H. KOMURA,
S. SUZUKI, N. SATO, T. OHTOMO, T. TAKADA, O. IIMURA 171

Ventricular Function in Elderly Hypertensive Patients:
A Radionuclide Assessment
M. PETITTO, V. LIGUORI, S. DI SOMMA, C. MAGNOTTA,
M. AUSIELLO, M. GALDERISI, M. BRIGNOLI, O. DE DIVITIIS 177

Distensibility of Large Arteries in Elderly Hypertensive Patients
After Chronic Treatment with Nicardipine SR
R. CARRETTA, M. BARDELLI, S. MUIESAN, F. VRAN, B. FABRIS,
F. FISCHETTI, L. CAMPANACCI 183

Effects of Nifedipine on Blood Pressure, Arterial Compliance and
Left Ventricular Mass in Elderly Patients with Isolated Systolic
Hypertension
S. NOVO, E. NARDI, G. NOTO, G. LICATA, A. STRANO 189

Long-Term (12-Month) Antihypertensive, Metabolic, and Renal
Hemodynamic Effects of Nifedipine and Nisoldipine
C. WITTENBERG, J.B. ROSENFELD 197

Long-Term Hemodynamic and Metabolic Effects of Nitrendipine
Vs Hydrochlorothiazide in Hypertensive Patients over 70 Years
of Age
R.W.M.M. JANSEN, H.J.J. VAN LIER, W.H.L. HOEFNAGELS 205

Complications and the Choice of Antihypertensive Drugs in
the Elderly
M. NAKAMARU, T. OGIHARA, H. MIKAMI, F. MASUGI,
J. HIGAKI, A. OTSUKA, T. HATA, Y. KUMAHARA 213

Quality of Life in the Treatment of Hypertension in the Elderly
H. MIKAMI, T. OGIHARA, M. NAKAMARU, F. MASUGI,
J. HIGAKI, A. OTSUKA, T. HATA, Y. KUMAHARA 219

Nisoldipine: A Replacement Therapy for Nifedipine and Other
Vasodilators in the Treatment of Moderate to Severe Hypertension
A. SHAMISS, E. GROSSMAN, M. BURSZTYN, T. ROSENTHAL 227

Panel Discussion

Concept of Antihypertensive Treatment in the Elderly 235

Author Index 247

Key Word Index 249

Session 1

Chairmen: C. Dollery (London)
T. Ozawa (Kochi)

Morbidity and Mortality of Elderly Hypertensives: Results from the Long-Term Prospective Study in Hisayama, a Japanese Community

Kazuo Ueda[1, 2], Teruo Omae[3], Yutaka Hasuo[1], and Masatoshi Fujishima[1]

Summary. The long-term prognosis and outcome study of elderly hypertensives was based on the 20-year prospective population survey conducted in a Japanese rural community, Hisayama; and the results were compared with those for younger subjects. The survival curves for the study population which were related to blood pressure levels decreased with the elevation of either systolic or diastolic pressure in both the younger and elderly groups. The survival curves decreased markedly beyond the 160 mmHg boundary for systolic pressure or the 100 mmHg boundary for diastolic pressure for those aged 40–59 years. There was however, no cut-off level for increased mortality in either systolic or diastolic pressure for those aged 60 or over. Mortality from stroke or heart disease was higher in diastolic or systolic hypertensives than in normotensives for the aged. However, the relative risk of death by stroke in either hypertensive group was attenuated compared to that for the younger subjects. Intracerebral hemorrhage and cerebral infarction occurred more frequently in diastolic hypertensives for both younger and elderly subjects, even though the imbalance of frequency in age, sex, electrocardiographic abnormalities and diabetes mellitus was corrected by Cox's Proportional hazard model. Systolic hypertension was strongly related to cerebral infarction in the aged and to myocardial infarction in both younger and elderly persons.

Key words: Elderly hypertension — Survival curves — Stroke — Myocardial infarction — Hisayama study

Introduction

To decide how elderly hypertensives should be treated, it is necessary to know the prognosis or outcome of different treatments of elderly persons in association with blood pressure levels. A long-term prognosis for hypertensives can be elucidated from several aspects. Firstly, an estimation of the life span for each individual in relation to blood pressure levels is a crucial procedure in determining the risk of hypertension. How hypertension influences an individual's survival should, however, be considered in proportion, since many factors might have an effect on life

[1] Second Department of Internal Medicine, Faculty of Medicine, Kyushu University, Fukuoka, Japan
[2] School of Health Science, Kyushu University, Fukuoka, Japan
[3] National Cardiovascular Center, Osaka, Japan

expectancy. Secondly, it is worth comparing morbidity and mortality from cardio-vascular disease between hypertensives and nonhypertensives. Hypertension has long been recognised as a major precursor of cardiovascular disease. Many risk factors other than hypertension could be associated with the development of cardiovascular disease; thus, they must be taken into consideration together with hypertension. In addition, superimposed conditions due to various degenerative factors on the normal aging processes may have great impact on the prognoses for elderly subjects.

In this paper, a long-term prognosis of elderly hypertensives is made on the basis of the prospective population survey conducted in the Japanese rural community, Hisayama. We initially examined the influence of systolic or diastolic pressure on total or cardiovascular mortality (taking other relevant risk factors into account), and then compared the results between those age 40–59 years and those 60 years or over. Secondly, the risk of death or the occurrence of cerebral stroke or heart disease is compared among blood pressure groups (diastolic, systolic, borderline hyperten-sive, and normotensive) in both the younger and elderly subjects.

Materials and Methods

The Hisayama prospective population study was initiated in 1961 to explore the epi-demiology of cardiovascular disease in a general population sample of 1 621 men and women age 40 years or older at entry. The subjects comprised about 90% of all the residents in this age group in the town of Hisayama. At entry, the following infor-mation was collected: medical or life history, a physical examination including anthropometric and blood pressure measurements, urinalysis for protein and sugar, electrocardiogram (ECG), findings of ocular fundi, and serum total cholesterol determination. In addition, the oral glucose tolerance test was performed on subjects who were found to have glycosuria, and consequently persons with diabetes mellitus (DM) were identified according to defined criteria [1]. Blood pressures were mea-sured 4 times in supine position of the standard sphygmomanometer after 5 min rest. The average value of the 3 consecutive readings from second to fourth was taken as an individual's blood pressure, on account of the variability of the first mea-surement.

Follow-up was complete, with only 0.1% of the sample lost during the 20-year period of follow-up. An outstanding feature of this study was that causes of death were verified by autopsy in more than 80% of the deceased. The autopsy rate for 20 years was 82.4%. Details of methods of examination and follow-up have been described elsewhere [1–5].

During the course of the prospective study, subjects who died of any cause, those who died of cardiovascular disease, and those who suffered cerebral stroke or myo-cardial infarction were analyzed in relation to blood pressure at the initial examina-tion. Cardiovascular diseases included all types of cerebral, stroke, coronary heart disease (CHD), congestive heart failure (CHF), and atherosclerotic disease, such as ruptured aortic aneurysum or intermittent claudication. The definition of systolic hypertension is diastolic pressure less than 95 mmHg and systolic pressure 160 mmHg or greater; diastolic pressure greater than or equal to 95 mmHg constitutes diastolic hypertension. In addition, subjects whose systolic pressure between 90 and 94 mmHg were defined as borderline hypertensives. The remainder were considered normotensives (WHO criteria [6]). To elucidate the net effect of hypertension while taking other relevant risk factors into account, Cox's proportional hazard model [7] was used to assess the relative influence of high blood pressure on the time-to-response incidence or mortality from cardiovascular disease, in which a couple of variables other than blood pressure components were controlled. The comparison among blood pressure groups with respect to the frequency of risk factors was tested by Mantel-Haenszel's chi-squared test, taking the imbalance in age and sex distribution into account [8].

Results

Survival curves for the cohort population according to systolic pressure levels were studied by Cox's proportional hazard model for those aged 40–59 and for those 60 or over. Subjects were divided into 5 groups at 20 mmHg intervals of systolic pressure, and the survival rate for each group was calculated after age and sex were controlled. Survival curves by each systolic pressure level for those 40–59 years are depicted in Fig. 1, and for those 60 years or over in Fig. 2. Survival curves tended to drop with the elevation of systolic pressure irrespective of age. However, there was a slight difference between the younger and elderly groups. For those aged 40–59, a clear distinction in decreasing survival rates was observed between those with systolic pressure over 160 mmHg and those below, especially in the later period of the follow-up (Fig. 1). On the other hand, the survival curve for those with systolic pressure of 140

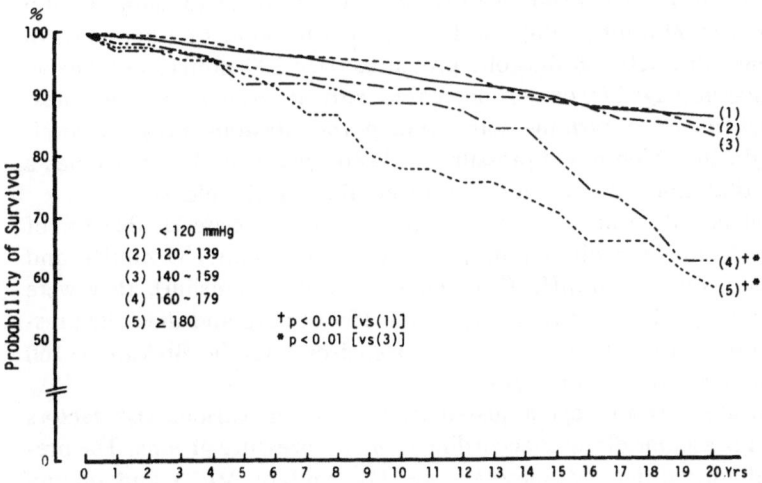

Fig. 1. Survival rate by systolic blood pressure levels using Cox's proportional hazard model (M and F; 40–50 years) in Hisayama

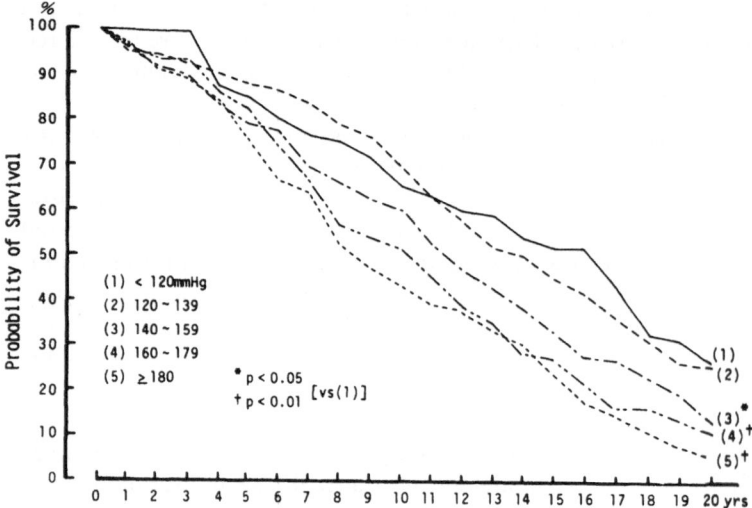

Fig. 2. Survival rate by systolic blood pressure levels using Cox's proportional hazard model (M and F; ≥ 60 years) in Hisayama

mmHg or over dropped significantly compared to that for those with systolic pressure of less than 120 mmHg. However, there was no cutoff point of systolic pressure beyond which survival curves dropped remarkably in the elderly group (Fig. 2).

A similar analysis was applied to diastolic pressure levels with a 10 mmHg interval. For the younger subjects, aged 40–59, survival curves for those with diastolic pressure of 100 mmHg or more fell significantly compared to those for subjects with diastolic pressure below 80 mmHg (Fig. 3). This seemed to point to a boundary of reduction in survival rates between diastolic pressures over 100 mmHg and below. Survival rates in the group aged 60 or over decreased with elevation of diastolic pressure, but there was no clear turning point among the diastolic pressure levels (Fig. 4). It is thought that high blood pressure for both systolic and diastolic has a greater impact on total mortality in younger subjects than in the elderly.

Subjects were divided into 4 blood pressure groups by WHO criteria. Because of the small number of subjects with systolic pressure greater than 159 mmHg and diastolic pressure less than 90 mmHg (isolated systolic hypertension), they were included in those with systolic pressure greater than 159 mmHg and diastolic pressure between 90 and 94 mmHg as systolic hypertensives (systolic pressure ≥ 160 mmHg and diastolic pressure < 95 mmHg).

Table 1 demonstrates sex-and age-adjusted frequencies in various risk factors associated with cardiovascular diseases according to blood pressure groups. The prevalence of ECG abnormalities (Minnesota code III_1 and/or VI_{1-3}) and obesity increased progressively in the order of normotension, borderline, systolic, and diastolic hypertension for those aged 40–59. The frequency of DM also tended to

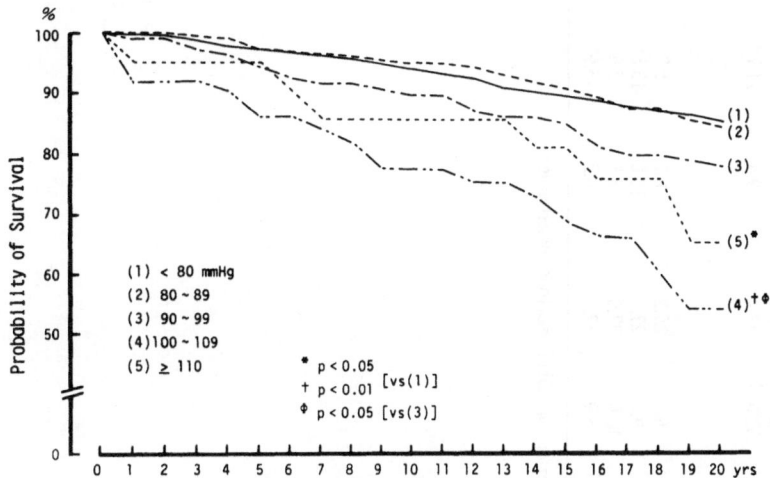

Fig. 3. Survival rate by diastolic blood pressure levels using Cox's proportional hazard model (M and F; 40–59 years) in Hisayama

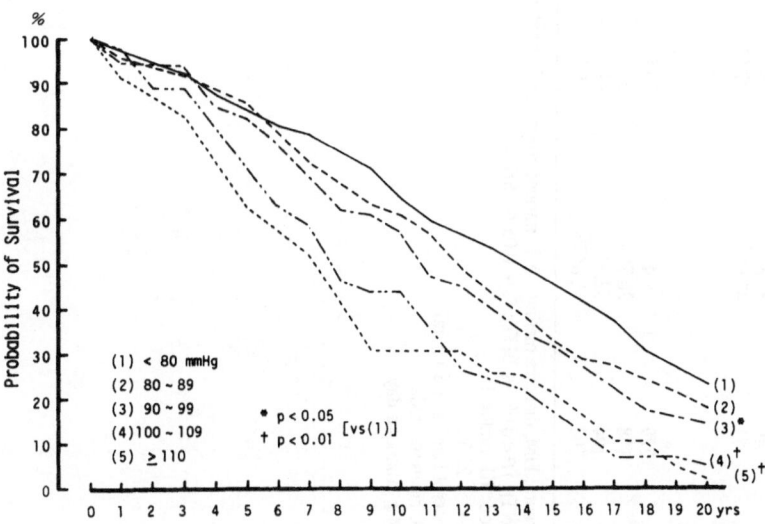

Fig. 4. Survival rate by diastolic blood pressure levels using Cox's proportional hazard model (M and F; ≥60 years) in Hisayama

Table 1. Frequency (%) of risk factors by blood-pressure groups (M and F; Hisayama, 1961)

Age and BP group	No. of subjects	E C G abnormalities[a]	Ocular fundi ≥ K W II	Proteinuria	DM	Obesity[b]	Hypercholesterolemia[c]	Smoking[d]	Drinking[e]
(40–59 years)									
N T	780	11.8	13.8	4.3	3.7	6.5	22.3	12.8	10.3
BHT	139	17.0	15.0	7.5	9.5*	13.1*	28.1	15.4	19.5*
SHT	40	33.8*†	18.8	14.2*	23.6*†	16.2	22.3	17.9	18.2
DHT	71	47.9*§	27.5*	9.8	18.7*	32.0*†	27.4	9.4	21.7*
(60+ years)									
NT	229	9.4	30.8	9.1	6.3	6.5	25.2	8.2	5.7
BHT	158	20.7*	35.8	9.4	8.8	9.8	27.6	11.0	13.8*
SHT	104	32.3*	41.6	19.7*†	13.3*	10.0	27.0	3.3	5.9
DHT	100	48.6*†§	50.7*	25.6*†	19.7*†	5.9	32.9	6.3	13.9*

BP, blood pressure; DM, diabetes mellitus; NT, normotension; BHT, borderline hypertension; SHT, systolic hypertension; DHT, diastolic hypertension

* $P<0.05$ (vs NT); † $P<0.05$ (vs BHT); § $P<0.05$ (vs SHT)

[a] Minnesota Code III, and/or IV$_{1,3}$

[b] Quetelet index > 25.3

[c] Plasma cholesterol level ≥ 1.8 mg/ml

[d] More than 10 cigarettes a day

[e] More than 34 g ethanol a day

Table 2. Average anual mortality from major diseases by blood pressure groups using Cox's proportional hazard model (M and F; Hisayama, 1961–81)

Age and blood pressure group	No. of subjects	Stroke	Heart disease	Malignant neoplasms
(40–59 years)				
NT	780	0.9 (1.0)	0.9 (1.0)	2.6 (1.0)
BHT	139	2.1 (2.3)	1.1. (1.2)	2.1 (0.8)
SHT	40	6.9 (7.7)[†]	1.9 (2.1)	4.5 (1.7)
DHT	71	9.3 (10.3)[†]	1.5 (1.7)	2.2 (0.8)
(60 + years)				
NT	229	7.0 (1.0)	4.7 (1.0)	15.8 (1.0)
BHT	158	16.4 (2.3)[†]	11.0 (2.3)[†]	12.2 (0.8)
SHT	104	22.6 (3.2)[†]	17.6 (3.7)[†]	8.5 (0.5)
DHT	100	14.4 (2.1)[†]	22.4 (4.8)[†]	19.4 (1.2)

Rate per 1000 years; ( ) relative risk
NT, normotension; BHT, borderline hypertension; SHT, systolic hypertension;
DHT, diastolic hypertension
[†]$P < 0.01$ (vs NT)
Age, sex, ECG abnormalities, and DM were corrected.

increase with the elevation of blood pressure, but was the highest in systolic hypertensives. For those aged 60 or over, ECG abnormalities, proteinuria, and DM increased in frequency in the same order; and ocular fundi $\geq$ KW II was most frequently observed in diastolic hypertensives.

Table 2 shows the average annual mortality from 3 major causes of death over the 20-year follow-up by blood pressure groups, representing the relative risk for the diastolic, systolic, or borderline hypertensive group as compared to the normotensive group. Mortality was calculated after controlling the imbalance of distribution of age, sex, ECG abnormalities, and DM in each group by the proportional hazard model. For those aged 40–59, mortality from cerebral stroke was about 8 times higher in systolic hypertensives and 10 times higher in diastolic hypertensives than in normotensives. Mortality from cerebral stroke was also significantly higher in borderline, systolic, and diastolic hypertensives than in normotensives for those aged 60 or over, but the relative risk to normotensives ranged between 2.0 and 3.0, approaching a lesser degree. Deaths by heart disease for elderly subjects occurred more in borderline, systolic, or diastolic hypertensives than in normotensives with a relative risk of 2.0–5.0. Deaths caused by malignant neoplasms increased in the elderly group irrespective of blood pressure levels, and there was no close relationship between mortality from malignant neoplasms and blood pressure for either age group.

Table 3 presents the relative risk of occurrence of 3 main cardiovascular diseases calculated after age, sex, ECG abnormalities, and DM were controlled by the proportional hazard model. For the younger age group, diastolic hypertension was

Table 3. Average annual incidence of intracerebral hemorrhage, cerebral infarction, and myocardial infarction by blood pressure groups using Cox's proportional hazard model (M and F; Hisayama, 1961–81)

Age and blood pressure group	No. of subjects	ICH	CI	MI
(40–59 years)				
NT	780	0.7 (1.0)	1.9 (1.0)	0.8 (1.0)
BHT	139	1.7 (2.4)	4.1 (2.2)*	0.6 (0.8)
SHT	40	2.3 (3.3)	4.0 (2.1)	3.5 (4.4)*
DHT	71	6.3 (9.0)†	9.2 (4.8)†	0.9 (1.1)
(60+ years)				
NT	229	1.1 (1.0)	11.6 (1.0)	1.5 (1.0)
BHT	158	1.5 (1.4)	17.5 (1.5)	5.3 (3.5)*
SHT	104	2.1 (1.9)	26.9 (2.3)†	10.0 (6.7)†
DHT	100	3.7 (3.4)*	17.0 (1.5)*	9.3 (6.2)†

Rate per 1000 years; ( ) relative risk
ICH, intracerebral hemorrhage; CI, cerebral infarction; MI, myocardial infarction;
NT, normotension; BHT, borderline hypertension; SHT, systolic hypertension;
DHT, diastolic hypertension
†$P<0.01$ (vs NT); *$P<0.05$ (vs NT)
Age, sex, ECG abnormalities, and DM were corrected.

strongly related to both intracerebral hemorrhage and cerebral infarction, with the relative risks being 9.0 and 4.8, respectively. Myocardial infarction was 4 times more frequent in systolic hypertensives than in normotensives for those aged 40–59. Meanwhile, intracerebral hemorrhage was 3 times more frequent in diastolic hypertensives than in normotensives, and both cerebral infarction and myocardial infarction more frequently occurred in systolic or diastolic hypertensives than in normotensives for those aged 60 or over. Also, the relative risk to systolic or diastolic hypertensives of myocardial infarction rather than cerebral infarction was much greater.

To examine the combined effect of hypertension with other risk factors, namely, cigarette smoking, hypercholesterolemia, and DM, on the occurrence of myocardial infarction, subjects were divided into low-and high-risk classes within each category of the 4 blood pressure groups (Table 4). For those aged 40–59, myocardial infarction most frequently occurred in systolic hypertensives, and more frequently in high-risk groups with respect to smoking and cholesterol than in low-risk groups; although there was little statistical difference because of the small number of cases. Myocardial infarction was also most frequently observed in systolic hypertensives for those aged 60 or over, but a higher incidence was seen only in the higher stratum for cholesterol in a comparison between high-and low-risk groups. When diastolic hypertensives, however, and smoking habits of more than 10 cigarettes a day, a cholesterol level greater than 1.8 mg/ml, or DM, the frequency of myocardial infarction significantly increased compared to normotensives with low-risk levels. There-

Table 4. Average annual incidence of myocardial infarction by blood pressure groups and 3 main risk factors (M and F; Hisayama, 1961–81)

Age and blood pressure group	Smoking		Cholesterol		DM	
	< 10[a]	≥ 10[a]	< 1.8 mg/ml	≥ 1.8 mg/ml	(−)	(+)
(40–59 years)						
NT	0.7	2.4	0.4	2.4	0.8	1.5
BHT	1.0	—	0.4	1.9	0.9	—
SHT	2.3	13.4	2.6	6.7	4.8*	—
DHT	1.1	—	—	4.5	1.0	—
(60+ years)						
NT	0.8	—	0.6	0.7	0.9	—
BHT	3.5*	—	4.4†	—	3.0	3.4
SHT	5.0†	—	4.5†	7.6	6.1†	—
DHT	3.1	10.2§	3.1†	3.4§Φ	2.0	8.8§

Rate per 1000 years
NT, normotension; BHT, borderline hypertension; SHT, systolic hypertension; DHT, diastolic hypertension
*$P<0.05$; †$P<0.01$ (vs NT with low risk); §$P<0.01$ (vs NT with low risk);
Φ$P<001$ (vs NT with high risk) using Mantel-Haenszel X^2
Age and sex were corrected.
[a] Cigarettes smoked per day.

fore, systolic hypertension can be considered to bear a risk of myocardial infarction for both the younger and elderly subjects, while diastolic hypertension for the elderly bears a risk of myocardial infarction, sustained by the contribution of other relevant risk factors.

Discussion

Blood pressure is a continuous variable, and the risk of morbidity and mortality increases in relation to pressure — there being no clear cutoff point for increased risk [9]. In the present study, however, there would be a clear boundary for an increased risk of death at systolic pressure of 160 mmHg or greater and at diastolic pressure of 100 mmHg or greater for those aged 40–59. For subjects aged 60 or over, systolic pressure of 160 mmHg or greater and diastolic pressure of 100 mmHg or more could indicate an increasing risk of mortality. However, the distinguishing line between high-and low-risk groups was less clear than that in the younger subjects. This may be partially explicable by the fact that the aging process, especially atherosclerotic changes, can have a relatively large effect on an individual's life span in the aged even for subjects with low blood pressure. At the same time, hypertension aggravates atherosclerosis and is the leading risk factor for cardiovascular diseases, especially thrombotic stroke and CHD. The majority of diastolic hypertension in the elderly possibly developed in middle age and might have persisted into later years, since elderly hypertensives frequently have hypertensive organ damage, which is considered evidence of long-term persistence of hypertension [10].

The Framingham data [9] clearly demonstrate the increased risk of cardiovascular disease associated with an increasing level of systolic pressure, especially for men over 50 years. Limited prospective information is available on mortality and morbidity among elderly individuals who have systolic hypertension [11, 12]. The risk of death due to all causes or cardiovascular disease was higher in individuals with systolic hypertension than in controls with blood pressure below 140/90 mmHg or in those with systolic pressure of 180 mmHg or more than in subjects with systolic pressure less than 160 mmHg. The incidence of stroke was 2.5–3.0 times higher in systolic hypertensives than in normotensives. In the present study, the risk of death due to stroke was 3 times greater in systolic hypertensives than in normotensives for those aged 60 or over. However, that for subjects aged 40–59 was 7.7 times greater in systolic hypertensives than in normotensives, although stroke mortality was more related to diastolic hypertension for younger subjects. This result was probably due to the higher incidence of intracerebral hemorrhage in diastolic hypertensives for those aged 40–59, and to that of cerebral infarction in systolic hypertensives for both groups aged 40–59 and 60 or over. Meanwhile, deaths due to heart diseases were 3.7 times greater in systolic and 4.8 times in diastolic hypertensives than in normotensives for those aged 60 or over. However, fatal or nonfatal myocardial infarction most frequently occurred in systolic hypertensives for both younger and elderly persons. Since systolic hypertension in the elderly is more or less associated in its etiology with the decreasing distensibility of the aorta due to atherosclerosis, systolic hypertension can be considered a form of existing systemic atherosclerosis.

Other reports [13, 14] revealed that pharmacological treatment of elderly hypertensives was effective for reducing cardiovascular mortality and stroke incidence, but less effective for reduction in CHD. Among prospective studies, only 1 report [11] showed that myocardial infarction occurred twice as frequently in those with elevated systolic pressure. In the present study, myocardial infarction for the elderly was associated with systolic hypertension alone, and tobacco smoking or DM did not accelerate the risk of myocardial infarction.

On the other hand, diastolic hypertension increased the risk of myocardial infarction with coexisting relevant risk factors. This suggests that systolic hypertension alone can have a more powerful impact on mycardial infarction in the aged, since myocardial infarction was almost equally found in both systolic and diastolic hypertension for those aged 60 or over.

It may be possible, however, that there is a racial difference in the type of cardiovascular disease. For example, a less frequent incidence of CHD and a more frequent incidence of stroke are observed among the Japanese population compared to that of the United States. In the Hisayama study, risk factors for myocardial infarction are somewhat different from those observed in the community studies of the United States. Namely, serum total cholesterol is less related [15]. In the present study, hypercholesterolemia was defined in those with a serum total cholesterol level of more than or equal to 1.8 mg/m — a much lower level than in the other study [9]. Nonetheless, hypercholesterolemia seemed likely to increase the risk of myocardial infarction in systolic hypertensives for both the younger and elderly subjects. This evidence is considered important, since the cholesterol level for the present-day Japanese population is expected to increase due to dietary or nutritional changes [5]. From the findings in the present study, it can be unequivocally stated that hypertension in the elderly is an important risk factor for cardiovascular disease due to atherosclerosis.

Acknowledgments. This research was supported in part by Research Grants for Cardiovascular Disease from the Ministry of Health and Welfare, Japan; facilitated by the Japan-U.S. Cooperative Agreement in the Cardiovascular Area by the Japanese National Cardiovascular Center and the National Heart, Lung, and Blood Institute, USA.

References

1. Omae T, Ueda K (1983) Diabetic nephropathy in a general adult population of Hisayama, Japan. In: Abe H, Hoshi M (eds) Diabetic microangiopathy. University of Tokyo Press, Tokyo, pp 317-328
2. Omae T, Ueda K, Kikumura T, Shikata T, Fujii I, Yanai T, Hasuo Y (1981) Cardiovascular deaths among hypertensive subjects of middle to old age: a long-term follow-up study in a Japanese community. In: Onesti G, Kim KE (eds) Hypertension in the young and old. Grune and Stratton, New York, pp 285-297
3. Ueda K, Omae T, Hirota Y, Takeshita M, Katsuki S, Tanaka K, Enjoji M (1981) Decreasing trend in incidence and mortality from stroke in Hisayama residents, Japan. Stroke 12: 154-160
4. Omae T, Ueda K (1982) Risk factors of cerebral stroke in Japan: Prospective epidemiological study in Hisayama community. In: Katsuki S, Tsubaki T, Toyokura Y (eds) Proceedings of 12th world congress of neurology. Excerpta Medica, Amsterdam, pp 119-135
5. Ueda K, Omae T (1985) Control of hypertension in a Japanese community. In: Bulpitt CJ (ed) Handbook of hypertension, vol 6. Epidemiology of hypertension. Elsevier, Amsterdam, pp 412-423
6. WHO (1987) Arterial hypertension. WHO technical report series no 628
7. Cox DR (1972) Regression model and life table. J Stat Soc 34: B187-B220
8. Mantel N, Haenszel W (1959) Statistical aspects of the analysis of data from retrospective studies of disease. J Natl Cancer Inst 22: 719-748
9. Kannel WB, Dawber TR, McGee DL (1980) Perspective systolic hypertension: the Framingham study. Circulation 61: 1179-1182
10. Omae T, Ueda K (1985) Epidemiological implications of blood pressure levels and changes in a Japanese population. Invited symposia of the 13 international congress of gerontology, New York (unpublished work)
11. Colandrea MA, Friedman GD, Nichman MZ, Lynd CN (1970) Systolic hypertension in the elderly: an epidemiological assessment. Circulation 41: 239-245
12. Dyer AR, Stamler J, Shekelle RB, Schoenberger JA, Farinaro E (1977) Hypertension in the elderly. Med Clin North Am 61: 513-529
13. European Working Party on High Blood Pressure in the Elderly (1985) Mortality and morbidity results from the European working party on high blood pressure in the elderly trial. Lancet 1: 1349-1354
14. Coope J, Warrender TS (1986) Randomised trial of treatment of hypertension in elderly patients in primary care. Br Med J 293: 1145-1151
15. Omae T, Ueda K (1983) Hypertension and other risk factors in cardiovascular diseases: the Hisayama study. In: Proceedings of two important symposia at the 8th Asian Pacific congress of cardiology. Excerpta Medica, Amsterdam, pp 12-19

Discussion

Dollery (London): Thank you very much, Professor Ueda. It is extremely interesting to have this data from Japan. I think we have time for about 2 questions.

Birkenhäger (Rotterdam): I think you ought to be congratulated together with Professor Omae on this unique study. I was particularly amazed to see that you had an autopsy rate of 82.4%, and, if I remember correctly, the Framingham group had no more than 25% on the record. So, you really know what you are talking about, whilst the Framingham people do not. Could you tell us how to achieve similar autopsy rates outside Kyushu? What is the secret of this high rate of autopsies?

Ueda (Fukuoka): I am not sure. This is just my data. But there would be no study with a high autopsy rate throughout Japan except for the Hisayama study.

Birkenhäger: You know, Professor Omae once confided to me that you had a Buddhist priest going around the rural population telling them that it was for their benefit to be autopsied. Would that be correct?

Ueda: That is correct.

Dollery: I am not sure that is a proper question!
   I think it is particularly interesting, Professor Ueda, to see this data on myocardial infarction, because myocardial infarction is a much less common event in Japan than it is in Europe or North America. Yet, you showed this very steep gradient in the elderly of the risk of myocardial infarction with blood pressure. I am not sure that I was able to dissect from your data what the influence of smoking was, but were there very few smokers in the older age group?

Ueda: The prevalence of smokers was almost 70% for the whole population — that is for males. So, we compared the prevalence of tobacco smokers during the study period. Unfortunately, the frequency did not decrease. So, I am not sure how tobacco smoking can contribute to the incidence of myocardial infarction. I suppose since among the Japanese the cholesterol level is not so high — an average of 1.8 mg/ml — this may be one of the reasons why myocardial infarction is not so prevalent among the Japanese.

Dollery: I think those of us in the West feel it is all the fish you eat that protects you from myocardial infarction! Well, thank you very much indeed, and we will all look forward to reading that paper in time.

Hypertension in the Elderly

A. AMERY, J. STAESSEN, R. FAGARD, and R. VAN HOOF[1]

Summary. The different intervention trials in elderly hypertensives are compatible with the hypothesis that hypotensive drug treatment can decrease cardiovascular mortality mainly by decreasing cerebrovascular mortality. A decrease in fatal and nonfatal cardiovascular event rate is mainly due to a decrease in cerebrovascular events. It is not established whether the hypotensive drug treatment is advisable in (1) symptomless patients with isolated systolic hypertension and (2) patients with uncomplicated hypertension over age 80. Sudden reduction in blood pressure should be avoided, but whether a progressive reduction of the systolic blood pressure below 140 mmHg and of diastolic blood pressure below 85 mmHg is dangerous or advantageous remains to be established.

Key words: Hypertension — Elderly — Antihypertensive therapy — Mortality — Epidemiology

Introduction

This paper will discuss the following topics:
1. The influence of antihypertensive therapy on morbidity and mortality observed in the trial of The European Working Party on High Blood Pressure in the Elderly (EWPHE).
2. Is the Influence of treatment on morbidity and mortality different in the various trials in elderly hypertensives?
3. Why is there a clear decrease in cerebrovascular events, but not in coronary event rate, in treated elderly hypertensives?
4. Could antihypertensive drug therapy be dangerous in certain subgroups of elderly hypertensive patients?

[1] Hypertension and Cardiovascular Rehabilitation Unit, Department of Pathophysiology, University of Leuven, Belgium

The European Working Party on High Blood Pressure in the Elderly Trial

Design of the Trial

The European Working Party on High Blood Pressure conducted a placebo-controlled double-blind trial in 840 patients from 18 centers in 10 European countries to assess the effects of antihypertensive drug treatment in patients aged 60 and above [1, 2].

Elderly hypertensive patients were admitted to the trial if they fulfilled certain criteria during a single-blind run-in period on placebo with a duration of at least 1 month, during which the patients were examined on at least 3 separate occasions. The inclusion criteria were: (1) age 60 years or more at admission to the study; (2) a sitting blood pressure on placebo during the run-in period within the limits 160–239 mmHg for systolic and 90–119 mmHg for diastolic pressure; and (3) the patient's willingness to give informed consent. The exclusion criteria were: (1) curable causes of hypertension; (2) certain complications of high blood pressure, such as retinopathy grade III or IV, congestive heart failure, and a history of cerebral or subarachnoid hemorrhage; and (3) concurrent diseases such as hepatitis, cirrhosis, gout, malignancy, and diabetes mellitus requiring insulin.

Patients were stratified in 8 categories on the basis of age, sex, and presence or absence of cardiovascular complications of hypertension and randomly allocated to either active treatment or placebo. At first, all patients received daily 1 diuretic capsule containing either 25 mg hydrochlorothiazide and 50 mg triamterene or a matching placebo. The daily dosage of the true or the placebo diuretic could be doubled to 2 capsules, but not before the patients had been on the study medication for a minimum of 2 weeks. If after 1 month the blood pressure remained high, methyldopa tablets, containing either 500 mg methyldopa or matching placebo, could be added to the diuretic regimen in the active treatment and placebo group, respectively. The starting dosage of methyldopa was half a tablet at night, but could eventually be increased to 4 tablets daily.

Of the randomized patients, 20% were recruited by population screening, 61% via outpatient clinics, and only 19% from sheltered housing or hospital wards. The placebo and active treatment groups were similar in sex ratio (70% women), age (average: 72 years), sitting blood pressure at randomization (182/101 and 183/101 mmHg, respectively), anthropometric characteristics, and prevalence of cardiovascular complications (35%) on admission to the trial.

Overall Results of the Trial of the European Working Party on High Blood Pressure in the Elderly

During the double-blind part of this trial, the blood pressure was lower ($P < 0.001$) in the actively treated patients than in those on placebo. One year after randomization, the difference in blood pressure between groups averaged 21/7 mmHg, while after 3 and 5 years a difference or respectively 23/9 and 21/10 mmHg was maintained.

In the report by the European Working Party on High Blood Pressure in the Elderly [1], both an intention-to-treat and a per protocol analysis of mortality were presented. The former analysis, based on the treatment groups to which the patients were randomized, included all fatal events which, irrespective of the actual treatment received, occurred during the double-blind part of the study, as well as during subsequent follow-up. The intention-to-treat analysis revealed a nonsignificant change in the total mortality (-9%), but a significant ($P = 0.037$) reduction in cardiovascular mortality. The latter was due to a reduction in cardiac mortality (-38%; $P = 0.036$) and a nonsignificant decrease in cerebrovascular mortality (-32%; $P = 0.16$). In the per protocol analysis, considering only the double-blind part of the trial, total mortality was not significantly reduced (-26%; $P = 0.077$). Cardiovascular mortality was significantly diminished in the actively treated group (-38%; $P = 0.023$) owing to a reduction in cardiac deaths (-47%; $P = 0.048$) and a nonsignificant decrease in cerebrovascular mortality (-43%; $P = 0.15$). The case-fatality rate from myocardial infarction was decreased (-60%; $P = 0.043$).

Owing to the difficulty in determining morbidity outside the period of double-blind follow-up, nonfatal events were analyzed only on a per protocol basis. Separate analyses were presented for (1) morbid study-terminative events, including cerebral hemorrhage, papilledema, and severe congestive heart failure; (2) non-morbid study-terminative events, including, among others, a severe rise in blood pressure; and (3) nonterminative cardiovascular events, including both cerebrovascular end points (cerebral thrombosis, embolism, transient ischemic attacks) and cardiac events (myocardial infarction, moderate congestive heart failure, arrhythmias, atrioventricular block).

Study-terminative, morbid cardiovascular events were significantly reduced by active treatment (-60%; $P < 0.007$). Also, study-terminative, non-morbid events occurred less frequently (-70%; $P < 0.001$) in the actively treated patients, mainly due to fewer cases of a severe rise in blood pressure on active treatment (-90%; $P < 0.001$). Nonterminative cerebrovascular events were reduced (-52%; $P = 0.026$), but the nonterminative cardiac events were not ($+3\%$; $P = 0.98$). Finally, the total cardiovascular event rate was computed, consisting of cardiovascular deaths plus the nonfatal, morbid cardiovascular terminative events and the nonterminative cardiovascular end points. Life-table analysis showed a significant reduction in the cardiovascular terminative (fatal and nonfatal) plus cardiovascular nonterminative events (-36%; $P < 0.002$). In the patients on active treatment, there were 29 fewer total cardiovascular events per 1 000 patient years than in the placebo group.

Subgroup Analyses of the Results of the EWPHE Trial

Table 1 shows three Cox proportional models. Cardiovascular mortality in the intention-to-treat analysis appears to be significantly decreased with treatment, increased with age, and significantly higher in men; it also related to the presence or absence of cardiovascular repercussion at randomization and increased with increasing systolic blood pressure at randomization. It was not related to diastolic blood pressure at randomization. For most variables, the interactions were not significant, but a bor-

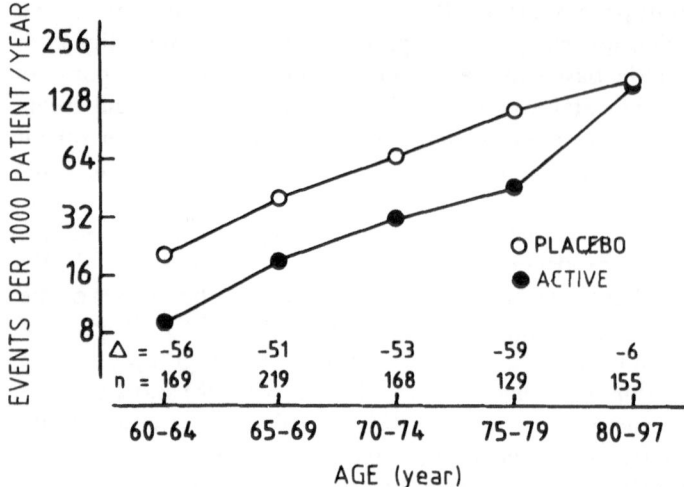

Fig. 1. Cardiovascular study-terminative events during randomized treatment (expressed in event rate per 1000 patient years) in 5 subgroups according to the *age* of the patients. Those on placebo are shown by *open circles* and actively treated patients by *closed circles*. △, difference in event rate for each subgroup between the placebo and actively treated patients; *n*, number of patients in each subgroup, combining the placebo and active-treatment groups. From Amery et al. [2]

derline significant interaction was observed between treatment and age. This is illustrated in Figs. 1–3.

Figure 1 shows the relationship between age and cardiovascular study-terminative event rate. The total population has been subdivided into 5 groups corresponding more or less to quintiles. In the placebo group, the event rate increased with age. In the actively treated group, the event rate was about 50% lower in the 4 younger quintiles, but above age 80 the two curves joined. The relative hazard rate model showed some tendency to interaction between age and treatment effect, the treatment being less effective at higher age. This does not prove that the effect of treatment is lacking because of the higher age. It could be related to other factors which are perhaps age-related, but which were not measured. The number of patients in each subgroup is rather small, and one hesitates to make general recommendations on the basis of the 155 patients in the highest age group.

Figure 2 shows the relationship between cardiovascular study-terminative event rate and systolic blood pressure at randomization. The patients are divided into 4 groups according to systolic pressure. In those on placebo, the event rate was higher with increasing pressure; and, in those actively treated, the event rate was lower for each level of systolic pressure.

Figure 3 shows that there was no relationship between entry diastolic blood pressure and cardiovascular study-terminative event rate in either those on placebo or those actively treated. However, for those actively treated, the event rate was lower than for those on placebo.

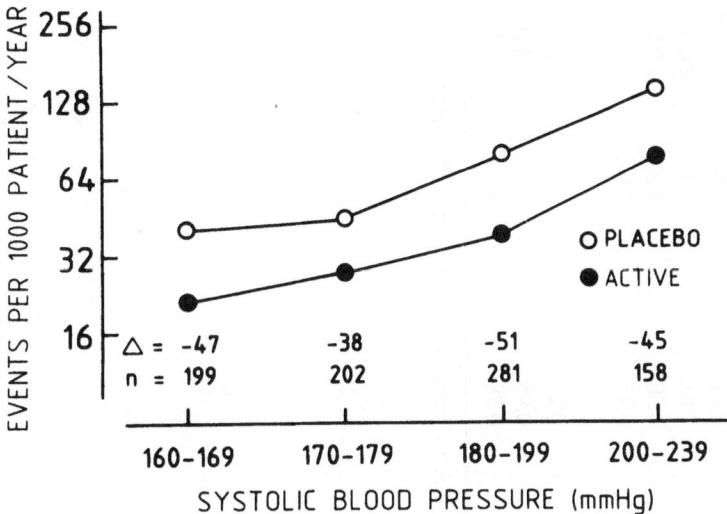

Fig. 2. Cardiovascular study-terminative events in 4 subgroups according to the *systolic blood pressure* at randomization. *Symbols* as in Fig. 1. From Amery et al. [2]

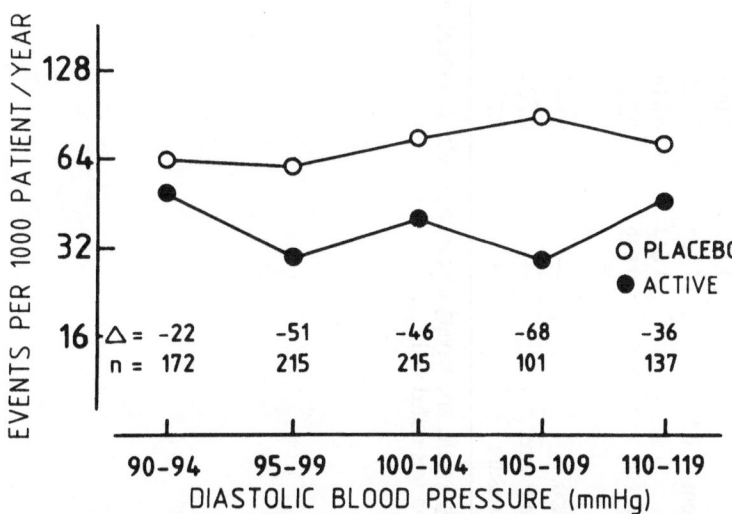

Fig. 3. Cardiovascular study-terminative events in 5 subgroups according to *diastolic blood pressure* at randomization. *Symbols* as in Fig. 1. From Amery et al. [2]

Figures 1–3 illustrate the crude event rates, but after correction for age (Table 1), the same general conclusions were reached. So, the EWPHE trial suggests that treatment effects were somewhat decreased with age. Whether this is caused by age per se, is not established.

Table 1. Three Cox proportional models. From Amery et al. [2]

	Cardiovascular death (intention-to-treat)		Cardiovascular death (on randomized treatment)		Cardiovascular study terminating events	
	RHR	P	RHR	P	RHR	P
Treatment (0,1)*	0.669	0.012	0.621	0.018	0.547	<0.001
Age (years)	1.107	<0.001	1.113	<0.001	1.094	<0.001
Sex (0,1)*	1.881	0.001	2.333	<0.001	1.814	0.005
Cardiovascular complications (0,1)*	1.435	0.025	1.647	0.013	1.771	<0.001
Systolic pressure (mmHg)	1.014	0.014	1.022	0.001	1.019	<0.001
Diastolic pressure (mmHg)	0.989	0.366	0.999	0.92	0.996	0.75
To enter into the model						
Treatment × age interaction	—	0.048	—	0.20	—	0.18
Treatment × diastolic pressure	—	0.208	—	0.95	—	0.80
Treatment × systolic pressure	—	0.80	—	0.78	—	0.95

* Placebo treatment, being female, and having no cardiovascular complication was coded as 0. Active treatment, being male, and hairing cardiovascular complication was coded as 1.
RHR, relative hazard rate.

Comparisons Between Different Trials in Elderly Hypertensives

Staessen et al. [3] performed a meta-analysis of different trials in elderly hypertensives. The randomized trials where only elderly patients were admitted included 2 double-blind trials (the small Japanese trial by Kuramoto et al. [4] and the EWPHE trial [1, 2]) and 2 open trials performed in general practice in England [5, 6]. Some trials included younger patients as well as patients over age 60; in these trials, the subgroup of patients above age 60 were considered: the Veterans trial [7], the Hypertension Stroke Cooperative study [8], the Australian trial [9], and the HDFP [10]. Unfortunately, data from the MRC trial [11] exclusively in patients over 60 years were not available.

Major problems arise when comparing or combining results from different trials. There is the difficulty of uniformity of diagnosis. For total mortality this is not a major difficulty, but for other items such as cerebrovascular event rate, there can be a major problem. Also, there are differences in recruitment, in treatment, and in the type of analysis (intention-to-treat analysis or not). We should be aware of these difficulties. Therefore, the results of the individual trials are presented together with the overall results, computed as described by Staessen et al. [12].

Mortality from All Causes Combined

Figure 4 illustrates the 95% confidence limits and the percentage difference between the actively treated group and the control group. When the number of events is high, the 95% confidence limits are small; when the number of events is small, the 95% confidence limits are large. Despite a tendency for total mortality to decrease in most trials, this tendency was never significant — neither in the individual trials nor when considering the overall results.

Cardiovascular Mortality

Cardiovascular mortality included cardiac, cerebral, and other vascular mortality. For some studies it was not possible to look at cardiovascular mortality, because the data were not given in a way suitable for this analysis. In general, there was a tendency to decrease in cardiovascular mortality except in the Japanese study. (Fig. 5). In most studies, except in the EWPHE trial ($P = 0.037$), this difference was not significant. Combining all trials on average, there is a decrease of 28%, which was significant at the 2% level.

Cerebrovascular Mortality

The data could be analyzed in only 2 trials (Fig. 6). In both trials there was a tendency to decrease, and this was significant in one and not in the other. If one combines the two, there is a decrease in cerebrovascular mortality of 41% ($P = 0.03$).

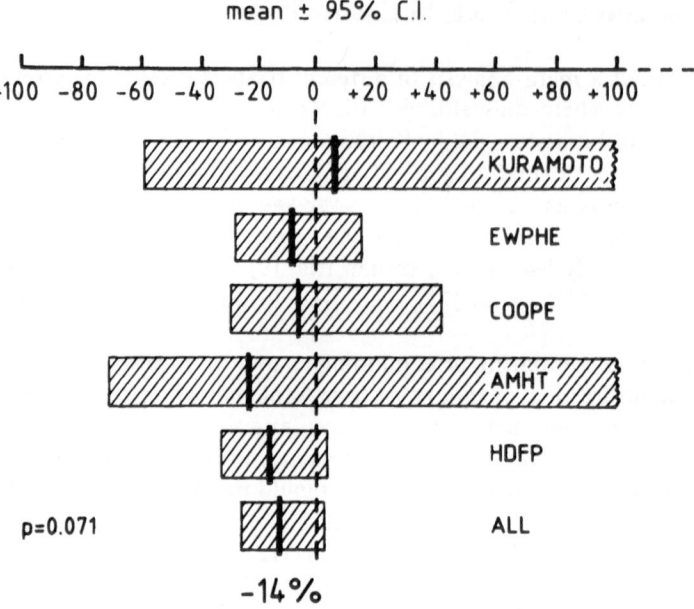

Fig. 4. Differences in mortality from all causes between the actively treated group and the control group is compared in different trials. For each trial, the difference and the 95% confidence limits (*C.l.*) are illustrated. When the *P*-value is higher than 0.05, it is not indicated. A negative sign means a decrease in events in the actively treated group compared to the control group. From Staessen et al. [3]

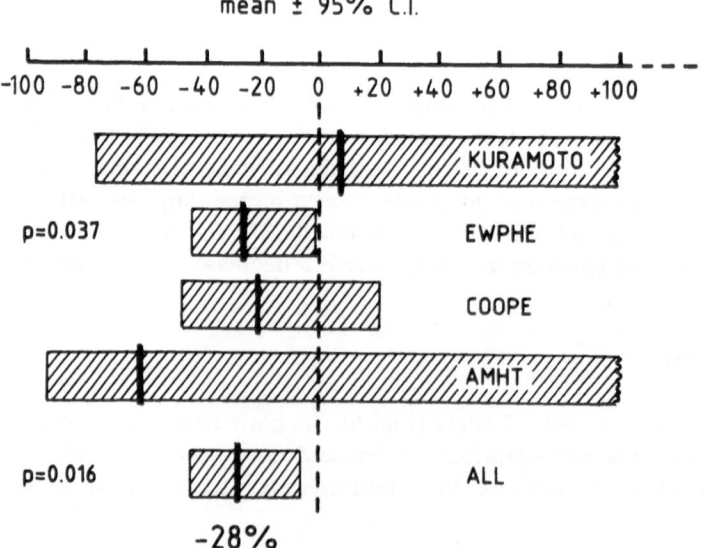

Fig. 5. Differences in cardiovascular mortality (see Fig. 4). From Staessen et al. [3]

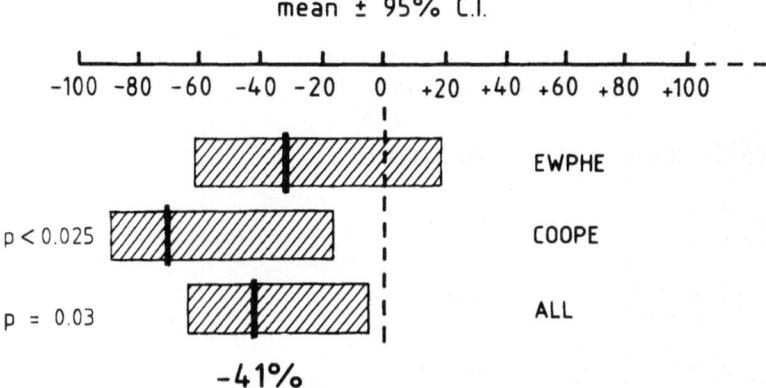

Fig. 6. Differences in cerebrovascular mortality (see Fig. 4). From Staessen et al. [3]

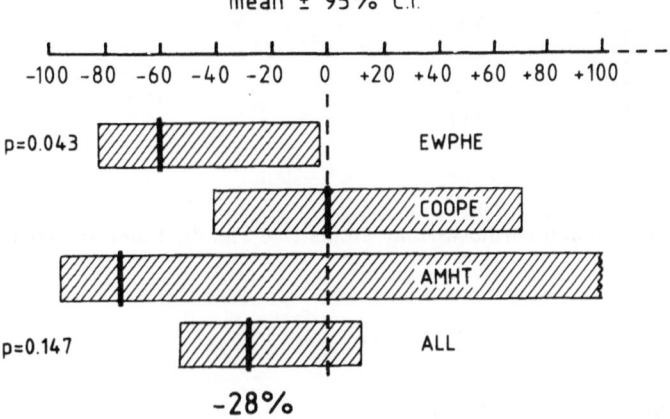

Fig. 7. Differences in coronary mortality (see Fig. 4).From Staessen et al. [3]

Coronary Mortality Including Sudden Death

Here there is a tendency to decrease in 2 trials and no difference in the other trial (Fig. 7). If one combines the 3 trials, there is a nonsignificant tendency to decrease.

Cardiovascular Fatal and Nonfatal Events

For every single trial, there was a decrease in cardiovascular events (Fig. 8). This decrease was significant in the trial of Kuramoto, but only when events such as increase in pressure in the placebo group were included in the analysis. The decrease was also significant in the EWPHE trial, in the trial of Coope and Warrender, and in the Veterans Administration Cooperative Study; in two other trials, the difference was not significant. Combining all trials, a difference of 41% was obtained, which was statistically significant.

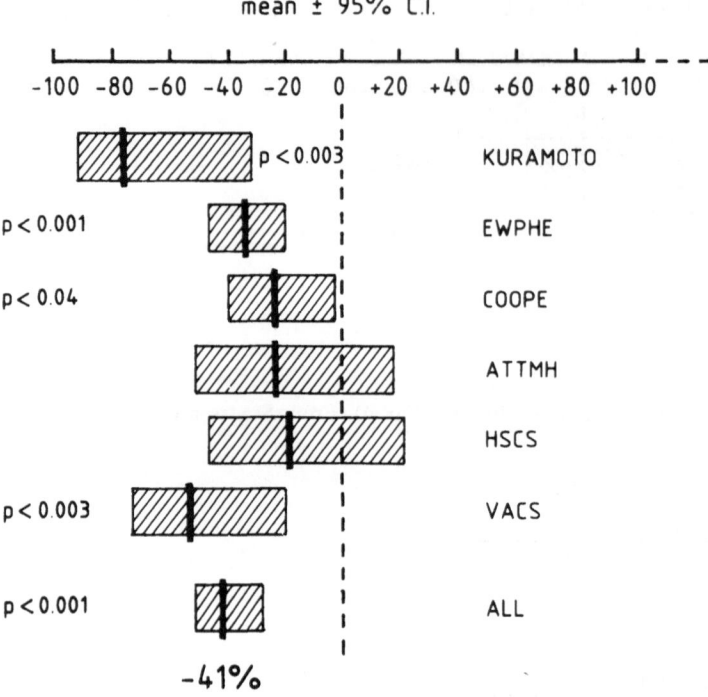

Fig. 8. Differences in fatal and nonfatal cardiovascular events (see Fig. 4). From Staessen et al. [3]

Cerebrovascular Event Rate

Cerebrovascular event rate tended to decrease in all trials (Fig. 9); this difference was significant in the trials with the highest number of events. Combining all trials, a significant decrease of 40% is observed.

Coronary Events

There are as many trials with a decrease as trials with an increase in coronary event rate (Fig. 10). When the trials are combined there is no indication of a decrease of coronary events.

Overall, the mortality data showed a nonsignificant tendency to decrease in total mortality but a significant decrease in cardiovascular mortality mainly due to the decrease in cerebrovascular mortality. Combining the fatal and nonfatal events, the following results were obtained: (1) a decrease in cardiovascular fatal and nonfatal events which was mainly due to the decrease in cerebrovascular events and (2) no significant decrease in the other events with the possible exception of congestive heart failure.

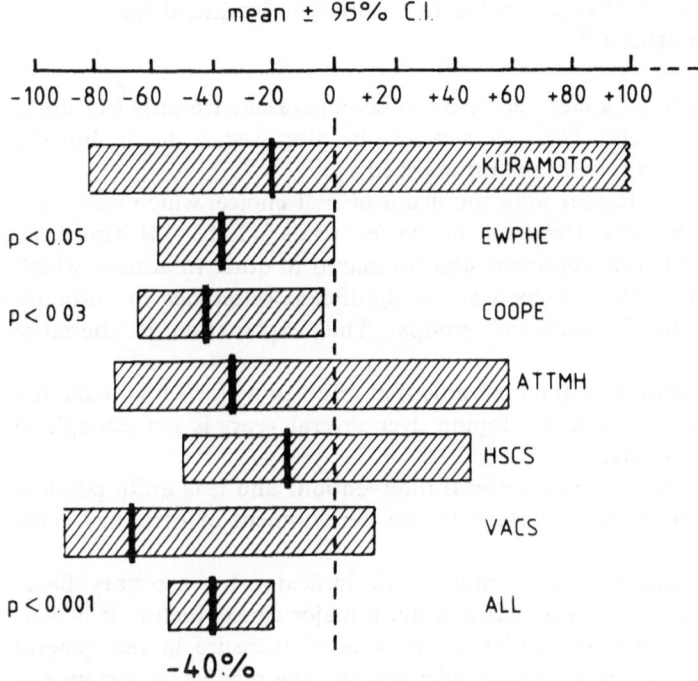

Fig. 9. Differences in fatal and nonfatal cerebrovascular events (see Fig. 4). From Staessen et al. [3]

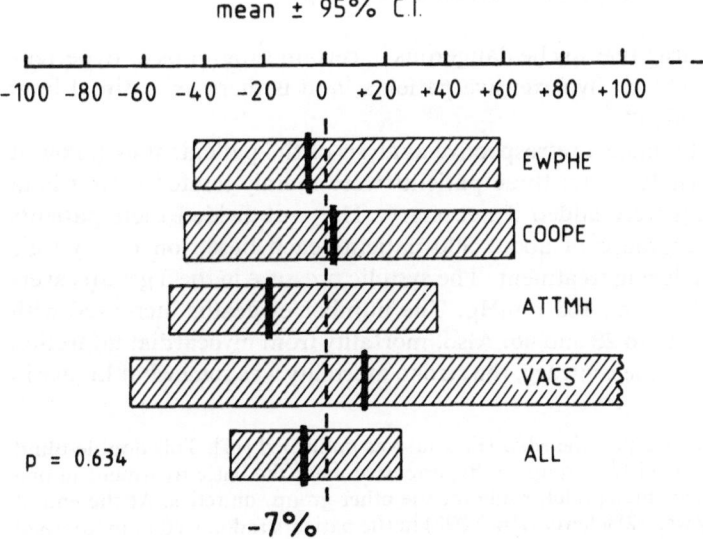

Fig. 10. Differences in fatal and nonfatal coronary events (see Fig. 4). From Staessen et al. [3]

Why is the Event Rate of Myocardial Infarction Not Reduced by Hypotensive Drug Treatment?

Why is there, in these elderly, a clear decrease in cerebrovascular events but not a decrease in coronary event rate? This point cannot be discussed in detail, but the possibilities which have been raised are summarized here:

1. In many of these trials, thiazides were the drugs of first choice, which may have affected the results adversely. However, in the few trials [11, 13, 14] where the effects of beta-blocker based treatment was compared to other treatment which consisted mainly of thiazides), there was no significant difference in coronary event rate between the 2 treatment groups. This explanation is therefore unlikely[1].
2. The trials were short-term. It is quite possible that intervening for a few years in a disease process which has been developing over several years is not enough to decrease coronary event rate.
3. The intervention was mainly a unifactorial intervention, and it is quite possible that other factors were more important in the development of coronary heart disease.
4. Finally, although hypertension is a major risk indicator for coronary heart disease, there is still the possibility that it is not a major causal factor. It is generally accepted that a pressure similar to the arterial pressure in the general circulation is necessary to develop atherosclerosis, but the relative importance of an increase in pressure in the development of atherosclerosis should be critically analyzed.

Danger of Hypotensive Drugs in Certain Subgroups

Could antihypertensive drug therapy be dangerous in certain subgroups of hypertensive patients, especially elderly hypertensive patients, and is there an optimal level for blood pressure reduction?

Cruickshank et al. [15] made a retrospective analysis of the patients they followed in their clinic for the last 10 years; these patients were mainly treated with a beta blocker, and other drugs were added if necessary. They subdivided their patients into 3 roughly equal subgroups of about 300 patients each based on the systolic blood pressure achieved during treatment. The systolic pressure in the 3 groups averaged respectively 129, 143, and 163 mmHg. The number of deaths increased with increasing pressure from 17 to 28 and 46. Also, mortality from myocardial infarction increased from 5 to 21. On the contrary, the stroke mortality was somewhat higher in

---

[1] Since the submission of this paper, the MAPHY trial was published [17]. This double-blind trial compared the outcome of two groups of hypertensive men; the basic treatment in one group was the beta blocker, metoprolol, while for the other group, diuretics. At the end of the study, total mortality was 22% lower ($P = 0.028$) in the patients radomized to metoprolol than in the patients randomized to diuretics; this was related to a decrease in cardiovascular mortality ($P = 0.012$), coronary mortality ($P = 0.048$), and stroke mortality ($P = 0.043$) in the metoprolol group. This important paper has been compared to the other three studies with a similar design, by Staessen et al. [18]. Additional data are needed to define to what extent this study differs from the other three and why.

the lowest systolic blood pressure group ($n = 7$); in the middle group it was only 3 and increased again to 11 in the highest group. The authors also mention that this so-called J-shaped curve was more clear in the elderly, but they did not present figures. There was no difference between the 3 groups in cancer mortality.

Cruickshank et al. also subdivided the same population according to the diastolic pressure during follow-up into 3 subgroups having a diastolic blood pressure around 80, 87, and 95 mmHg. They suggested that myocardial infarction mortality shows a J-shaped curve: the mortality being high in the lower group, lower in the middle group, and highest in the highest blood pressure group. The number of deaths from myocardial infarction was rather small: 12, 7, and 21, respectively. Based on the same population, Cruickshank et al. presented [16] the coronary mortality expressed per 1000 patient years rather than in absolute numbers. Although no statistical analysis is presented, it is obvious that the differences between the lower and the middle subgroup are not significant.

Does the risk of treatment depend on age? The total group of 900 patients [16] was divided into those below age 60 and those 60 years and over. If anything, the risk was highest in the younger, and certainly not in the older patients; but, again, these differences are not significant. They also subdivided the patient population by patients with and without ischemic disease. Ischemic disease was defined here as patients who had, before randomization, an infarction, ECG abnormalities, claudication, or angina pectoris. They further subdivided the patients with and without ischemic disease into 3 subgroups according to diastolic blood pressure during treatment. They showed that the J-shaped curve, if it exists, was mainly present in the patients with ischemic disease.

It should be noted that these curves were based on a total number of deaths from myocardial infarction of 12, 7, and 21 patients, respectively, in the 3 diastolic pressure subgroups. In addition, the nature of this trial should be kept in mind when interpreting these results; it is a retrospective study, there is no control group, and the blood pressure of the patients was reduced, but not intentionally to a middle or low range. The J-shaped curve was not seen for the relationship between systolic blood pressure and myocardial infarction, and it was also not seen for diastolic blood pressure and stroke. Neither the statistical significance of the results nor the power of such a study was clearly indicated.

Moreover, the chicken and the egg argument is not completely resolved; it is still possible that those patients with a diseased myocardium had both a lower pressure and a higher mortality. Therefore, definite conclusions should not be drawn from these data until other studies have been analyzed in the same way. In fact, the IPPPSH study [13] was also analyzed according to similar criteria and no J-shaped curve was obtained. There is a suggestion in the HAPPHY trial [14] that such a J-shaped curve could appear, but we should wait for full publication of the data.

All clinicians would agree that it is dangerous to decrease the blood pressure in the elderly too quickly, and it is best to try to lower the blood pressure progressively.

Whether it is beneficial to treat isolated systolic hypertension in elderly patients is still not proven by intervention trials. Therefore, the European Working Party is considering a new trial with the purpose to establish whether antihypertensive drug treatment in elderly patients with systolic hypertension reduces morbidity and mortality while preserving the quality of life.

References

1. Amery A, Birkenhäger W, Brixko P, Bulpitt C, Clement D, Deruyttere M, De Schaepdryver A, Dollery C, Fagard R, Forette F, Forte J, Hamdy R Henry JF, Joossens JV, Leonetti G, Lund-Johansen P, O'Malley K, Petrie J, Strasser T, Tuomilehto J, Williams B, (1985) Mortality and morbidity results from the European working party on high blood pressure in the elderly trial. Lancet 1: 1349–1354
2. Amery A, Birkenhäger W, Brixko R, Bulpitt C, Clement D, Deruyttere M, De Schaepdryver A, Dollery C, Fagard R, Forette F, Forte J, Hamdy R Henry JF, Joossens JV, Leonetti G, Lund-Johansen P, O'Malley K, Petrie JC, Strasser T, Tuomilehto J, Williams B, (1986) Efficacy of antihypertensive drug treatment according to age, sex, blood pressure, and previous cardiovascular disease in patients over the age of 60. Lancet 2: 589–592
3. Staessen J, Fagard R, Van Hoof R, Amery A (1988) Mortality in various intervention trials in elderly hypertensive patients. A review. Eur Heart J 9: 215–222
4. Kuramoto K, Matsushita S, Kuwajima I, Murakawi M (1981) Prospective study on the treatment of mild hypertension in the aged. Jpn Heart J 22: 75–85
5. Sprackling ME, Mitchell JRA, Short AH, Watt G (1981) Blood pressure reduction in the elderly: a randomized controlled trial of methyldopa. Br Med J 283: 1151–1153
6. Coope J, Warrender TS (1986) Randomized trial of treatment of hypertension in elderly patients in primary area. Br Med J 293: 1145–1151
7. Veterans Administration Cooperative Study Group on Antihypertensive Agents (1972) effect of treatment on morbidity in hypertension. Circulation 45: 991–1004
8. Hypertension-Stroke Cooperative Study Group (1974) Effect of antihypertensive treatment on stroke recurrence. JAMA 229: 409–418
9. Report by the Management Committee (1980) The Australian therapeutic trial in mild hypertension. Lancet 1: 1261–1267
10. Hypertension Detection and Follow-up Program Cooperative Group (1979) Five-year findings of the hypertension detection and follow-up program. JAMA 242: 2562–2571
11. Medical Research Council Working Party on Mild to Moderate Hypertension (1985) MRC trial of treatment of mild hypertension; principal results. Br Med J 291; 97–104
12. Staessen J, Van Hoof R, Fagard R, Amery A, (1989) Epidemiology of untreated versus treated hypertension in elderly patients. (Handbook of hypertension, vol XII) Elsevier pp 320–351
    patients. Elsevier (Handbook of hypertension, vol XI) (accepted for pulication)
13. The IPPPSH Collaborative Group (1985) Cardiovascular risk and risk factors in a randomized trial of treatment based on the beta-blocker oxprenolol: The International Prospective Primary Prevention Study in Hypertension (IPPPSH). J Hypertens 3: 379–392
14. Wilhelmsen L, Berglund G, Elmfeldt D, Fitzsimons T, Holzgreve H, Hosie J, Hörnkvist PE, Pennert K, Tuomilehto J, Wedel H, (1987) Beta-blockers versus diuretics in hypertensive men: Main results from the HAPPHY trial. J Hypertens 5: 561–572
15. Cruickshank JM, Pennert K, Sörman AE, Thorp JM, Zacharias FM, Zacharias FJ (1987) Low mortality from all causes, including myocardial infarction, in well-controlled hypertensives treated with a beta-blocker plus other antihypertensives. Hypertens 5: 489–498
16. Cruickshank JM, Thorp JM, Zacharias FJ (1987) Benefits and potential harm of lowering high blood pressure. Lancet 1: 581–584
17. Wikstrand J, Warnold I, Olsson G, Tuomilehto J, Elmfeldt D, Berglund G; on behalf of the Advisory Committee (1988) Primary prevention with metoprolol in patients with hypertension: mortality results from the MAPHY study. JAMA 259 (13): 1976–1982
18. Staessen J, Fagard R, Amery A (1988) Primary prevention with metoprolol in patients with hypertension: letter to the editor. JAMA 260: 1713-1714

Discussion

Zanchetti (Milan): May I ask you about the last slide you showed where the relation of morbidity and mortality to blood pressure before starting treatment was given? Do you have any data analyzed in terms of in-treatment blood pressure to see if there is some correlation of that, with in-treatment blood pressure? There must be, for instance, some very nice data correlating morbidity and mortality with that.

Amery (Leuven): I think that is a very important question, especially in relation to the recent publications on the U-shaped curve. We are, in fact, preparing that paper, and I hope it will be accepted by the publication committee soon.

Safer (Paris): Tony (Amery), do you think it would be possible to show — I do not know if it is exact — that for a given systolic pressure the risk would be higher when diastolic blood pressure is lower?

Amery: Well, from the Cox analysis, you can see that at a given systolic blood pressure, diastolic blood pressure at randomization is not an independent risk indicator.

Clinical Pharmacological Considerations in the Treatment of Hypertension in the Elderly

C.M. NEWMAN and C.T. DOLLERY[1]

Summary. There are few, if any, fundamental differences in the action of antihypertensive agents in older hypertensive patients compared with those in middle age. Nonetheless, there are many detailed considerations which may influence the efficacy and side effects of anti-hypertensive medication in the elderly, and some knowledge of these is useful when deciding upon treatment. Four aspects are of particular interest:
1. The magnitude of the pharmacodynamic response. Diuretics are slightly more effective and beta-blockers less effective hypotensive agents in older patients.
2. Drug kinetics may be different in the elderly. Mild reduction of glomerular filtration rate is common as age advances and may be further impaired by use of high doses of diuretics. Drugs excreted unchanged by the kidney may show an exaggerated effect. Drugs metabolism is little changed by advancing age.
3. Side-effect patterns alter with age. Drugs that cause sedation, unsteadiness or orthostatic hypotension may cause greater problems in the elderly, while headache caused by vasodilators is less common.
4. Older patients are often multiply ill. The presence of other serious illness such as heart failure may influence both the selection and response to treatment.

Key words: Elderly — Pharmacokinetics — Antihypertensive medication — Hypotensive response

The Pharmacodynamic Response

Since inter-patient variations in drug response are considerable at all ages, it is impossible to predict precisely the hypotensive effect of a given dose of drug in any particular individual. Even so, a knowledge of the likely pattern of response in a particular type of patient is useful in making a rational choice of first-line agent. Elderly hypertensive patients, for example, differ from younger patients in several ways that may influence drug response:
1. Plasma renin activity decreases progressively with age in both normotensive and hypertensive subjects.
2. Plasma noradrenaline rises slightly with age.
3. Responsiveness to catecholamine stimulation is impaired.

---

[1] Department of Medicine, Royal Postgraduate Medical School, Ducane Road, London, United Kingdom

4. Beta-adrenoceptor number and sensitivity may be reduced.
5. Baroreflex function is impaired.
6. Pretreatment (particularly systolic) blood pressure is often higher in elderly hypertensives.

Despite these theoretical considerations, there are very few studies in the literature which specifically examine the hypotensive effects of any given treatment regime in hypertensive patients of different ages. In fact, such comparisons are often derived from subgroup analysis of studies primarily concerned with other issues, such as the Medical Research Council trial of treatment of mild hypertension [1], or by inference from the results of separate studies of similar design but performed in different age groups — a practice fraught with possible errors.

Diuretics and Beta-Adrenoceptor Antagonists

Benzothiadiazine diuretics and beta-adrenoceptor antagonists are widely used as first-line antihypertensive agents in all age groups. Both have the practical advantage of a flat dose-response curve which reduces the probability of major variations in hypotensive response between individual patients, regardless of age.

The available evidence suggests that the hypotensive effects of benzothiadiazine diuretics may increase slightly with advancing age, whereas the reverse may apply to beta-adrenoceptor antagonists. At least 2 studies have directly compared the hypotensive effects of benzothiadiazine diuretics and beta-adrenoceptor antagonists and have performed subgroup analysis by age [1, 2]. One of these, performed by the Veterans Administration Cooperative Study Group on Antihypertensive Agents involved a prospective trial of hydrochlorothiazide or propranolol in the treatment of 683 patients aged 21–65 years with diastolic blood pressures off treatment between 95 and 144 mmHg. Over a 10 week titration period, one or the other drug was given in increasing doses until the target diastolic pressure of 90 mmHg was obtained or the maximum dose allowed in the protocol design had been reached (200 mg hydrochlorothiazide or 740 mg propranolol daily). The mean fall in blood pressure (systolic/diastolic) during hydrochlorothiazide therapy was significantly greater in hypertensives aged 55–65 than in the younger patients (22/13 vs 16/12 mmHg, respectively), whereas an identical analysis for propranolol showed no significant differences between these 2 age groups (11/11 vs 10/11 mmHg). The mean hypotensive response to the diuretic was greater in black than in white patients, including patients aged 55–65 (26/14 mmHg for black patients, 18/12 mmHg for white patients). Finally, patients aged 55–65 treated with hydrochlorothiazide were more likely to achieve goal diastolic BP during the study (72%) than the younger patients (59%). No such relationship was found for patients treated with propranolol.

Subgroup analysis of the MRC trial in mild hypertension [3], in which over 17000 patients aged between 35 and 64 were followed for 5 years, also suggests that the effects of benzothiadiazine diuretics are greater in older patients and that this effect of age persists beyond the early months of treatment. Thus, a greater proportion of the older patients initially randomized to treatment with bendrofluazide had attained target diastolic blood pressure at any given time point within the 5-year study period when compared to the younger patients within the same group, and less of these had required supplementary antihypertensive medication to do so. No comparable trend was observed in those patients initially randomized to receive propranolol as starting medication, and indeed the hypotensive potential of this agent appeared to diminish somewhat with increasing age. Whilst sub-group analysis is an imperfect means of assessing the effects of age on hypotensive efficacy, the comparison of similar but separate studies involving patients in different age-groups is often an unhelpful and even misleading exercise, since between-study variations may outweigh any effect of age per se.

A reduction in the hypotensive response to beta-adrenoceptor antagonists with increasing age has been noted in other studies. For example, Buhler et al. [4] claimed that only 20% of hypertensive patients over the age of 60 will respond satisfactorily to beta-adrenoceptor antagonists alone, though the exact conditions of this study are unclear. In contrast, however, other studies have shown beta-adrenoceptor antagonists to be effective in all age groups.

The intrinsic alpha-blocking potential of labetalol confers some theoretical advantage for the treatment of elderly hypertensives in whom peripheral resistance is particularly elevated, and several studies have shown this agent to be effective.

In summary, it appears that any age-related changes in the pharmacodynamics of benzothiadiazine diuretics and beta-adrenoceptor antagonists are likely to be of little clinical importance, and the choice of first-line antihypertensive agent for elderly patients will depend much more upon individual susceptibility and the likelihood of adverse effects.

Other Agents

Several trials have demonstrated that calcium antagonists are effective hypotensive agents in elderly hypertensives. Buhler has claimed a strong positive correlation between age and the hypotensive response to verapamil [5], but there was no correlation for nifedipine in the study conducted by Erne et al. [6]. Most other studies using calcium antagonists in which comparisons between "old" and "young" hypertensives have been made indicate at best a weak link, or commonly, no such relationship. As with all hypotensive agents, the interpretation of these data must consider the fact that the starting blood pressure in the elderly is often higher than in younger patients, and bigger absolute falls in blood pressure may be similar to those seen in younger patients when expressed in terms of percentage of the starting pressure. Such analyses are not always performed, although the relationship of percentage fall in blood pressure with verapamil was still positively correlated with age in the study by Buhler et al. [5]. A significant negative correlation between hypotensive response and plasma renin concentrations has been noted in some [6], but by no means all studies involving the use of calcium antagonists.

The lower circulating renin levels in the elderly could theoretically reduce the efficacy of angiotensin-converting enzyme (ACE) inhibitors in this age group. Previous studies have shown, however, that the long-term hypotensive effect of these drugs is poorly correlated with pretreatment renin levels [7]. It is not surprising, therefore, that monotherapy with ACE inhibitors can achieve adequate blood pressure control in the majority of elderly patients with an efficacy similar to benzothia-diazine diuretics and beta-adrenoceptor antagonists. Some studies have even sug-gested an increased effectiveness of ACE inhibitors in older patients, particularly with respect to systolic blood pressure, but this may simply represent a combined effect of the higher starting pressures in this age group and some changes in enalapril pharmacokinetics with age.

Centrally acting sympatholytic agents such as methyldopa, clonidine, and guanfacine are widely used as second-or third-line antihypertensive agents in middle-aged hypertensives. Reduced beta-adrenoceptor mediated cardiovascular responses in the elderly and consequent unopposed alpha-adrenoceptor mediated vasoconstric-tion would suggest an increased hypotensive response to a drug induced reduction in central sympathetic outflow, particularly in the presence of depressed baroreflexes. Methyldopa may itself depress the reactive vasoconstrictor and heart rate responses to a reduction in carotid baroreceptor activity. Studies which directly compared the hypotensive effects of such drugs in young and older hypertensives are not available, but the available evidence from short-term studies would suggest a similar efficacy in all age groups. Methyldopa was used successfully as a second-line agent throughout the 12 years of the EWPHE trial [8] and is a recommended second-line agent for elderly hypertensives in the United States.

Similar theoretical considerations apply to alpha-1 adrenoceptor antagonists, and to some extent direct-acting vasodilator agents such as hydralazine but again, studies concentrating on the elderly are scarce and within-study comparisons with younger patients virtually non-existent. Nonetheless, these agents seem to be effec-tive in lowering blood pressure in the elderly, and their usage should be governed by factors other than pharmacodynamic potency.

In summary, antihypertensive drugs from different pharmacological classes appear to be capable of lowering the blood pressure in young and elderly patients to a broadly similar degree. The small differences that have been reported, e.g., slightly greater efficacy of benzothiadiazine diuretics and calcium antagonists in the elderly, are as much of theoretical as practical interest.

Pharmacokinetic Considerations in the Elderly

Theoretically at least, changes in drug pharmacokinetics with age could explain some of the differences between drug pharmacodynamics in young and elderly patients. There are relatively few data on the pharmacokinetics of antihypertensive agents in old age. Nonetheless, age-related changes in body composition and organ system function may considerably affect the absorption, distribution, and elimina-tion of these and other drugs.

Body weight falls with advancing age. Thus, the same dose of drug given to an elderly patient will often be higher on a dose per unit body weight basis than in a younger individual.

Body composition alters with age. For example, total body water decreases by 10%–15% between the ages of 30 and 80 years. Moreover, lean body mass declines and adipose tissue mass increases in relation to total body weight in the elderly. Such changes in body composition may have significant effects on the elimination half-life and peak plasma concentration of administered drugs but have little effect on steady state plasma concentrations during multiple dosing.

Average renal function declines gradually with age, although inter-individual variations are much greater than the effect of age per se. Glomerular filtration rate may fall by as much as 50% from young adulthood to extreme old age, and renal plasma flow falls predictably by about 1.9% per year after the age of 30. For drugs whose elimination is dependent on renal excretion, the rate at which the body is cleared of the drug will decline with age in proportion to the rate of decline of renal function.

Some aspects of hepatic function decline with age. Many drugs are converted into pharmacologically inactive and/or water-soluble metabolites by the action of hepatic microsomal enzymes. The increased water solubility of such metabolites facilitates subsequent elimination by the kidneys. There is some evidence that microsomal enzyme function declines with age, but most studies have not taken into account differences in the number of cigarette smokers and the extent to which drug metabolising activity is inducible at different ages. Tobacco smoking induces the synthesis of some forms of hepatic cytochrome p450 and thereby increases the rate of metabolism of drugs which are substrates for these forms. There is some evidence that the degree of inducibility declines with age, and this tends to reduce the effect of smoking on the rate of drug metabolism in older individuals. In addition, the percentage of patients who smoke decreases with age as such patients have a much higher mortality rate at all ages than non-smokers.

Hepatic blood flow is considerably reduced in the elderly. Total liver blood flow may be 40%-45% lower in elderly patients than that observed in young adults. This change reflects both the smaller liver size and the reduced cardiac output of elderly patients, which may be further reduced in the presence of cardiac failure. Changes in hepatic blood flow will particularly affect the pharmacokinetics of drugs that have a high extraction ratio in the liver.

Despite these not inconsiderable changes in bodily function and composition, studies which specifically examine the effect of age on the pharmacokinetics of antihypertensive drugs are relatively uncommon.

The action of many antihypertensive drugs is terminated by hepatic metabolism. Propranolol is one such drug whose pharmacokinetics have been studied in patients of all ages, largely because propranolol is a good model of presystemic metabolism within the liver. At least 2 studies [9, 10] have shown that the systemic bioavailability and peak/steady state plasma levels of propranolol are increased in the elderly, both after single and multiple doses, whereas systemic clearance is reduced. The best explanation for these findings appeared to be a reduction in the rate of propranolol metabolism in the liver, both on first pass and at steady state. Other studies have not always found such a difference [79]. There appear to be at least two factors which may explain these discrepancies. Firstly, some studies have involved healthy patients only [11], whereas others have included long-stay inpatients in the elderly subgroup [9, 10]. Secondly, it appears that the smoking habits of the patients involved are of critical importance. For example, Vestal et al. [12] demonstrated that propranolol kinetics were similar in nonsmokers of all ages. Healthy young subjects who smoked, however, appeared to induce hepatic metabolism of propranolol, since peak concentrations were approximately half those of nonsmokers and the half-life was shorter. The same rate of tobacco smoking by healthy elderly subjects appeared to have less effect on hepatic enzymes so that propranolol kinetics in the older smokers were similar to those of nonsmokers. Combining the data from smokers and nonsmokers at each age showed a higher peak concentration and prolonged half-life of propranolol in older patients.

Notwithstanding these problems of interpretation, similar pharmacokinetic changes with age particularly increased bioavailability, increased peak and steady state plasma concentrations, decreased clearance, or some combination of these have also been noted for other antihypertensive agents extensively metabolised in the liver, e.g., verapamil, nifedipine, nicardipine, and labetalol. The effects of age on the metabolism of agents such as metoprolol and diltiazem appear to be less striking.

A number of other important antihypertensive drugs such as hydrochlorothiazide, atenolol, and enalapril are mainly excreted unchanged via the kidney. Digby et al. [13] reported that the renal clearance of atenolol is reduced in elderly patients, although one group could not establish a direct correlation between creatinine and atenolol clearances [14]. As far as benzothiadiazine diuretics are concerned, no changes relating to aging per se have been documented and excretion is related colsely to renal function.

Reid et al. [15, 16] have studied the effect of age on the pharmacokinetics of enalapril, both after a single dose and after 8 days of treatment with 10 mg daily. Clearance of enalapril was lower in older subjects and was positively correlated with creatinine clearance.

In practical terms, the effects of age on the pharmacokinetics of various antihypertensive drugs are unlikely to necessitate major changes in dosage schedules for elderly patients. Indeed, inter-individual and between sex differences in drug pharmacokinetics are likely to be of greater magnitude than any alternations due to age itself. In addition, the dose response curves for the most commonly prescribed antihypertensive agents, namely benzothiadiazine diuretics and beta-adrenoceptor antagonists, are so flat that moderate overdose due to altered pharmacokinetics in the elderly would be of little consequence. Perhaps the most important aspect of drug pharmacokinetics concerns the frequency at which various drugs must be administered. If at all possible, drugs requiring once daily administration should be used in order to maximize patient compliance and minimize the risk of confusion caused by complicated drug regimes, particularly since many elderly patients will require specific therapy for more than one condition.

In summary, it is sensible practice to institute therapy at the lowest recommended dose and highest dose interval, increasing by small increments at infrequent intervals until control of hypertension is achieved.

Adverse Reactions in the Elderly

There have been few systematic studies of changes in symptomatic drug side effects with age. Studies in this area are difficult to perform in a meaningful fashion since factors other than age per se may have profound effects on the incidence and reporting of adverse reactions. For example, in a study of 1160 hospital inpatients, Hurwitz [17] found that whilst drug reactions occurred most frequently in patients over 60, there was also a significant correlation with the total number of drugs given and with a history of previous drug reactions. Since the elderly often require multiple drugs to treat several coexistent diseases and have had more opportunity to experience drug reactions, these factors are unlikely to be entirely independent. Other confounding factors may also complicate the interpretation of apparent age-related changes in the incidence of adverse reactions, e.g., age-related differences in the response to direct questioning for the presence of side effects, etc.

As far as antihypertensive drugs are concerned, Bulpitt, Dollery, and Carne [18] reported a study in which a postal symptom questionnaire was circulated to 374 hypertensive outpatients. Four symptoms were positively correlated with age, namely, impotence, slow walking pace, nocturia, and postural hypotension. In contrast, headache, depression, and sleepiness were negatively correlated with age. In the absence of an age-matched control group, these changes may largely reflect the effects of aging per se. Nonetheless, it is interesting that the same symptoms were significantly more common in treated hypertensives than in untreated normotensive controls, implying an effect of either hypertension per se or, more likely, antihypertensive medication. (It was not possible to assess the effect of age on this phenomenon due to the relatively small size of the control group [78 normal subjects]). In contrast, the Hypertension Detection and Follow-up Program showed a small decrease in the 5 year incidence of total side effects in older age groups [19].

Whilst the overall incidence of adverse reactions to antihypertensive drugs may be little affected by age, certain clinical characteristics more common in elderly patients may increase the likelihood of side effects in particular individuals:

1. Older patients are more likely to have an orthostatic fall in blood pressure before antihypertensive treatment. It is interesting that the results of most studies referenced in this article would suggest a very low incidence of either objectives or symptomatic postural hypotension. This may reflect the fact that study investigators are particularly aware of the importance of measuring the standing blood pressure as part of the initial and dose titration assessments.
2. Older patients are more likely to have occlusive vascular disease in brain and heart, which makes a rapid fall in blood pressure undesirable.
3. Older patients are less steady on their feet.
4. Older patients are more susceptible to drugs which impair intellectual performance.

Diuretics and Beta-Adrenoceptor Antagonists

Since any age-related pharmacodynamic differences between benzothiadiazine diuretics and beta-adrenoceptor antagonists are likely to be more of theoretical than practical concern, the side effect profile of these agents is of particular importance in the choice of first-line drugs in elderly hypertensives. It has been suggested that benzothiadiazine and related diuretics are relatively unsuitable for use in the elderly hypertensive, as such patients may be particularly likely to develop and/or suffer the consequences of drug-induced metabolic abnormalities.

Hypokalemia. Some degree of hypokalemia occurs in virtually all patients treated with benzothiadiazine diuretics alone [2, 3], but there is no convincing evidence that elderly patients are biochemically more severely or frequently affected than other age groups despite the added problems of poor dietary intake and possibly low total body potassium. Hypokalemia due to therapy with benzothiadiazines and related diuretics may largely be avoided by the use of relatively low doses, since the dose response curve for hypotensive effect is flatter than that for the development of hypokalemia. If higher doses are required for some reason, perhaps due to the coexistence of hypertension with peripheral edema, then there is some evidence that indapamide may have a lesser tendency to cause persistent hypokalemia than other diuretics. The combination of a benzothiadiazine with a potassium sparing agent, e.g. amiloride or triamterene, is, however, an effective and considerably cheaper alternative. In contrast, potassium supplements are not generally unpleasant to take, but have their own hazards and often fail to restore potassium balance.

Whilst severe hypokalemia can undoubtedly cause lethargy and muscle weakness, there is no evidence that diuretic-induced hypokalemia is commonly severe enough to cause such symptoms. In addition, the effects of mild hypokalemia on mortality are still a subject of much controversy. There is certainly no hard evidence that the elderly fare any less well than other age groups in this regard, at least not in the absence of complicating factors such as concomitant therapy with digitalis compounds.

Glucose intolerance. Benzothiadiazine diuretics can exacerbate establish maturity onset diabetes mellitus [20, 21]. There are also many reports that these agents lead to impairment of glucose tolerance in patients who are not diabetic. There is no firm evidence that elderly patients are more susceptible to the diabetogenic effects of benzothiadiazine diuretics. In the EWPHE trial, the fasting blood sugar of patients on active treatment (based on 25–50 mg hydrochlorothiazide and 50–100 mg triamterene daily) was about 4 mg/dl higher than that of the placebo group at the end of the 1st year [22]. Over the next 2 years of the study, the fasting blood sugar rose in both groups, but the active-placebo difference remained at 40–50 mg/ml. Thus, the progressive increases in blood sugar in the placebo group appeared to be due to aging, whereas the effect of the diuretic was established within the 1st year of treatment and did not increase as the patients got older.

One particularly interesting speculation is that the incidence and degree of glucose intolerance in this study was kept artificially low by the routine use of the potassium sparing agent, triamterene, in the actively treated group (with the result that serum potassium fell by only 0.2 mmol/l overall during the trial), since several authors have noted a direct correlation between the degree of hypokalemia and severity of glucose intolerance. Such a correlation might also explain why another long-term study, this time using a low-dose thiazide/potassium chloride regime (2.5 mg bendrofluazide +0.57 g potassium chloride) failed to demonstrate any significant degree of hypokalemia or glucose intolerance over a 5-year period [23]. In addition, prevention of potassium depletion during treatment with benzothiadiazines may prevent the development of glucose intolerance [24]. In summary, the predictable, albeit small, and fixed degree of glucose intolerance attributable to benzothiadiazine diuretics may be sufficent to precipitate frank diabetes mellitus in elderly patients with particularly depleted pancreatic function, and such problems may be reduced by the use of small doses, possibly combined with a potassium sparing agent.

Others metabolic problem. Hyperuricemia, hyponatremia, hypomagnesemia, and lipid abnormalities all occur during therapy with benzothiadiazine diuretics, but information concerning the relative incidence of these problems in elderly vs young hypertensives participating in the same trial is not available. Nonetheless, elderly patients are likely to be more susceptible to the effects of metabolic abnormalities such as hyponatremia, leading to a toxic confusional state.

Two other adverse reactions to diuretic therapy are important. Firstly, the MRC trial showed that men taking bendrofluazide developed impotence nearly 4 times more often than those taking propranolol [25]. This factor could be of importance to older men in whom sexual function is already declining. Secondly, the use of loop diuretics, whilst causing less carbohydrate intolerance and hypokalemia in otherwise healthy hypertensive patients, is more likely to cause incontinence in elderly patients due to the sudden rush of urine after each dose in the presence of detrusor instability and/or prostatism. There is also a small risk of hypovolemia and its various consequences.

Analysis of trials in which elderly hypertensive patients have been treated with beta-adrenoceptor antagonists suggests that the incidence of side effects is no different from younger age groups. While this may be true for otherwise healthy elderly patients, the conditions which commonly exclude patients from entry into these trials such as heart failure, cardiac conduction defects, peripheral vascular disease, and chronic lung disease are much more common in the elderly. The oft-quoted concern over the precipitation of heart failure in otherwise healthy elderly patients appears to be overstated, since many studies have failed to demonstrate this to be a major problem. Part of the reason may be that any negative inotropic action is offset by the advantages of decreased ventricular afterload and the increased filling time of the stiff hypertensive, elderly ventricle resulting from drug-induced bradycardia. Beta-adrenoceptor antagonists with intrinsic sympathomimetic activity have theoretical advantages in elderly patients since they may be less negatively inotropic than other beta-adrenoceptor antagonists and have a lesser trendency to precipitate sinus node dysfunction. As in younger individuals, water-soluble agents such as atenolol are effectively excluded from the central nervous system and are therefore less likely to cause nightmares and sleep disturbance than lipid-soluble agents such as propranolol.

Calcium Antagonists

The use of calcium antagonists as monotherapy in "young" hypertensives is often associated with side effects directly referable to peripheral vasodilatation (headache, flushing, peripheral edema). Similar symptoms occur in elderly patients. One side effect of verapamil, namely constipation, may be particularly troublesome in elderly patients, in whom gastrointestinal motility is already impaired. The overall incidence of side-effects ranges from as low as 5% to as high as 90%, and an incidence greater than 30% is commonplace. Some studies even suggest an increased incidence of side effects in the elderly but in one large study using nicardipine, the withdrawal rate due to side effects was not age dependent [26].

On the positive side, calcium antagonists may have a lesser tendency to cause reflex tachycardia in elderly patients due to age-related changes in compensatory baroreflex mechanisms and chronotropic responses to autonomic stimuli, in addition to direct cardiac actions of drugs such as verapamil and diltiazem on cardiac conducting tissue. There is some evidence for this suggestion from clinical studies using nicardipine and verapamil, though nitrendipine and diltiazem have little effect on heart rate in any age group, and heart rate still tends to increase in elderly patient treated with nifedipine, at least in the early stages, although not sufficiently to cause symptoms. Other possible advantages of calcium antagonists include the lack of secondary metabolic abnormalities during treatment.
malities during treatment.

Angiotensin-Converting Enzyme (ACE) Inhibitors

ACE inhibitors reduce blood pressure without causing a reflex tachycardia in any age group, probably as the result of the removal of angiotensin II mediated vagal inhibition and sympathetic potentiation. These agents appear to be well tolerated in elderly patients. Indeed, there is evidence that a sense of well-being may be associated with the use of these agents. It is likely, however, that this sense of well-being is a consequence of the fact that the ACE inhibitors may have less side effects than the antihypertensive drugs that such patients had previously been given [27]. There is no evidence that ACE inhibitors have an intrinsic euphoric effect in previously untreated patients, despite theoretical reasons why this might be the case. Mental performance appears to be unaffected by ACE inhibitors, which is of particular importance in relation to elderly patients. ACE inhibitors are not entirely devoid of side effects, however. One of particular concern in the elderly is the first-dose hypotensive effect, which, although more common in patients with heart failure or those taking diuretics, may occur in the absence of such factors. A rapid drop in blood pressure may have particularly deleterious effects on the renal, coronary, and cerebral circulations of elderly patients with extensive atheroma. Other side effects such as rash, gastrointestinal upset, taste disturbance, and cough are probably no more frequent in older vs younger patients.

Other Agents

Drugs such as methyldopa and clonidine appear to be reasonably well tolerated in elderly subjects, but dry mouth, sedation, and dizziness are particularly unpleasant side effects which may lead to poor compliance. This is particularly dangerous with clonidine in view of possible rebound hypertension. As with the calcium antagonists, side effects tend to occur early in the course of treatment and may show some tendency to subside with time; therefore, supervision must be particularly vigilant during this period. Long-acting transdermal clonidine preparations are now available, but may have an unacceptable propensity to cause skin reactions. Postural hypotension does not appear to be a major problem with the use of these agents in the elderly. Despite the impression that these agents are no more prone to cause side effects in the elderly subgroup as a whole, the fact that their action is mediated at a central level would suggest that they should not be used in patients with any prior history of intellectual impairment. Similar side effects also occur in patients treated with alpha-adrenoceptor antagonists. Indoramin has significant effects on the central nervous system and should probably be avoided in the elderly. Reflex tachycardia appears uncommon in elderly patients treated with prazosin or indoramin. Additional side effects include first-dose hypotension, edema, and sexual dysfunction, although the frequency of these and other side effects in the elderly vs younger patients is not known.

The Importance of Intercurrent Diseases

Since there are no major differences in the average expected effect of any antihypertensive drug between different age groups, the choice of antihypertensive agent in the elderly should be determined primarily by the clinical characteristics of individual patients. In this regard, the presence of intercurrent diseases which may modify drug kinetics, dynamics, or adverse effects are an important consideration, not least because they may require specific treatment themselves, thereby increasing the chance of drug interactions. The coexistence of other diseases may also modify the choice of antihypertensive agent in a rather more positive manner in the sense that many antihypertensive drugs are also useful in the treatment of other conditions common amongst the elderly. Some examples may illustrate these points:

Heart failure. This is a common complication in elderly hypertensive patients. Beta-adrenoceptor antagonists are absolutely contraindicated in advanced heart failure, calcium antagonists must be used with caution, whereas diuretics are still the mainstay of treatment. ACE inhibitors have been shown to produce a moderate increase in the life expectancy of patients with severe heart failure but considerable care is required. Diuretic dosage should be reduced to render the patient less angiotensin dependent before the ACE inhibitor is administered, and the blood pressure should be checked frequently following the first dose. Patients with heart failure requiring high dose diuretics are particularly likely to develop hypotension and/or acute renal failure with ACE inhibitors, and a number of deaths have been reported, particularly in elderly patients [28]. Centrally acting vasodilators such as methyldopa are not contraindicated in heart failure, and alpha receptor antagonists have been used in the treatment thereof. All vasodilator agents may, however, exacerbate pre-existent ankle edema, which may necessitate the introduction of or an increased dose of diuretics.

Osteoarthritis. The incidence of this condition rises progressively with age, and the use of nonsteroidal anti-inflammatory drugs (NSAID) by elderly patients is very common. The administration of NSAID to treated hypertensive patients may also lead to a deterioration in blood pressure control, the mechanisms of which are complex. Since a comprehensive drug history is often difficult to obtain from elderly patients, this problem may go unnoticed. In addition, these agents have recently been implicated in the pathogenesis of some cases of renal failure following the administration of ACE inhibitors to elderly patients with heart failure and hypertension [28].

Atheromatous vascular disease. Hypertension and age are both risk factors for coronary, cerebral, and peripheral vascular disease, and it is therefore not surprising that one or more of these conditions may coexist in the elderly hypertensive. The choice of antihypertensive agent in such patients somewhat depends on which vascular territory is most severely affected. Thus, hypertensive patients with predominant angina may particularly benefit from the use of beta-adrenoceptor antagonists or calcium antagonists.

Diabetes mellitus. Pancreatic function deteriorates progressively with age and consequently benzothiadiazine diuretics are more likely to precipitate diabetes mellitus rather than mild glucose intolerance. Beta-adrenoceptor blockade reduces the reactive glyemic response to hypoglycemia, but, unless elderly patients with maturity-onset diabetes are taking insulin or inappropriately large doses of sulphonylurea agents, particularly chlorpropamide, this is unlikely to pose a greater problem in the elderly vs younger diabetic population. Both ACE inhibitors and calcium antagonists are suitable alternatives in such patients, and ACE inhibitors may reduce proteinuria in diabetic patients with renal impairment [29, 30].

Chronic lung disease. Moderate or severe airways disease is a contraindication to the use of beta-adrenoceptor antagonists, although some authors suggest that agents with intrinic sympathomimetic activity, e.g., pindolol, or cardioselectivity, e.g., atenolol, may be tolerated in patients with mild disease.

Concluding Remarks

Elderly patients whose only medical problem is hypertension appear to respond similarly, though not identically, to all the hypotensive agents commonly used in younger patients. At all ages, the degree of variation in response between individuals exceeds the effect of age itself. Elderly patients, however, are much more likely to suffer from an intercurrent disease which may indicate or contraindicate one of the main classes of antihypertensive drugs. A good working knowledge of the pharmacology and side effects of many different antihypertensive drugs is therefore essential. In deciding upon a drug regime for these patients, it should be remembered that the incidence of side effects will be minimized if drugs are introduced at the smallest dose, in the smallest number, and with the longest acceptable dose interval. This parsimony of prescribing is important at any age, but in the elderly it is vital.

References

1. Medical Research Council Working Party (1985) MRC trial of treatment of mild hypertension: principal results. Br Med J 291: 97-104
2. Veterans Administration Cooperative Study Group on Antihypertensive Agents (1982) Comparison of propranolol and hydrochlorothiazide for the initial treatment of hypertension. Results of short-term titration with emphasis on racial differences in response. JAMA 248: 1996-2003
3. Miall W, Greenberg G (1987) Mild hypertension — is there pressure to treat? Cambridge University Press
4. Buhler F, Burkart F, Lutold B, Kung M, Marbet G, Pfisterer M (1975) Antihypertensive betablocking action as related to renin and age: a pharmacological tool to identify pathogenetic mechanisms in essential hypertension. Am J Cardiol 36: 653-669
5. Buhler F (1983) Age the cardiovascular response adaptation. Determinants of an antihypertensive treatment concept primarily based on beta-blockers and calcium entry blockers. Hypertension 5 (Suppl III): 94-100
6. Erne P, Bolli P, Bertel O, Hulthen U, Kiowski W, Muller F, Buhler F (1983) Factors influencing the hypotensive effects of calcium antagonists. Hypertension 5 (Suppl II): 97-102.
7. Wenting G, DeBruyn J, Man In't Veld A, Woittez A, Derkx F, Schalekamp M (1982) Hemodynamic effects of captopril in essential hypertension, renovascular hypertansion and cardiac failure: correlations with short- and long-term effects on plasma renin. Am J Cardiol 49: 1453-1459
8. Amery A, Birkenhager W, Brixko R, Bulpitt C, Clement D, Deruyttere M, De Schaepdryver A, Dollery C, Fagard R, Forette F, Forte J, Hamdy R, Henry J, Joossens J, Leonetti G, Lund-Johansen P, O'Malley K, Petrie J, Strasser T, Tuomilehto J, Williams B (1986) Efficacy of antihypertensive drug treatment according to age, sex, blood pressure and prior cardiovascular disease in patients over the age of 60. Lancet 2: 589-592
9. Castleden C, Kaye C, Parsons R (1975) The effect of ageing on plasma levels of propranolol and practolol in man. Br J Clin Pharmacol 2: 303-306
10. Castleden C, George C (1979) The effect of ageing on the hepatic clearance of propranolol. Br J Clin Pharmocol 7: 49-54
11. Schneider R, Bishop H, Yates R (1980) Effect of age on plasma propranolol levels. Br J Clin Pharmacol 10: 169-171
12. Vestal R, Wood A, Branch R, Shand D, Wilkinson D (1979) Effects of age and cigarette smoking on propranolol disposition. Clin Pharmacol Ther 26: 8-15
13. Digby J, Scott A, Hawksworth G, Petrie J (1985) A comparison of the pharmacokinetics of atenolol, metoprolol, oxprenolol and propranolol in elderly hypertensive and young healthy subjects. Br J Clin Pharmacol 20: 327-331
14. Rubin P, Scott P, McLean K, Pearson A, Ross D, Reid J (1982) Atenolol disposition in young and elderly subjects. Br J Clin Pharmacol 13: 235-237
15. Hockings N, Ajayi A, Reid J (1986) Age and the pharmacokinetics of angiotensin converting enzyme inhibitors enalapril and enalaprilat. Br J Clin Pharmacol 21: 341-348
16. Lees R, Reid J (1987) Age and the pharmacokinetics and pharmacodynamics of chronic enalapril treatment. Clin Pharmacol Ther 41: 597-602
17. Hurwitz N (1969) Predisposing factors in adverse reactions to drugs Br Med J 1: 536-539
18. Bulpitt C, Dollery C, Carne S (1974) A symptom questionnaire for hypertensive patients. J Chronic Dis 27: 309-323
19. Curb J, Borhani N, Blaszkowski T (1985) Long-term surveillance for adverse effects of antihypertensive drugs. JAMA 253: 3263-3268
20. Goldner M, Zarowitz H, Akgun S (1960) Hyperglycemia and glycosuria due to thiazide derivatives administered in diabetes millitus. N Engl J Med 262: 403-405
21. Hicks B, Ward J, Jarrett R (1973) A controlled study of clopamide and clorexolone and hydrochlorothiazide in diabetes. Metabolism 22: 101-109

22. Amery A, Birkenhager W, Brixko P, Bulpitt C, Clement D, Deruyttere M, De Schaep-
    dryver A, Fagard R, Forette F, Forte J, Hamdy R, Leonetti G, O'Malley K, Murphy M,
    Petrie J, Tuomilehto J, Webster J, Williams B (1986) Glucose intolerance during diuretic
    therapy in elderly hypertensive patients. A second report from the European working
    party on high blood pressure in the elderly (EWPHE). Postgrad Med J 62: 919-924
23. Berglund G, Andersson O (1981) Beta-blockers or diuretics in hypertension? A six-year
    follow-up of blood pressure and metabolic side effects. Lancet 1: 744-747
24. Helderman J, Elahi D, Andersen D, Raizes G, Tobin J, Shocken D, Andres R (1983)
    Prevention of the glucose intolerance of thiazide diuretics by maintenance of body potas-
    sium. Diabetes 32: 106-111
25. MRC Trial (1981) Report of medical research council working party on mild to moderate
    hypertension. Adverse reactions to bendrofluazide and propranolol for the treatment of
    mild hypertension. Lancet 2: 539-542
26. Dubois C, Blanchard D, Loria Y, Moreau M (1987) Clinical trial of a new antihyper-
    tensive drug, nicardipine: efficacy and tolerance in 29 104 patients. Curr Ther Res
    42: 727-736
27. Hill J, Bulpitt C, Fletcher A (1985) Angiotensin converting enzyme inhibitors and quality
    of life: the European trial. J Hypertens 3 (Suppl II): S91-S94
28. Speirs C, Dollery C, Inman W (1988) Post-marketing surveillance of enalapril, part II.
    Investigation of the potential role of enalapril in deaths with renal failure. Br Med J (in
    press)
29. Taquma Y, Kitamoto Y, Futaki G, Ueda H, Monma H, Ishizaki M, Takahashi H,
    Sekino H, Sasaki Y (1985) Effect of captopril on heavy proteinuria in azotemic diabetics
    N Engl J Med 313: 1617-1620
30. Bjorck S, Nyberg G, Mulec H Granerus G, Herlitz H, Aurell M (1986) Beneficial effects
    of angiotensin converting enzyme inhibition on renal function in patients with diabetic
    nephropathy. Br Med J 293: 471-474

Discussion

Birkenhäger (Rotterdam): One comment — I completely agree with you that the attenuating effect of indomethacin is a more general one than has been supposed by some. Still, the prostaglandin story pops up all the time. Could you think of an alternative explanation? I myself, was thinking about mild chronic sodium retention and the influence of that kind of drugs. What do you think?

Dollery (London): I did not mean to imply, Wilhelm, that prostaglandins are not important in blood pressure regulation. I simply meant that I did not think that they played a unique role with ACE inhibitors. I went to a very interesting meeting in America about a year ago, where we discussed at great length these issues with Mike Dunn from Cleveland; and the conclusion we reached then was the effect of non-steroidals on blood pressure is probably a combination of two factors. One is that they do tend to increase the peripheral vascular resistance, and that may be due to an attenuation of presynaptic receptor effects of PGE_2. The other thing is, as you said, they do tend to cause retention of sodium with an average weight gain of about 1.5 kg. Our conclusion in that meeting was that the combination of those two things was probably the reason the blood pressure went up. It is worth making the point that blood pressure will go up with indomethacin without the patient being on any antihypertensive drug; in other words, it will push the blood pressure up per se.

Takeda (Osaka): Whenever I consider the treatment of elderly hypertension, I usually keep in mind that older patients have had a longer history of management. For instance, some patients have had more than a quarter of a century of receiving antihypertensive drugs. Sometimes they began with taking rauwolfia for more than 10 years; then added with thiazides; and then began the beta-blockers and Ca antagonists. So some patients will continue for more than 20 years with diuretics; some will switch to other drugs with other mechanisms. in the case of patients treated for more than 10 or 20 years with rauwolfia, they have long-term depletion of internal catecholamine content. For many people, the cross-sectional view was a matter most, but we must always consider the longtitudinal effect of every patient's history of continued long-term treatment with various drugs. What do you think?

Dollery: I think it is a very important question, Dr. Takeda. One of the reasons we did the withdrawal study and the MRC trial, which I have spoken about before at this meeting, was that we wanted to have better data about what would happen if one stopped treatment after a long period. We concluded from that that the blood pressure would go up again to the previous level. Therefore, if there was a good reason for treating someone earlier in their life, then it seems unwise in most cases to stop the treatment. Fortunately, treatment usually gets somewhat easier during the first 5 years of treatment rather than more difficult, presumably because of the reversal of cardiovascular hypertrophy. If I can quote to you the last two or three sentences of the manuscript I submitted for this meeting, I said that in the treatment of the elderly one should try to use the lowest doses and at the longest intervals of the antihypertensive drugs. It probably didn't matter too much which one you used, as long as the patient responded to it. I went on to say that that parsimony of prescribing — I am not sure whether parsimony is an English word that would be well understood in Japan, but it means, if you like, sort of "economy" of prescribing — is important at any age group, but in the elderly it is vital.

Kuramoto (Tokyo): You mentioned that drug metabolism is little changed by advancing age; it has a very small influence. However, drugs metabolized or excreted from the liver such as calcium antagonists still have a higher blood concentration in old age than in younger age groups. How do you account for this kind of difference, and how would you differentiate the liver factor or metabolic factor from the renal factor?

Dollery: That is correct. I think the point I was trying to make is at any age group, if you take a drug that is metabolized, you are likely to find at least a five-fold range of half-lives in the normal population (if you take the mean and two plus a minus two standard deviations of the half-life) That variation at any age is actually greater than the change that takes place with aging itself. So, although it may be true that the average dose requirement is lower in elderly people, knowing that someone is elderly is of very limited help in telling you what the appropriate dose of the drug may be. It may turn out that they are a relatively rapid metabolizer, although elderly; and conversely a young person may be a relatively slow metabolizer. So, although what you say is true, when you are facing a patient across the office desk, it is of limited help.

Zanchetti (Milan): I think you rightly made a point of the effects of the nonsteroidal inflammatory drugs in blunting most of the antihypertensive medication's effects. You mentioned the certainly large use and abuse of these drugs in the elderly. My point is whether there is any evidence that the use of these drugs in clinical practice, mostly in hypertensive patients, is going to be different in terms of doses and duration than the one in the trial you showed. So, the intermittent doses, which very often the patients, (the elderly) are taking, are these going to give the same effect that you got in your trials? Is these evidence available from the EWPHE trial, for instance?

Dollery: You would have to ask Tonery, Alberto. I can answer the question indirectly because I have been reviewing with Dr. Inman in England the study he did in monitoring enalapril. Now that was a study mainly in heart failure, although quite a few of the patients were hypertensive, and we were interested in the provocation of renal failure in patients on enalapril. And the first thing we found was that most of those who seemed to have drug-related renal failure were elderly. The mean age was 72 years. The second thing was that almost all of those episodes of renal failure were related to inappropriate drug therapy, i.e., too high a dose of the ACE inhibitor itself; most commonly the use of high doses of diuretics. In, I think, four instances that were reasonably well documented, a patient who was in stable mild renal failure while on treatment with enalapril was then given a nonsteroidal antiinflammatory drug on top of that; and their blood pressure deteriorated, and their renal function deteriorated at the same time.

Session 2

Chairmen: W.H. Birkenhäger (Rotterdam)
T. Ogihara (Osaka)

Hemodynamics in Treatment with Calcium Antagonists

Per Lund-Johansen and Per Omvik[1]

Summary. The hemodynamic mechanisms responsible for increased blood pressure in the elderly differ greatly from the hemodynamic situation in younger patients. Recent data from our 20-year follow-up study on central hemodynamics in essential hypertension show that in elderly hypertensive subjects (aged 60-69 years with mean arterial blood pressure (MABP) of 113 mmHg), cardiac index (CI) was 42% lower than in young hypertensives (17-29 years) with the same MABP. Total peripheral resistance was 69% higher. During exercise, the blood pressure increased more steeply in the older group.

The hemodynamic changes induced by 5 different calcium antagonists were studied invasively at rest and during exercise in 76 patients aged 19-64 years with mild to moderate essential hypertension. *Acute* studies (nisoldipine and tiapamil) demonstrated that the initial fall in blood pressure was due to a marked decrease in total peripheral resistance and was associated with reflex tachycardia and an increase in cardiac output. During long-term treatment the reflex tachycardia disappeared. *Chronic* studies with verapamil ($n = 9$), tiapamil ($n = 18$), diltiazem ($n = 16$), nifedipine ($n = 15$), and nisoldipine ($n = 17$) demonstrated that all compounds reduced blood pressure 10%-17% at rest and during exercise. In all drug therapy, the fall in blood pressure was associated with reduction in total peripheral resistance. No reduction in heart pump function at rest or during exercise was seen. Exercise heart rate was reduced on verapamil, diltiazem, and tiapamil, but was compensated with an increase in stroke volume.

Since calcium antagonists induce few biochemical side effects, do not disturb pulmonary function, and maintain total and regional blood flow, they are well suited for treatment of hypertension in the elderly. Due to a rapid initial effect, however, the first dose should be small.

Key words: Hypertension — Hemodynamics — Exercise — Calcium antagonists — Nifedipine — Nisoldipine — Verapamil — Diltiazem — Tiapamil

Introduction

The hemodynamic mechanisms behind increased blood pressure may differ widely. In elderly subjects—who often have been hypertensive for decades—the flow/resistance pattern is generally very different from that seen in young and middle-aged subjects and is characterized by higher vascular resistance, considerably lower cardiac output and regional blood flow, and a steeper rise in blood pressure during exercise [1].

[1] Section of Cardiology, Medical Department, University of Bergen School of Medicine, Bergen, Norway

Antihypertensive agents affect the hemodynamics of hypertension in various ways and differ greatly in their ability to normalize central hemodynamics [2]. While beta-blockers generally induce a permanent reduction in the blood flow both at rest and during exercise and an increase in the arteriovenous oxygen difference, the more modern antihypertensive agents—like the calcium antagonists—lower blood pressure through different and more physiological mechanisms.

This paper will describe briefly the major hemodynamic abnormalities in elderly hypertensive subjects, and then, discuss how the various calcium antagonists effect these hemodynamic disturbances.

Hemodynamics in Elderly Hypertensives

Data on the hemodynamics of the aging cardiovascular system are insufficient and many controversies still exist in normotensive as well as in hypertensive populations.

In *normotensive* subjects, most studies based on invasive methods have demonstrated a fall in cardiac output and a slight increase in blood pressure and total peripheral resistance with normal aging [3]. However, in recent years a large study from Baltimore, based on non invasive methods, has indicated that in carefully selected subjects (without any signs of heart diesease), cardiac output at rest and during exercise did not fall with aging, the fall in heart rate (HR) being compensated by an increase in stroke volume [4].

In *hypertensive* populations, many cross-sectional and some longitudinal studies have demonstrated a fall in cardiac output and stroke index (SI) with aging — at rest as well as during exercise. Total peripheral resistance increases markedly. The dimension of these alterations can be illustrated by some results from our 20-year follow-up study on central hemodynamics in hypertensive patients.

This study, which started in 1967, has followed central hemodynamics at rest and during exercise by invasive methods: blood pressure through catheter in brachial artery and cardiac output by dye dilution method (Cardiogreen). Recordings have been made at rest, supine, and sitting and during 50, 100, and 150 w steady state exercise loads [5].

Table 1 shows the results in 14 subjects, age 17–29 years when studied in 1967, and in 19 subjects, age 60–69 years when studied in 1987. The older group had been hypertensive for at least 20 years. (The group had been on antihypertensive treatment, but was taken off drugs a short time before the 20-year hemodynamic follow-up re-examination. The table shows that the 2 groups have approximately the same MABP (114.1 vs 113.0 mmHg); but the systolic blood pressure (SP) is 11 mmHg higher in the older group, and the diastolic blood pressure (DP) is 7.3 mmHg lower.

When the older group is compared to the younger, it is seen that CI is only 2.17 vs 3.72 l/min m² or 42% lower, and total peripheral resistance index (TPRI) is 69% higher.

During 100 w exercise, CI in the older group is 36% lower than in the younger, partly due to lower HR and partly due to lower SI. TPRI is 78% higher in the older group (Table 2). The rise in SP from rest to exercise is approximately 10 mmHg higher in the older group, and the rise in MAB is 25.9 mmHg vs only 9.8 mmHg in the younger group.

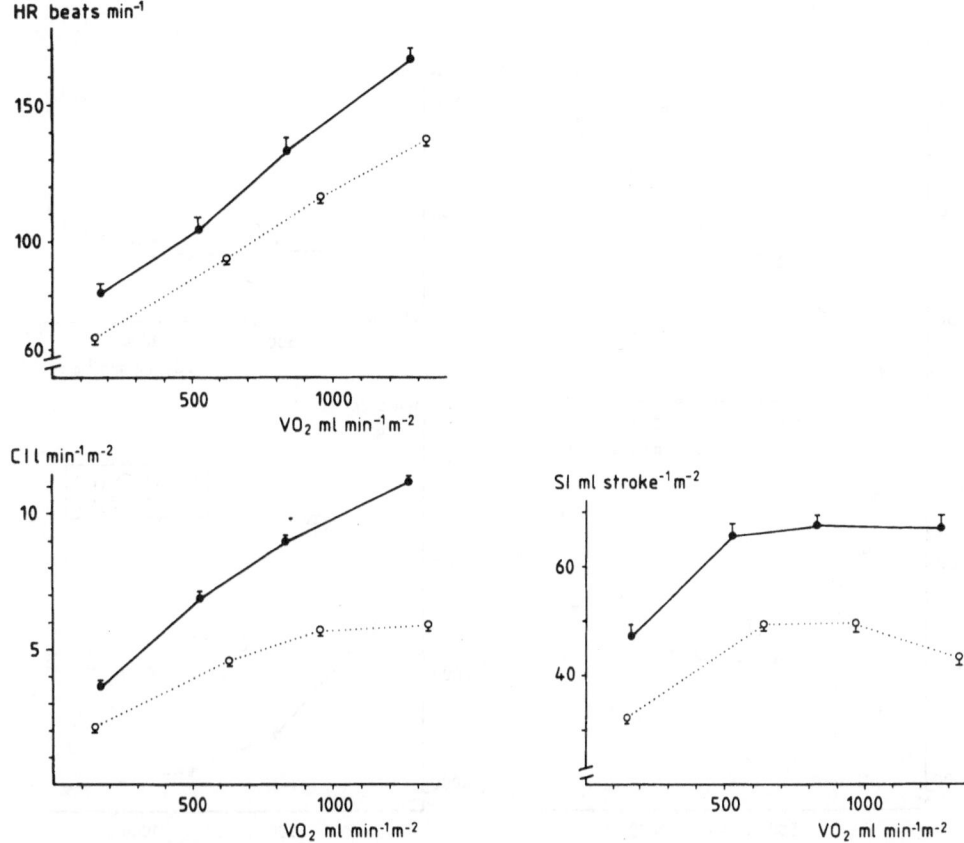

Fig. 1. Hemodynamics in 19 elderly (60-69 years) (⋯⋯⋯) and 14 young (17-29 years) (——) hypertensive subjects. Mean values; *CI*, cardiac index; *SI*, stroke index; VO_2, oxygen consumption

Figures 1 and 2 illustrate the differences between central hemodynamics in these 2 age groups. Note that SI is falling in transition from mild to severe exercise in the oldest group — indicating incipient heart failure.

Like TPRI, aortic rigidity also increases with age. Figure 3 shows that it was much higher in the older group, and increased with aging in both age groups.

A few studies from even older subjects (studied at rest only) have shown results rather similar to ours, a fall in CI and an increase in TPRI with aging [6, 7]. The reduction in the heart pump function at rest and during exercise with aging is generally associated with left ventricular hypertrophy and reduced compliance of the left ventricle. Reduction in compliance is already seen at an early stage, and it has been shown that peak filling rate at rest and during exercise decreases with advancing age [8, 9]. There are few large systematic studies on regional blood flow in hypertensive subjects in different ages; but, in general, it seems that the reduction in cardiac output with aging is reflected as reduced blood flow to the kidneys, the splanchnic area, the myocardium, and the brain [1].

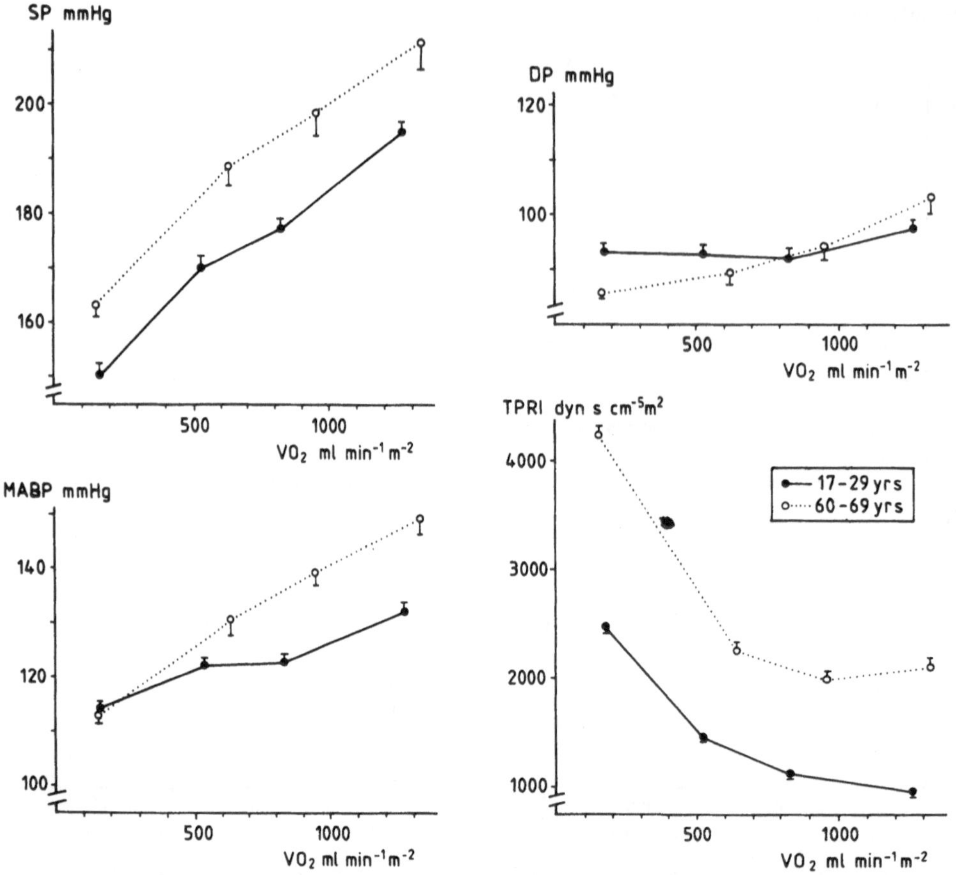

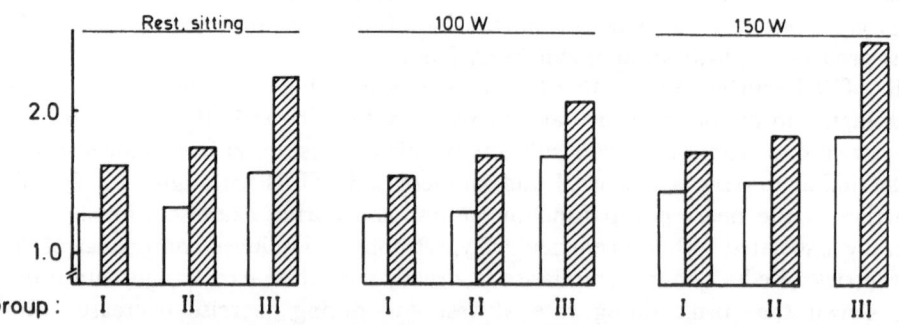

Fig. 2. Hemodynamics in old (60–69 years; $n = 19$)(··········) versus young (17–29 years; $n = 14$) (——) hypertensive subjects. Systolic (*SP*), diastolic (*DP*), and mean arterial (*MABP*) blood pressure and total peripheral resistance index (*TPRI*) at rest and during exercise. Mean values and SEM

Fig. 3. Aortic rigidity index in hypertensive subjects on first examination in 1967 (□) and on reexamination in 1987 (▨). Age group I (17–29 years), age group II (30–39 years), and age group III (40–49 years) at first study in 1967. Note the increase in aortic rigidity with aging in all age groups

Hemodynamic Effects of Calcium Antagonists in Hypertension

Although the calcium antagonists have been used for treatment of hypertension in patients covering a large age span, most of the data on the hemodynamics are unfortunately obtained in middle-aged subjects.

Our own studies have been performed in patients with mild to moderately severe essential hypertension, aged 19–64 years. Central hemodynamics have been studied invasively at rest and during exercise, and the following calcium antagonists have been studied: nifedipine ($n = 15$), nisoldipine ($n = 17$), verapamil ($n = 9$), tiapamil ($n = 19$), and diltiazem ($n = 16$).

The number of patients in each drug study, their age distribution, basic blood pressures, body surface area (BSA), and dosage are seen in Table 3. Generally, the starting dosage was approximately half of the later daily maintaining dosage. The aim of treatment was a basic blood pressure — 140/90 mmHg (sitting, after at least 10 min rest) without side effects. No patients had to be withdrawn due to side-effects in any of the series, but temporary flushing, palpitations, and restlessness appeared in 7 patients in the dihydropyridine derivative series. Ankle edema was seen in 4 patients on nisoldipine. In the other series fewer side effects were seen.

Hemodynamic Results

The Dihydropyridine Derivatives (Nifedipine and Nisoldipine)

The *acute* effect was studied only in the nisoldipine series [10]. The immediate effects (at rest, supine) are seen in Fig. 4. One h after 10 mg orally, there was a fall in TPRI of 19% ($P < 0.001$). The fall in blood pressure was partly counteracted by reflex tachycardia (HR increase of 9%) and an increase in CI of 12%. Due to the marked effect on total peripheral resistance, the net effect was a fall in MABP of 9% ($P < 0.001$). TPRI fell in all but one patient. During the following hours the effect leveled off.

After the acute study, the patients continued on nisoldipine orally, the dose gradually being increased to maximally 40 mg daily. With continued treatment the reflex tachycardia disappeared. Fig. 4 shows that *1 year* after treatment was started, HR and CI had practically returned to pretreatment levels at rest, supine. The fall in MABP (14%; $P < 0.001$) was due to reduction in TPRI of about 20%–18% ($P < 0.001$) at rest, supine and sitting. The reductions in SP, DP, and MABP were blood pressure similar. During exercise the relative fall in blood pressure was 12%, mainly due to fall in TPRI.

Thus, nisoldipine, acutely as well as chronically, reduced blood pressure through vasodilatation and reduction in TPRI. No reduction in heart pump function at rest (measured as CI) was seen. Details of our nisoldipine series have been published recently [10].

Table 1. Hemodynamics at rest (sitting) in patients with essential hypertension

Age (years)	Systolic pressure (mmHg)	Diastolic pressure (mmHg)	Mean arterial blood pressure (mmHg)	Cardiac index (l/min m²)	Stroke index (l/stroke m²)	HR (beats/min)	Total peripheral resistance index (dyn s/cm⁵ m²)
17–29 (n = 14)	151.8 ± 13.3	93.3 ± 7.3	114.1 ± 7.9	3.72 ± 0.59	46.5 ± 7.7	81.1 ± 13.5	2499 ± 377
60–69 (n = 19)	162.8 ± 15.9	86.0 ± 4.4	113.0 ± 8.1	2.17 ± 0.27	34.2 ± 5.0	64.2 ± 8.1	4223 ± 589

Means values ± SD

Table 2. Hemodynamics at 100 w exercise on ergometer bicycle in patients with essential hypertension

Age (years)	Systolic pressure (mmHg)	Diastolic pressure (mmHg)	Mean arterial blood pressure (mmHg)	Cardiac index (l/min m²)	Stroke index (l/stroke m²)	HR (beats/min)	Total peripheral resistance index (dyn s/cm⁵ m²)
17–29 (n = 14)	177.8 ± 15.7	92.9 ± 8.7	123.9 ± 8.9	8.95 ± 0.79	67.5 ± 8.2	134.0 ± 17.4	1112 ± 100
60–69 (n = 19)	197.4 ± 27.5	94.5 ± 12.3	138.8 ± 16.4	5.70 ± 0.72	49.2 ± 6.9	116.7 ± 15	1977 ± 303

Means values ± SD

Table 3. Patient parameters before and during calcium antagonist therapy

Group	n	Age (years) Range	Mean	Casual blood pressure (mmHg) Before	During	Body surface area (m²)	Dosage (mg) Range	Mean
Verapamil	9	35–55	(45)	166/106	143/92	2.01	120–240	(220)
Diltiazem	16	38–64	(52)	174/106	144/86	1.99	180–360	(278)
Tiapamil	19	19–64	(45)	166/106	148/92	1.97	600–1200	(980)
Nifedipine	15	20–64	(44)	160/104	140/94	1.99	40–80	(52)
Nisoldipine	17	29–61	(43)	167/108	141/88	2.01	10–40	(25)

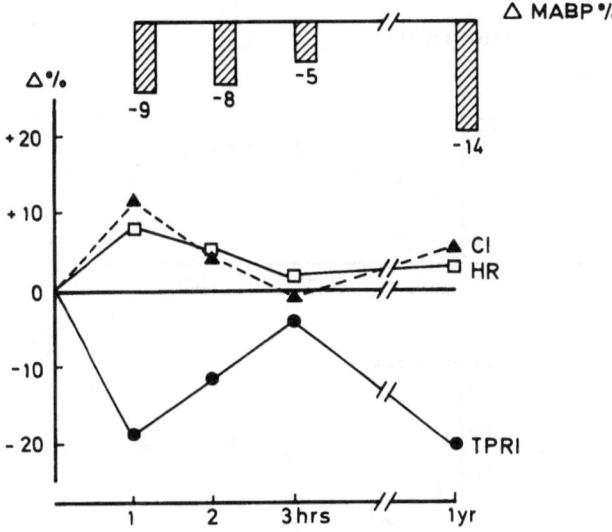

Fig. 4. Acute and chronic (1 year) hemodynamic changes induced in 19 hypertensives (21–69 years) by nisoldipine treatment. Note reflex tachycardia the first hours after initial dose. *MABP*, mean arterial blood pressure; *CI*, cardiac index; *TPRI*, total peripheral resistance index. With permission from J Hypertens [10]

Nifedipine

Studies from other laboratories have shown that nifedipine given *acutely* induces hemodynamic changes very similar to those observed in our nisoldipine series [11, 12].

Nifedipine was studied only on *long-term* basis. We used long-acting nifedipine tablets (40–80 mg daily) [13]. All 15 patients studied achieved some reduction in blood pressure. The fall in MABP was approximately 17% during rest and 11%–15% during exercise. The changes in SP, DP, and MABP were similar. The fall in blood pressure was entirely due to reduction in TPRI of approximately 17%. During chronic treatment, there were no changes in HR, CI, or SI. The long-term hemodynamic profile of nifedipine at rest and during exercise is shown in Fig. 5. Note that the CI, SI and HR values before and after treatment overlap and that no reflex tachycardia was seen. Recording were made 2–4 h after the last dose.

The group has continued on nifedipine for 6 years. There has been no indication of tachyphylaxis, and the blood pressure control over 6 years has been satisfactory.

Calcium Antagonists with Electrophysiological Effects (Verapamil, Diltiazem, and Tiapamil)

All three compounds have important electrophysiological effects and may induce bradycardia and increase atrio-ventricular conduction time [14, 15] — essential facts to remember when elderly hypertensives are to be treated.

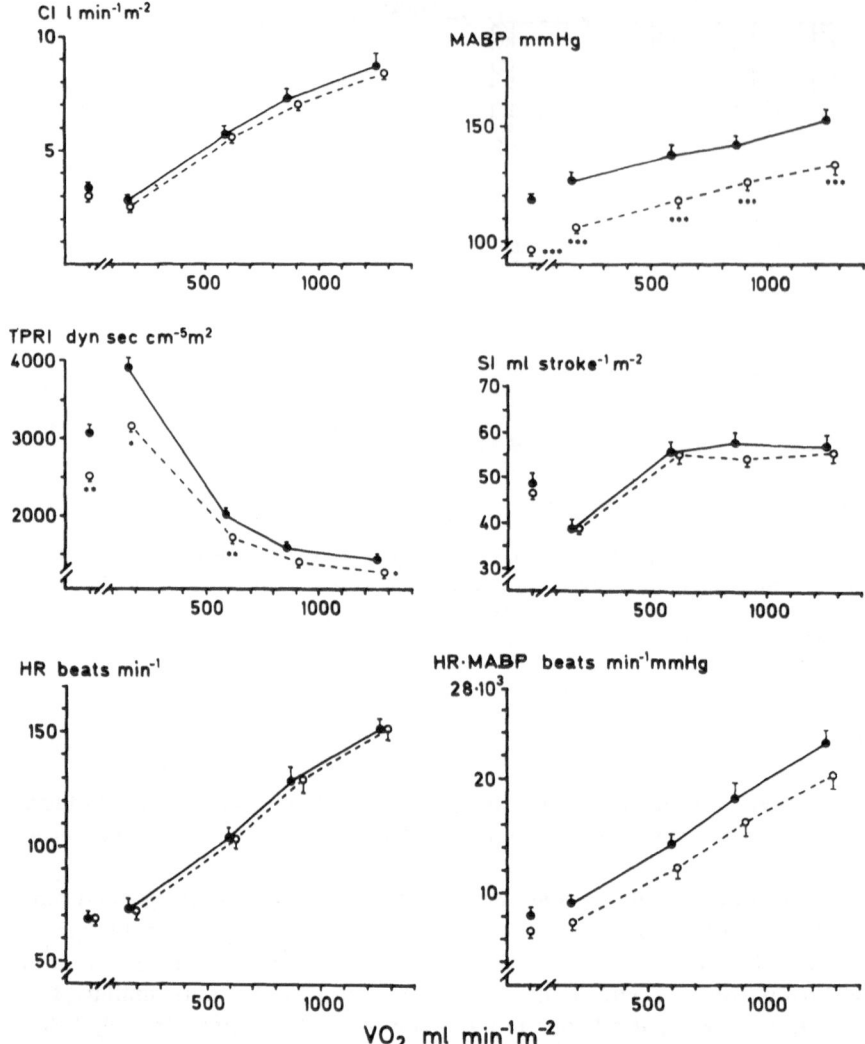

Fig. 5. Hemodynamic profile of chronic treatment with nifedipine. 14 hypertensives (20–64 years) before (——) and after (·····) *CI*, cardiac index; *SI*, stroke index; *MABP*, mean arteria blood pressure; *TPRI*, total peripheral resistance index. From Hypertens [13] with permission

Verapamil

In our verapamil series (daily dosage 120–240 mg; 1 year follow-up) blood pressures (SP, DP, and MABP) were reduced about 10% at rest and slightly less during exercise. The blood pressure reduction was due to significant reduction in TPRI at rest, sitting, (14%, $P < 0.001$). During exercise the reductions in resistance and blood pressure were less. In contrast to nifedipine, verapamil induced a reduction in exercise HR of approximately 8%–11%. However, the reduction in HR was compensated by an increase in SI, and CI was practically unchanged, at rest as well as during exercise. Thus, exercise blood flow was maintained undisturbed. No side effects were seen in this small group of 9 patients.

Diltiazem

The 16 patients participating in the diltiazem study had somewhat higher blood pressures and TPRI values than patients participating in other series. At the first hemodynamic study, the intra-arterially recorded values at rest, sitting, were: SP/DP, 183/108 mmHg; MABP, 137 mmHg; CI, 2.43 l/min. m²; and TPRI, 4613 dyn s/cm⁵. m².

Diltiazem retard was given twice daily (120–360 mg, mean 278 mg). After 1 year, the group was reevaluated. No side effects were reported. The reductions in blood pressures (SP, DP, and MABP) were 13%–16% at rest and 12%–14% during exercise. TPRI was reduced by 19% ($P < 0.001$) at rest, sitting, and slightly less during muscular exercise. Like verapamil, diltiazem also induced a fall in exercise HR. During 50, 100, and 150 w exercise, the reductions were 10% ($P < 0.001$) in all situations. The reduction in exercise HR was compensated completely by an increase in SI, and CI was practically unchanged. No patient developed bradycardia, however. Exercise time on 150 w exercise was not reduced, and SI during 150 w did not decline from the 7th to the 20th of exercising.

Tiapamil

In the *acute* study, 600 mg tiapamil was given orally, and central hemodynamics were studied over 3 h. A 21% reduction in TPRI was seen after 1 h. This was counteracted by increases in HR and CI of 7% and 11%, respectively; but due to the marked fall in TPRI, the net effect was a decrease in SP, DP, and MABP of approximately 14%. The effect leveled off during the following 3 h.

During *chronic* treatment (600–1200 mg daily, mean 980 mg), basic blood pressure fell in all 18 patients who were reexamined — from 166/106 mmHg after the placebo period to 148/92 mmHg shortly before the hemodynamic reevaluation. However, the long-term reduction in TPRI on tiapamil was less than that induced by diltiazem, nifedipine, and nisoldipine — only approximately 5%–6%. There was no reduction in HR during rest, but post-treatment exercise HR was reduced approximately 8%. The fall in blood pressure was a modest 8%–10%. Thus, in our long-term series, tiapamil induced less reduction in TPRI and less satisfactory blood pressure control than the other calcium antagonists studied.

Discussion

Cross-sectional as well as longitudinal studies have shown that the central hemo-dynamics in essential hypertension change over the years from a "high-flow normal-resistance" pattern in the starting phase towards a "low-flow high-resistance" pattern in established and late hypertension [1]. Thus, in elderly hypertensives, cardiac output at rest and during exercise is considerably lower than in middle-aged and young hypertensive subjects. The arteriovenous oxygen difference is increased, particularly during exercise, and signals decrease in the pumping reserve of the heart [3]. From a pathophysiological point of view, the logical way to treat hypertension in the elderly would be to reduce vascular resistance without further compromising blood flow, at rest or during exercise.

Although chronic use of thiazide diuretics reduce total peripheral resistance, these compounds do not cause a complete normalization of the circulatory system. They also induce a permanent reduction in plasma volume and frequently cause unwanted biochemical side effects [2].

It is well established that the beta-blockers tend to reduce cardiac output in the majority of patients with essential hypertension, at rest and in particular during exercise. Although beta-blockers with strong intrinsic sympathomimetic activity (ISA) may not reduce cardiac output at rest in the relaxed state [16], reduction in cardiac output during exercise may also be induced with these compounds [17]. In elderly hypertensives (without coronary heart disease), further reduction in the abnormally low blood flow may induce decreases in the regional circulation in different vascular beds. In clinical practice, the beta-blockers frequently induce reduction in peripheral blood flow in the extremities and cause complaints of cold hands and feet. The results obtained on the calcium antagonists studied in our series clearly differ from what has been achieved with beta-blockers in similar groups of patients studied with the same protocol. All the calcium antagonists studied induced reduction in blood pressure through vasodilatation and reduction in total peripheral resistance. There was no depression in heart pump function measured as cardiac output, at rest or during exercise.

It is important to note the differences between the dihydropyridine derivatives on one hand and verapamil, diltiazem and tiapamil on the other. The latter induce about 10% reduction in HR during exercise and sometimes also during rest conditions. It has been claimed that combination of such drugs and beta-blockers may induce substantial bradycardia in some patients and should therefore be used with caution or not used at all [14, 15, 18].

In contrast, the dihydropyridine derivatives do not effect HR during chronic use; and they may be combined with beta-blockers, which may be an advantage in subgroups of elderly patients. The dihydropyridine derivatives (used in capsule preparation) reduce blood pressure very quickly and should be used with some caution — particularly in elderly subjects. With respect to nifedipine, a starting dose of 5 mg might be appropriate. Even if the blood pressure does not fall to levels lower than desired, a pronounced reflex tachycardia may be bothersome; consequently, some patients might be reluctant to continue using the drug. Since orthostatic hypotension is also common in elderly patients, it is important that these very potent antihypertensive agents should be used properly. For chronic use, the long-acting (or slow-release) forms are preferable [19]. In our own series nifedipine was used in tablet preparation, and complaints of tachycardia and palpitations were rare. During long-term use, the reflex tachycardia tends to disappear in most patients.

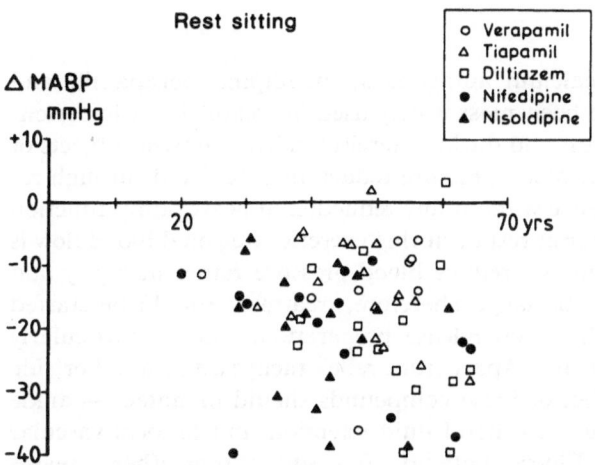

Fig. 6. Changes in mean arterial blood pressure ($\Delta MABP$) during chronic therapy in relation to patient age. All 74 patients on 5 different calcium antagonists are shown. Note that the calcium antagonists are effective in patients of all ages

Studies from other laboratories on regional circulation have shown that calcium antagonists in general induce vasodilatation [18, 19]. Vasodilatation has been demonstrated both in the large and small arteries. Although hard, long-lasting physical exercise is not commonly practised by most elderly patients, it should be stressed that the calcium antagonists do not reduce cardiac output or work performance — even during prolonged physical exercise [20–25]. This is in great contrast to beta-blockers, where reduction in physical endurance has been demonstrated [26, 27].

It has been much debated whether the calcium antagonists are more effective in elderly than in younger hypertensives with respect to the fall in blood pressure induced [28, 29]. Most of the published data show that the calcium antagonists are able to reduce blood pressure in adult hypertensive patients of all ages [Fig. 6. 30]. Figure 6 shows the pooled data from our 74 patients on chronic therapy, and they support this view.

In the debate about the drug of first choice in hypertensive patients in general, and in the elderly in particular, it should be stressed that other classes of antihypertensive agents are also able to induce reduction in blood pressure without a fall in heart pump function. Alpha-receptor blocker such as prazosin and doxazosin also reduce blood pressure through vasodilatation without reduction in heart pump function either at rest or during exercise [2]. Likewise, angiotensin-converting enzyme (ACE) inhibitors (like enalapril and captopril) reduce blood pressure through vasodilatation without fall in heart pump function. In recent years, these compounds have been used extensively in patients with heart failure, with or without hypertension. For this subgroup of patients, the ACE inhibitors are particularly useful and are preferable to the calcium antagonists [2].

Conclusion

It is well established that the calcium antagonists, (nifedipine, verapamil, and diltiazem) (which until now have been most widely used in treatment of hypertension), reduce blood pressure (at rest and during exercise) in hypertensive subjects of all ages including the elderly. The blood pressure reduction is achieved through reduction in total peripheral resistance without any reduction in heart pump function (measured as cardiac output) either at rest or during exercise. Regional blood flow is maintained. Most calcium antagonists reduce blood pressure rather abruptly and tend to induce reflex tachycardia initially. Therefore, treatment should be started with a low dose, preferably with a slow-release preparation. This is particularly important in the elderly hypertensive. Apart from reflex tachycardia, another side effect related to the vascular effect of these compounds should be noted — ankle edema. This side effect is not due to general fluid retention, but to local vascular effect and hydrostatic pressure. Elderly patients often suffer from other diseases which may limit the selection of suitable antihypertensive agents. The lack of biochemical side effects or unwanted effects on the airways are additional factors that would seem to make calcium antagonists an attractive choice when treating hypertension in the elderly [31, 32].

References

1. Lund-Johansen P (1983) The hemodynamics of essential hypertension. In: Robertson JIS (ed) Handbook of hypertension. Vol 1: Clinical aspects of essential hypertension. Elsevier, Amsterdam, pp 151–173
2. Lund-Johansen P (1988) Hemodynamic effects of antihypertensive agents. In: Doyle AE (ed) Handbook of hypertension. Vol 5: Clinical pharmacology of antihypertensive drugs. Elsevier, New York, pp 41–72
3. Lund-Johansen P (1988) The hemodynamics of the aging cardiovascular system. J Cardiovasc Pharmacol 12 (Suppl VIII): S20–S30
4. Rodeheffer RJ, Gerstenblith G, Becker LC, Fleg JL, Weisfeldt ML, Lakatta EG (1984) Exercise cardiac output is maintained with advancing age in healthy human subjects: cardiac dilatation and increased stroke volume compensate for a diminished heart rate. Circulation 69: 203–213
5. Lund-Johansen P (1967) Haemodynamics in early essential hypertension. Acta Med Scand 181 (Suppl 482): 1–101
6. Sato I, Tazumi K, Kato K, Kato S, Aoki K, Niimi T, Maeda K (1977) Significance of haemodynamic and electrocardiographic changes in elderly hypertension. Nippon Ronen Igakkai Zasshi 14: 99–109
7. Terasawa F, Kuramoto K, Ying LH, Suzuki T, Kuramochi M (1972) The study on the haemodynamics in old hypertensive subjects. Acta Gerontol Jpn 56: 47–55
8. Manvari DE, Patterson Ch, Johnson D, Belenkie I, Anderson P, Melendez L, Cape R (1985) Left ventricular diastolic function in a population of healthy elderly subjects. J Am Geriatr Soc 33: 758–767
9. Marcomichelakis J, Withers R, Newman GB, O'Brien K, Emanuel R (1983) The relation of age to the thickness of the inter-ventricular septum, the posterior left ventricular wall and their ratio. Int J Cardiol 4: 405–415
10. Omvik P, Lund-Johansen P, Haugland H (1988) Nisoldipine. Central haemodynamics at rest and during exercise in essential hypertension: acute and chronic studies. J Hypertens 6: 95–103

11. Kiowski W, Erne P, Bertel O, Bolli P, Bühler F (1986) Acute and chronic sympathetic reflex activation and anti-hypertensive response to nifedipine. J Am Coll Cardiol 7: 344–348
12. Aoki K, Sato K, Kawaguchi Y (1985) Increased cardiovascular responses to norepinephrine and calcium antagonists in essential hypertension compared with normotension in humans. J Cardiovasc Pharmacol 7 (Suppl VI): S182–S186
13. Lund-Johansen P, Omvik P (1983) Haemodynamic effects of nifedipine in essential hypertension at rest and during exercise. J Hypertens 1: 159–163
14. Halperin AK, Cubeddu LX (1986) The role of calcium channel blockers in the treatment of hypertension. Am Heart J 111: 363–382
15. Eichelbaum M, Echizen H (1984) Clinical pharmacology of calcium antagonists: a critical review. J Cardiovasc Pharmacol 6 (Suppl VII): S963–S967
16. Man in 't Veld AJ, Schalekamp MADH (1982) How intrinsic sympathomimetic activity modulates the haemodynamic responses to beta-adrenoceptor antagonists. A clue to the nature of their antihypertensive mechanism. Br J Clin Pharmacol 13: 245–257
17. Lund-Johansen P (1983) Central haemodynamic effects of beta-blockers in hypertension. A comparison between atenolol, metoprolol, timolol, penbutolol, alprenolol, pindolol and bunitrolol. Eur Heart J 4: D1–D12
18. Opie LH (1984) Calcium antagonists and cardiovascular disease. Ravan Press, New York
19. Lund-Johansen P (1987) Clinical use of calcium antagonists in hypertension: update 1986. J Cardiovasc Pharmacol 10 (Suppl X): S29–S34
20. Herpin D, Amiel A, Boutaud P, Wajman A, Demange J (1985) Effect of a calcium antagonist: verapamil on resting blood pressure and pressor response to dynamic exercise. Acta Cardiol 40: 277–290
21. Cody RJ, Kubo SH, Covit AB, Müller FB, Lopez-Ovejero J, Laragh JH (1986) Exercise hemodynamics and oxygen delivery in human hypertension. Response to verapamil. Hypertension 8: 3–10
22. Yamakado T, Oonishu N, Nakano T, Takezawa H (1985) Effects of nifedipine and diltiazem on hemodynamic responses at rest and during exercise in hypertensive patients. Jpn Circ J 49: 415–421
23. Klein W, Brandt D, Vrecko K, Härringer M (1983) Role of calcium antagonists in treatment of essential hypertension. Circ Res 52 (Suppl I): 174–181
24. Pool PE, Seagren SC, Salel AF, Skalland ML (1985) Effects of diltiazem on serum lipids, exercise performance and blood pressure: randomized, double-blind, placebo-controlled evaluation for systemic hypertension. Am J Cardiol 56: H86–H91
25. Franz I-W, Wiewel D (1984) Antihypertensive effects on blood pressure at rest and during exercise of calcium antagonists, beta-receptor blockers, and their combination in hypertensive patients. J Cardiovasc Pharmacol 6 (Suppl VII): S1037–S1042
26. Kaiser P (1984) Physical performance and muscle metabolism during beta-adrenergic blockade in man. Acta Physiol Scand 536 (Suppl I): 1–44
27. Lundborg P, Aström H, Bengtsson C, et al. (1981) Effect of beta-adrenoceptor blockade on exercise performance and metabolism. Clin Sci 61: 299–305
28. Bühler FR (1983) Age and cardiovascular response adaptation. Determinants of an antihypertensive treatment concept primarily based on beta-blockers and calcium entry blockers. Hypertension (Suppl III): 94–100
29. Bühler FR, Bolli P, Erne P, et al. (1985) Position of calcium antagonists in antihypertensive therapy. J Cardiovasc Pharmacol 7 (Suppl IV): S21–S27
30. Chalmers JP, Smith SA, Wing LMH (1988) Hypertension in the elderly: The role of calcium channel blocking drugs. J Cardiovasc Pharmacol (Suppl) (in press)
31. Brouwer RML, Follath F, Bühler FR (1985) Review of the cardiovascular adversity of the calcium antagonist betablocker combination: Implications for antihypertensive therapy. J Cardiovasc Pharmacol 7 (Suppl IV): S38–S44
32. Trost BN, Weidmann P (1984) Effects of nitrendipine and other calcium antagonists on glucose metabolism in man. J Cardiovasc Pharmacol 6 (Suppl VII): S1063–S1066

Discussion

Di Somma (Naples): Do you think that the diuretic effect of dihydropyridine derivative could be useful for hypertensive patients with a tendency to left ventricle impairment? In other words, what do you think of the possibility that dihydropyridine derivatives such as those Professor Zanchetti and Professor Leonetti have showed influencing this? Is a dihydropyridine derivative a good choice for hypertension and congestive heart failure? In other words, do you think that the diuretic effect of dihydropyridine derivatives could be an additive or positive effect for these kinds of drugs?

Lund-Johansen (Bergen): Well I am not aware of comparisons between, say, dihydropyridines and ACE inhibitors and/or diuretics in patients with heart failure. Obviously if the patient has a very poor heart, like in the study from Packer which I have shown, it might be dangerous to use these compounds. I do not think that any of us would recommend these compounds for patients with very severe heart failure. We would obviously use a diuretic which has a much greater diuretic effect; and I think that we would all — for this subgroup of patients — rather select an ACE inhibitor, which, as I guess you all know, have been shown to be very effective in patients with heart failure and have also prolonged life (the so-called Consensus trial).

Weidmann (Bern): I found it interesting and also refreshing that you did not see any relationship between the blood pressure level and the effects of some calcium antagonists and age, as was discussed before for the beta-blockers. Taking it from there, I was somewhat surprised that you concluded that the calcium antagonists may be valuable first-line drugs for treating the elderly. I thought, looking at your data, they would suggest as other data do that in fact calcium antagonists may be as useful in the young as in the elderly. However, you say that there might be other disadvantages particularly relevant to the young.

Lund-Johansen: Well, my impression and my own experience show that these compounds work in all ages; the shortcoming of my studies is that we have very few elderly subjects. I think the oldest subject was 68 years of age. So, we have no data which can really tell you about the elderly. In the young and in the middleaged, these compounds certainly are useful, they certainly lower blood pressure, and they certainly do not decrease cardiac output; So, I think that in young subjects also they might have many favorable charactersitics. Still, I think that if you have a young subject with an increased HR, those who are "nervous" with HRs around 80–85 at basic blood pressure recording; I would not recommend a dihydropyridine, because I think you would be asking for trouble. I would use either a beta-blocker or another compound, or, if a Ca antagonist, one which rather tended to reduce the heart rate, based on the hemodynamic characteristics.

Amery (Leuven): You showed that these was a decrease during exercise in the mean pulmonary artery pressure. Was it a decrease in the pulmonary artery resistance or wedge pressure?

Lund-Johansen: This was not one of my studies; it was a study by Leishman, where I just showed a simplified presentation of data. It was definitely a decrease in the filling pressure. I do not recall the pulmonary resistance values. I think this was also reduced.

Antihypertensive Drugs and Cerebral Circulation

Yoshihiro Kuriyama, Tohru Sawada, and Teruo Omae[1]

Summary. In elderly hypertensive patients, long-standing hypertension associated with occlusive cerebrovascular disease (CVD) might impair cerebral blood flow (CBF) autoregulation. The clinical significance of CBF autoregulation and the effects of antihypertensive drugs; on cerebral circulation are discussed. In the hemodynamic transient ischemic attack (TIA) cases we studied, the appearance of TIA was closely connected to the occurrence of moderate reduction in blood pressure as well as to the existence of advanced cerebral arteriosclerosis and to the hemoconcentration. In the ischemic CVD patients, the lower limits of CBF autoregulation were shifted to a higher pressure level, and shifts were proportional to the severity of the arterial occlusion. The effects of orally administered antihypertensive drugs on the cerebral circulation were investigated by the argon inhalation method. Calcium antagonists effectively reduced blood pressure without inducing orthostatic hypotension or effecting CBF autoregulation. Enalapril, a converting enzyme inhibitor, corrected CBF autoregulation. Carteorol, a beta-blocking agent, corrected orthostatic hypotension. Clinicians must take care not to induce the acute lowering of blood pressure normal in the treatment of elderly hypertensive patients, especially those with advanced cerebral arteriosclerosis. The initial goal should be within 15%–20% of the pretreatment blood pressure level. When choosing antihypertensive drugs, care must be taken not to induce hemoconcentration and not to aggravate orthostatism in order to prevent cerebral ischemia.

Key words: Hypertension — Hemodynamic TIA — Antihypertensive drugs — Cerebral circulation — CBF autoregulation

Introduction

In the face of normal variations in blood pressure, CBF is maintained fairly closely to the resting level. In normotensive subjects, the lower limit of CBF autoregulation has been reported to be in the range of 60 mmHg [1] mean arterial blood pressure (MABP) [1]. The most important feature of CBF in hypertension is the change that occurs in CBF autoregulation: increased cerebrovascular resistance (CVR) causes both the lower and upper limits of CBF autoregulation to be situated at higher pressure levels [1]. In the treatment of elderly hypertensive patients, longstanding hypertension and associated occlusive CVD have the potential to impair CBF autoregulation. The clinical problems of to what extent antihypertensive therapy should

---

[1] Department of Internal Medicine, National Cardiovascular Center, Osaka, Japan

be undertaken in elderly hypertensive patients and the effects of orally administered antihypertensive drugs on the cerebral circulation have not been adequately explored. To clarify these problems, the CBF autoregulation and effects of various antihypertensive drugs on the cerebral circulation were examined in clinical cases.

Clinical Significance of Cases with Large Vessel Occlusion and Transient Hypotension

Cases of hemodynamic TIA which showed transient focal neurological symptoms following moderate hypotension were investigated, and the clinical significance of reducing the blood pressure level in cases with large vessel occlusion of the brain was assessed.

Case Report

A 58-year-old right-handed man was admitted to a hospital in February 1983 for examinations to evaluate transient right hemiparesis and speech disturbance. On standing up after a bath, he had experienced sudden right hemiparesis and difficulty in speaking, which he described as stuttering and knowing what he wanted to say, but being unable to say it. He went to bed and after 30 min the neurological symptoms disappeared. Subsequent to these events, he had frequently experienced

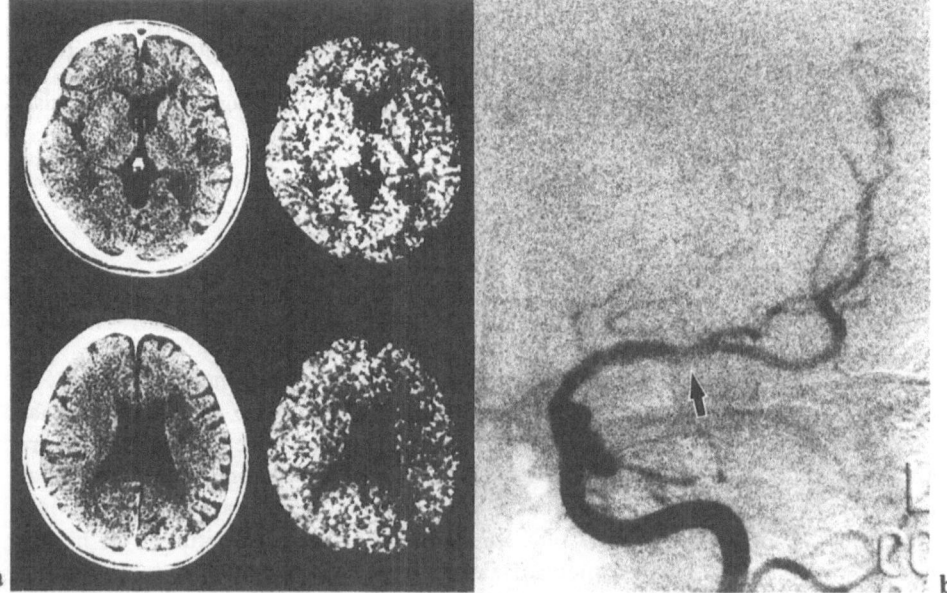

Fig. 1a. Computerized tomography (CT) and the local-CBF map by use of cold-xenon-CT, and **b** left carotid angiography in case-1. CT revealed left watershed infarction. Left carotid angiography revealed severe stenosis of the stem of the middle cerebral artery. Flow map showed hypoperfusion in the left cerebral hemisphere

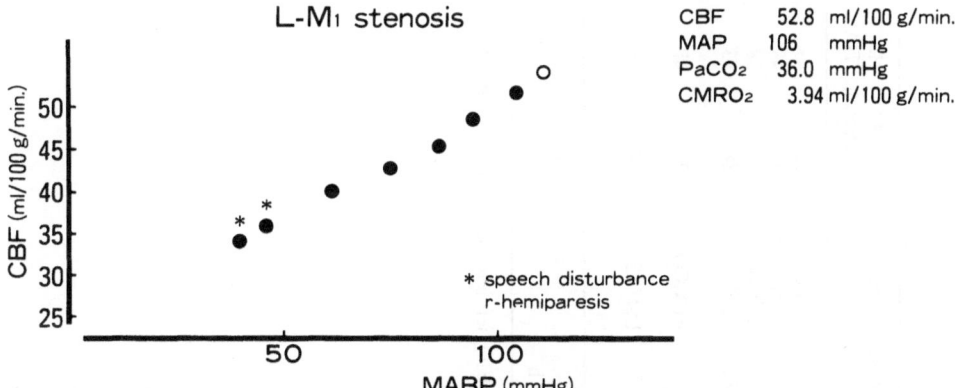

Fig. 2. A relationship curve between %change of cerebral blood flow (*CBF*) and mean arterial blood pressure (*MABP*) in case 1 (58 years; male) shows a dysautoregulation pattern, which indicates CBF falls following blood pressure fall and the plateau of autoregulation disappeared. Below the level of 50 mmHg of MABP (indicated by *), aphasia and right hemiparesis appeared. *MAP*, mean arterial pressure; *PaCO₂*, arterial carbon dioxide tension; *CMRO₂*, cerebral metabolic rate for oxygen

transient right hemiparesis and speech disturbance especially just after standing up, although the symptoms disappeared on squatting and/or on assuming a supine position. Neurological examinations on admission revealed a single anomalous error among 15 objects and reduced right arm swing. Blood pressure was 120/74 mmHg supine, without postural change. An electroencephalogram was normal. A computerized axial tomography (CT) brain scan revealed low-density areas in the left border zones between anterior and middle cerebral arteries. Left carotid angiography demonstrated severe stenosis in the horizontal portion of the left middle cerebral artery (Fig. 1). After angiography, his pulse rate dropped to 40 beats per min, his blood pressure fell to 76/40 mmHg, and he became aphasic. Spontaneous speech was unintelligible, with stuttering and paraphasia. Repetition and comprehension were impaired and he could not follow verbal commands. He was unable to raise his right arm or leg. After intravenous injection of 0.5 mg atropine sulfate and 10 mg etilefrine HC1, blood pressure rose to 170/80 mmHg and the aphasia and right hemiparesis resolved over a period of 10 min. Three-dimensional display of the local CBF by the cold xenon-CT method revealed widespread low-flow areas in the left cerebral hemisphere (Fig. 1). The relationship curve relating CBF and mean arterial blood pressure (MABP) showed loss of autoregulation (Fig. 2).

Details of Cases with Hemodynamic TIA

Data for 6 cases of hemodynamic TIA which showed transient focal neurological symptoms following moderate hypotension are presented in Table 1. The mean age of 4 male and 2 female cases was 73 years. The causes for hypotension at the time of the appearance of the focal neurological symptoms were vasovagal reflex in 1 case, complete atrioventricular conduction block in 2 cases, orthostatic hypotension in 1

Table 1. Clinical cases of hemodynamic TIA

Case	Age	Sex	Blood pressure (mmHg) (Habitual)	Blood pressure (mmHg) (TIA)	Causes	Symptoms	Duration	Angiography	Ht (%) (Habitual)	Ht (%) (TIA)
1	58	M	120/74	76/40	Vasovagal reflex	Right hemiparesis	10 min	Lt-MCS	37	41
2	76	M	160/100	130/80	complete AV block	Right hemiparesis	12 h	Arterio-sclerosis	44	48
3	72	M	170/100	128/70	complete AV block	Right hemiparesis	3 h	Lt-ICO	35	38
4	79	M	160/90	120/70	Nitroglycerin Sitting	Left hemiparesis	10 min	Rt-ICS	38	43
5	76	F	150/90	120/70	Fever Diuretics	Left hemiparesis Hemianopsia	6 h	Rt-MCO	38	48
6	74	F	180/100	160/80	Diuretics	Right hemiparesis Aphasia	12 h	Lt-MCS	34	45
Mean	73 ±7		157/92 (113)	122/68 (86)			5.5 ±5.4 h		38 ±4	44 ±4

TIA, transient ishemic attack; AV, atrioventricular; Ht, hematocrit; Lt-MCS, left middle cerebral artery stenosis; Lt-ICO, left internal carotid artery occlusion; Rt-ICS, right internal carotid artery stenosis; Rt-MCO, right middle cerebral artery occlusion

case, and diuretic therapy in the other 2 cases. Cerebral angiography revealed large vessel occlusion or severe stenosis in five of the 6 cases and advanced arteriosclerotic changes in the other one. The mean value of the habitual MABP was 113 mmHg, and the mean value of MABP at the time of the attacks was 83 mmHg. A 23% fall in MABP thus occurred at the time of the attacks. The mean hematocrit value at the time of the attacks was 44% and was significantly elevated compared to the value in the interictal state (38%).

Comments

These findings suggest that the occurrence of hemodynamic TIA was closely connected to the occurrence of moderate reducation in blood pressure as well as to the existence of large vessel occlusion and to the hemoconcentration. It should be emphasized that in the treatment of elderly hypertensive patients initial antihypertensive therapy which might induce more than a 20% blood pressure fall and which will induce hemoconcentration must be avoided.

CBF Autoregulation in Clinical Cases

The relationship between CBF autoregulation and the type of cranial artery occulsion in cases with occlusive CVD was examined.

Materials and Methods

CBF was measured by argon inhalation method [2]. Hemoglobin (Hb) and oxygen saturation were estimated with a Hemoximeter (Radiometer, Denmark). Arterial oxygen tension (PaO_2), arterial carbon dioxide tension ($PaCO_2$), and pH were measured by use of ABL2 (Radiometer, Copenhagen). Arterial blood pressure was determined by the direct method. The cerebral circulation parameters were calculated as follows. CBF was calculated according to the method of Kety and Schmidt [3]. The cerebrovascular resistance (CVR) was obtained by dividing the MABP by the CBF. The cerebral metabolic rate for oxygen ($CMRO_2$) was obtained by multiplying the arteriovenous (A-V) oxygen difference by CBF. CBF autoregulation was evaluated by stepwise reduction of the blood pressure by combined use of trimetaphan camsylate infusion and tilting head up. CBF changes at various pressure levels were estimated from the changes in cerebral $(AV)O_2$. The lower limit of autoregulation was the pressure level below which CBF began decreasing, and the range of autoregulation was obtained from the habitual blood pressure minus the lower limit of autoregulation.

The subjects comparised 86 patients: 11 cases without a history of CVD and 75 cases with histories of cerebral ischemic episodes. The 11 non-ischemic cases were divided into a control group with hypetension alone (CONT: 5 cases) and those with occulsions of the aortic main branches and extracranial collateral circulation (AORT: 6 cases). Of the 75 cases with cerebral ischemic episodes, 47 (CIT) had cerebral thrombosis without arterial occlusion, and 28 (IMO) had aerteriosclerotic occlusion of either the internal carotid artery or the stem of the middle cerebral aetery with intracranial collateral circulation.

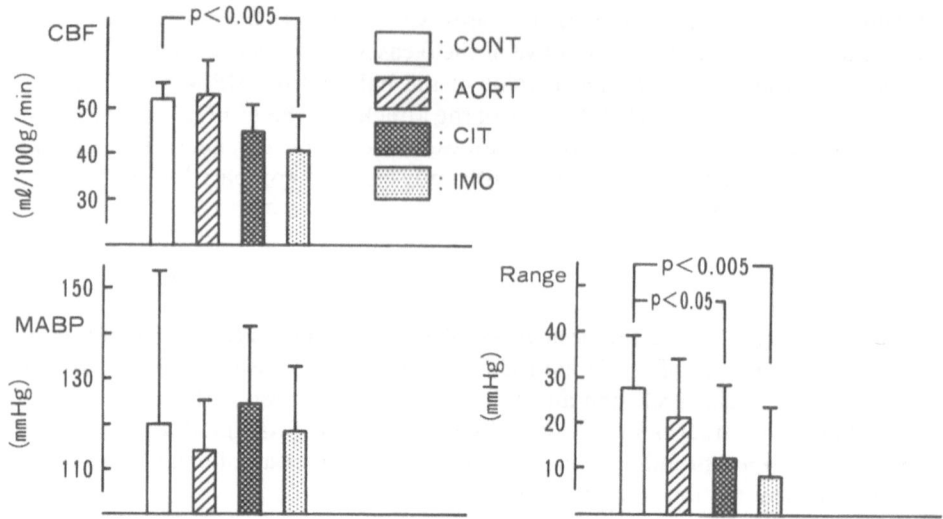

Fig. 3. *CBF* (cerebral blood flow), *MABP* (mean arterial blood pressure), and RANGE (range of autoregulation) in 5 control cases (*CONT*), 6 cases of occlusion of the aortic main branches with extracranial collateral circulation (*AORT*), 47 cases of cerebral thrombosis without arterial occlusion (*CIT*), and 28 cases of cerebral thrombosis with occlusion of either the internal carotid or the stem of middle cerebral artery with intracranial collateral circulation (*IMO*)

Results

CBF, MABP, and Range of Autoregulation

The mean CBF values in the 4 groups were (in ml/100 g per min): 52.3 ± 2.9 (CONT), 53.1 ± 8.7 (AORT), 45.0 ± 10.3 (CIT), and 41.6 ± 7.0 (IMO) (Fig 3). The CBF in IMO was significantly decreased compared to that of CONT ($P < 0.005$). The mean MABP values were 119 ± 33.9 mmHg (CONT), 114 ± 11.2 mmHg (AORT), 124 ± 17.4 mmHg (CIT), and 119 ± 13.5 mmHg (IMO). The average values for range of autoregulation were 28.0 ± 11.4 mmHg (CONT), 21.8 ± 12.3 mmHg (AORT), 12.9 ± 15.3 mmHg (CIT), and 8.3 ± 12.1 mmHg (IMO). The average ranges of CBF autoregulation were significantly decreased in CIT ($P < 0.05$) and IMO ($P < 0.005$), as compared to that of CONT.

Relationship Between Lower Limit of Autoregulation and Habitual Blood Pressure

Fig. 4 shows the relationships between the lower limit of autoregulation and habitual blood pressure in 11 non-CVD cases (5 control cases and 6 cases with occlusions of aortic main branches), 47 cases of cerebral thrombosis without arterial occulsion, and 28 cases of cerebral thrombosis with arterial occlusion. Positive linear correlations ($P < 0.001$) were noted in each of the 3 groups (r = 0.867 in the non-CVD cases, r = 0.792 in the cases of cerebral thrombosis without aertial occulsion, and r = 0.720 in the cases of cerebral thrombosis with arterial occlusion).

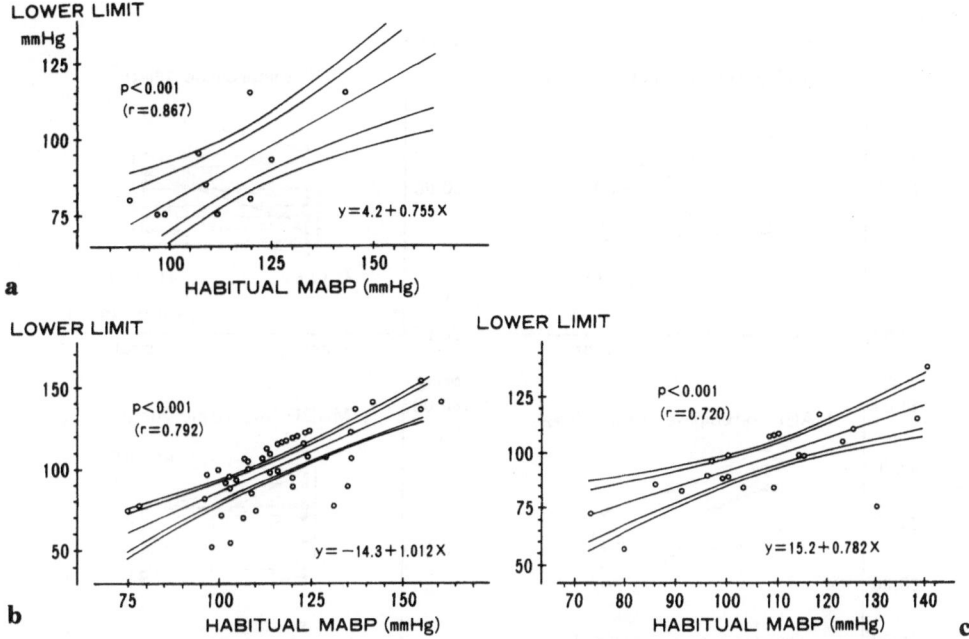

Fig. 4a-c. The relationship between *LOWER LIMIT* of autoregulation and *HABITUAL MABP* (mean arterial blood pressure) in **a** 11 non-CVD (cerebrovascular disease) cases (5 control and 6 cases with occlusion of aortic main branches), **b** 47 cases of cerebral thrombosis without arterial occlusion, and **c** 28 cases of cerebral thrombosis with main artery occlusion

Table 2. Lower limit of autoregulation in clinical cases

	Lower limit/habitual mean arterial blood pressure
Non-cerebrovascular disease ($n = 11$)	79.7%
Cerebral thrombosis without arterial occlusion ($n = 47$)	86.9%
Cerebral thrombosis with arterial occlusion ($n = 28$)	93.4%

Comments

The CBF value was significantly decreased in cases of cerebral thrombosis with arterial occlusion, and the CBF autoregulatory mechanisms were feebler in ischemic CVD cases than in non-CVD cases. The diminutions of the CBF autoregulation were closely connected to be level of aortocranial aertery occlusion and the history of cerebral ischemic episodes. The lower limits of CBF autoregulation expressed as percentages of habitual blood pressure were 79.7% in the non-CVD cases, 86.9% in the cases of cerebral thrombosis without arterial occlusion, and 93.4% in the cases of cerebral thrombosis with arterial occlusion (Table 2). In the ischemic CVD patients, the lower limit of CBF autoregulation was shifted to a higher pressure level, and the shift was proportional to the severity of arterial occlusion.

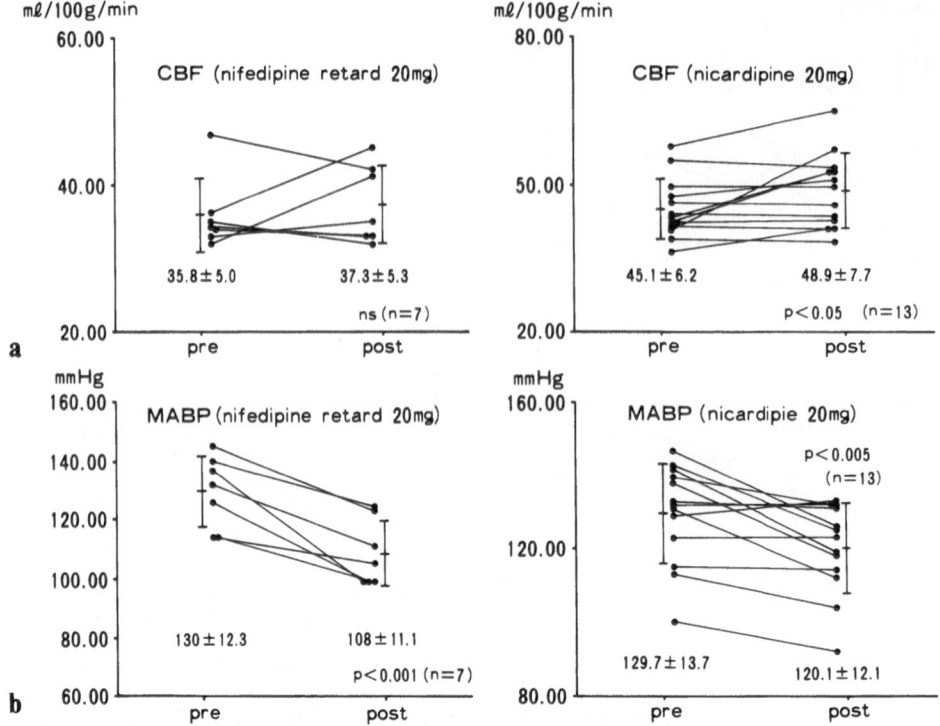

Fig. 5a, b. The effects on *CBF* (cerebral blood flow) and *MABP* (mean arterial blood pressure) following single oral administration of 20 mg of **a** nifedipine retard and **b** nicardipine

Effects of Antihypertensive Drugs on Cerebral Circulation

The effects of orally administered antihypertensive drugs on the cerebral circulation were investigated by the argon inhalation method. In addition to measuring cerebral circulation parameters, such as CBF, $CMRO_2$, CVR, MABP, and $PaCO_2$, the auto-regulation index and MABP on tilting head up ($\Delta MABP$) were estimated. The autoregulation index was calculated as the ratio between the CBF change and the MABP change on transition from the supine position to 35-degree head up tilting. The subjects studied consisted of hypertensive patients with old CVD, and the measurements were made 2 h after breakfast.

Calcium Antoagonists

Acute Effects of Calcium Antagonists

The effects of single oral administration of 20 mg nifedipine retard and of 20 mg nicardipine were studied in 7 and 13 hypertensive cases with old CVD, respectively. One hour after the initial measurement, a second measurement was made. The rela-

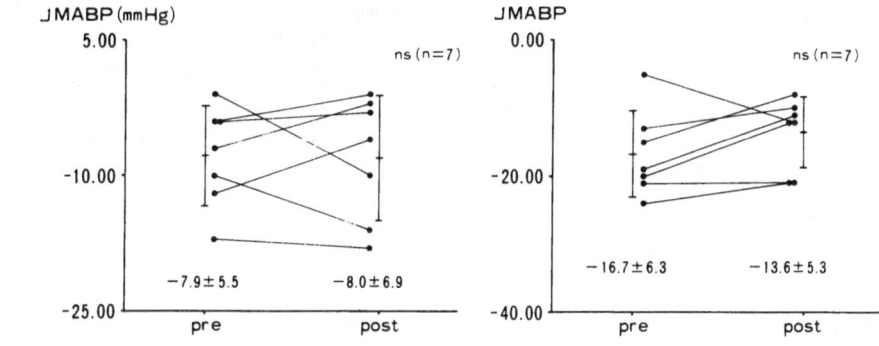

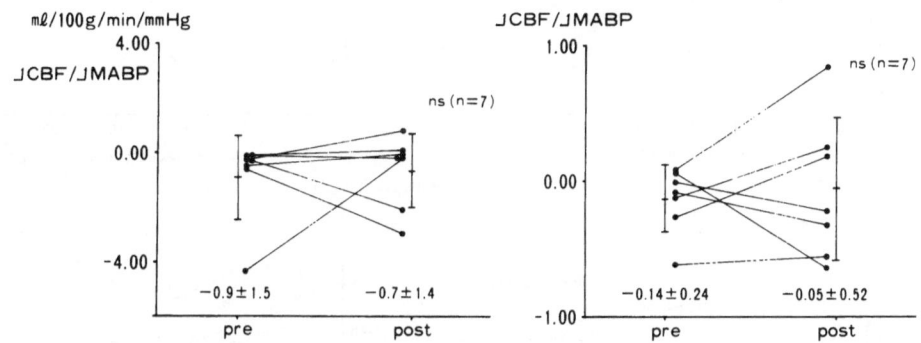

Fig. 6a, b. The effects on **a** $\Delta MABP$ (MABP on tilting head up) and **b** autoregulation index ($\Delta CBF/\Delta MABP$) following single oral administration of 20 mg nifedipine retard (*left*) and 20 mg nicardipine (*right*)

tionships between the plasma concentrations of the 2 calcium antagonists and the changes of cerebral circulation parameters such as CBF, MABP, and CVR were studied.

The mean CBF values were significantly increased after administration of nicardipine ($P < 0.05$), but not after nifedipine retard. The mean MABP values were significantly decreased after administration of the 2 calcium antagonists (nifedipine retard, $P < 0.001$; nicardipine, $P < 0.005$) (Fig. 5). The mean values of $\Delta MABP$ on tilting head up and the mean values of the autoregulation index were not significantly changed after administration of nifedipine retard and nicardipine (Fig. 6). Following administration of nifedipine retard, a significant linear correlation was noted in the relation between the plasma concentration and the change in MABP on tilting head up ($\Delta MABP$). On the other hand, following administration of nicardipine, the relations between the CBF change and plasma concentration and between the CVR change and plasma concentration were significant; but that between $\Delta MABP$ and the plasma concentration was not (Fig. 7).

Mostly, nifedipine retard exerted its influence in reducing the blood pressure, and nicardipine, in reducing CVR.

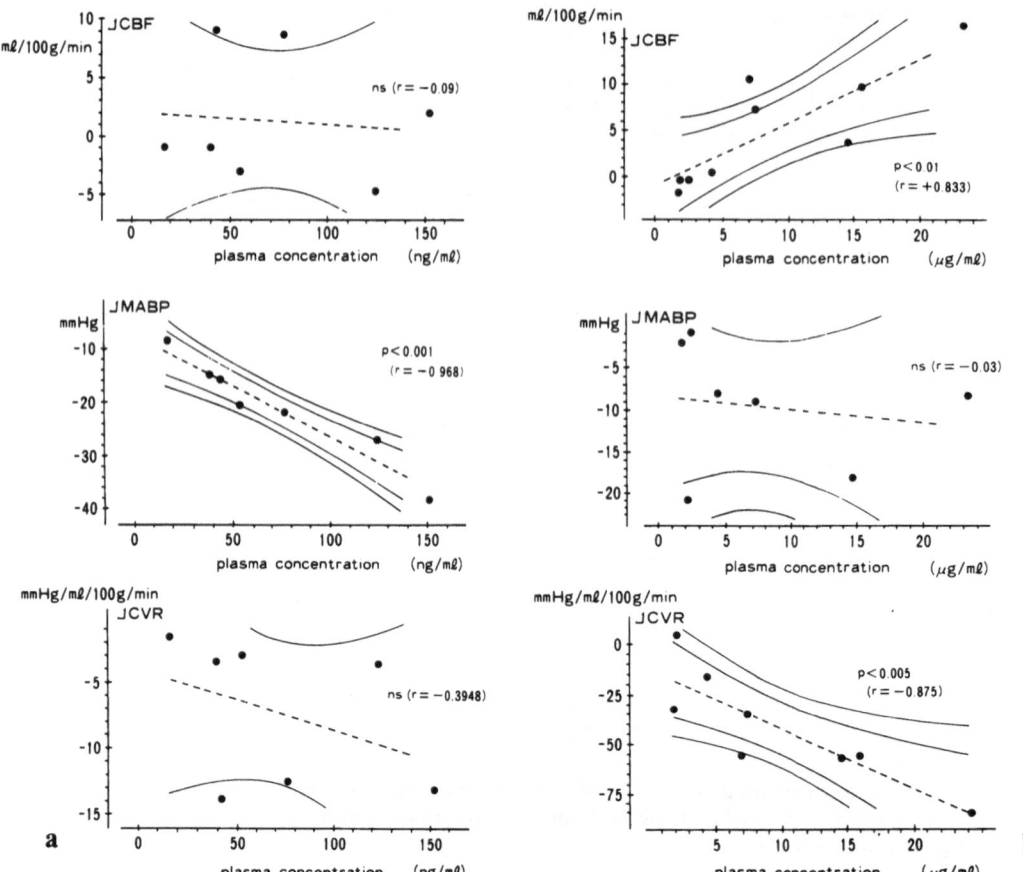

Fig. 7a, b. Relationships between cerebral circulation parameters and the *plasma concentration* of the calcium antagonists, **a** nifedipine retard and **b** nicardipine following single oral administration of 20 mg

Subacute Effects of Calcium Antagonists

The effects of 2-week administration of 40 mg/day nifedipine retard, 60 mg/day nicardipine, and 180 mg/day diltiazem were studied in 8, 6, and 8 hypertensive cases with old CVD, respectively.

The mean CBF values were not significantly changed by the 3 types of calcium antagonists. The changes in MABP and CVR, however, were significant with all 3 calcium antagonists. The percent change in MABP was -15.9% for nifedipine retard ($P < 0.001$), -15.7% for nicardipine ($P < 0.001$), and -7% for diltiazem ($P < 0.05$) (Fig. 8).

Two-week administration of nifedipine retard, nicardipine, and diltiazem induced significant reductions in MABP without decreasing the CBF. The effects in reducing blood pressure were most potent in the cases of 40 mg/day nifedipine retard and weakest with 180 mg/day diltiazem.

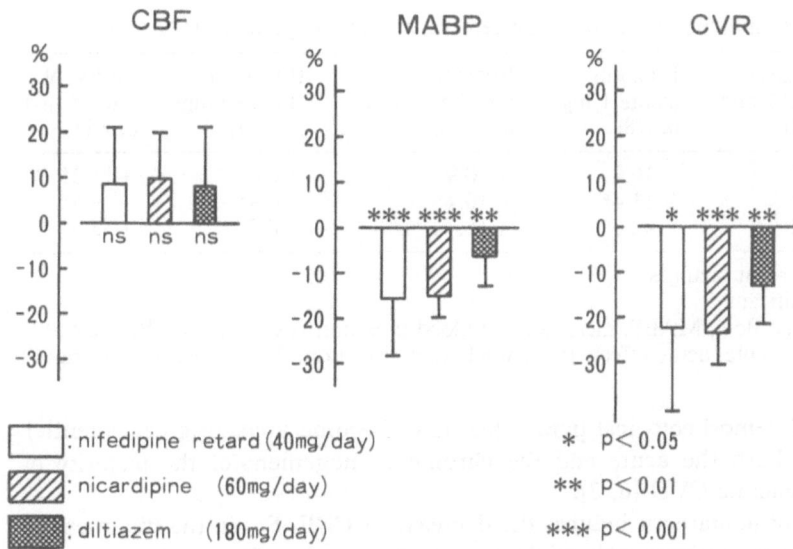

Fig. 8. Effects of 2 weeks administration of *nifedipine retard*, *nicardipine*, and *diltiazem* on the cerebral circulation parameters: *CBF* (cerebral blood flow), *MABP (mean arterial blood pressure)*, and *CVR* (cerebrovascular resistance)

Other Antihypertensive Drugs and Cerebral Circulation

Percentage figures of the changes in CBF, MABP, and ΔMABP after administration of the other antihypertensive drugs are shown in Table 3. Two types of α_1-blocking agents were studied. Following single oral administration of 1 mg bunazosin, a significant decrease was noted in MABP, but not in CBF and the MABP change after tilting head up. On the other hand, single oral administration of 1 mg prazosin induced significant decreases in MABP and increased the MABP change after tilting head up. Subacute effects after administration of 2.5–5.0 mg/day enalapril and 180 mg/day buderacin showed significant decrease in MABP. Two-week administration of 15 mg/day carteorol induced a mild but significant decrease in MABP. Moreover, carteorol improved the blood pressure response to tilting the head up.

Discussion

A syndrome of orthostatic transient ischemic attacks has been reported by several authors[4, 5]. This syndrome illustrates the importance of collateral blood supply. When a large vessel is occluded, if collateral supply is inadequate, infarction occurs. If the supply is sufficient, neurological dysfunction is temporary or absent. If collateral supply is marginal, recurrent orthostatic TIAs may occur. In such patients, collateral vessels are already maximally dilated, leaving no autoregulatory reserve to prevent clinical ischemia when mild hypotension occurs. The medical evaluation and

Table 3. Effects of antihypertensive drugs on cerebral circulation parameters

	Bunazosin (acute 1 mg) ($n = 8$)	Prazosin (acute 1 mg) ($n = 8$)	Enalapril (2w 2.5–5.0 mg) ($n = 13$)	Buderacin (1w 180 mg) ($n = 11$)	Carteorol (2w 15 mg) ($n = 11$)
CBF	+ 0.5	− 10.8	+ 0.9	+ 6.6	+ 11.2*
MABP	− 10*	− 11.4*	− 10.4*	− 6.9*	− 9.6*
△MABP	− 2.2	− 42.0*	+ 15.4	− 8.2	+ 55.5*

Values indicate percent changes.
* Statistically significant
CBF, cerebral blood flow; MABP, mean arterial blood pressure; △MABP, MABP change
on head-up tilting; acute, acute effect; 1w, 1 week administration; 2w, 2 week administration

manipulation of hemorheological parameters have become areas of great potential with respect to both the acute and the chronic management of the majority of patients with ischemic CVD [6, 7].

The increase of hematocrit induces the decrease of CBF. So, in the treatment of elderly hypertensive patients who might have large vessel occlusion, care must be taken not to induce more than a 15%–20% blood pressure fall and not to aggravate hemoconcentration.

In chronic hypertension, CBF autoregulation is adapted to high pressure, and the lower end of the autoregulation curve is shifted towards high pressure [8, 9]. Even though structural changes in the resistance vessels improve tolerance to high pressure, they impair tolerance to hypotension, presumably because autoregulatory vaso-dilatation is compromised by wall thickening and luminal narrowing. These vascular changes cause a shift of the lower limit of autoregulation to a higher pressure, with the shift being proportional to the severity of the hypertension [8].

The schematic presentation of the effects of various antihypertensive drugs on cerebral circulation, which was studied by the same method and same kind of subjects as described for subacute effects of calcium antagonists, was presented in Table 4. Calcium antagonists effectively reduced blood pressure without inducing orthostatic hypotension and without changing autoregulation. However, prazosin, an α_1-blocking agent, induced orthostatic hypotension and reduced CBF autoregulation. Carteorol, a β-blocking agent, had a positive effect on improving orthostatic hypotension.

The question of whether, and to what extent, the shift in CBF autoregulation can be reversed by chronic treatment of the hypertensive patient has not been conclusively studied. Some clinical studies, however, suggest that chronic treatment can restore the lower limit to normal or reduce CVR [8, 10, 11]. So, patients should be given a period of time to allow for readaptation of their cerebral vessels to normal blood pressure.

In conclusion, clinicians should be careful not to induce acute lowering of the blood pressure norm when treating elderly hypertensive patients, especially those with large vessel occlusion. The initial goal in blood pressure reduction should be within 15%–20% of the pretreatment blood pressure level. When choosing antihypertensive drugs, care must be taken not to induce hemoconcentration and not to aggravate orthostatic hypotension in order to prevent cerebral ischemia.

Table 4. Effects of antihypertensive drugs on cerebral circulation parameters in hypertensive cases with cerebrovascular disease

Drug	Dosage	CBF	MABP	ΔMABP	Autoregulation index
Nifedipine	20 mg (acute)	→	↓	→	→
retard	40 mg/day (2 week)	→	↓	→	→
Nicardipine	20 mg (acute)	↗	↓	→	→
	60 mg/day (2 week)	→	↓	→	→
Diltiazem	180 mg/day (2 week)	→	↘	→	→
Bunazosin	1 mg (acute)	→	↓	→	→
Prazosin	1 mg (acute)	→	↓	↘	↘
Enalapril	2.5-5.0 mg/day (2 week)	→	↓	→	↗
Carteorol	15 mg/day (2 week)	↗	↘	↗	→
Buderacin	180 mg/day (1 week)	→	↘	→	→

CBF, cerebral blood flow; MABP, mean arterial blood pressure; ΔMABP, MABP change on head-up tilting; →, no change; ↗, slight increase; ↘, slight decrease; ↓ decrease.

References

1. Strandgaad S, Olesen J, Skinhoj E (1973) Autoregulation of brain circulation in severe hypertension. Br Med J 1: 507–510
2. Pevsner PH, Bhushan C, Walker AE (1971) Cerebral blood flow and oxygen consumption. An on-line technique. Johns Hopkins Med J 128: 134
3. Kety SS, Schmidt CF (1945) The determination of cerebral blood flow in man by use of the nitrous oxide in low concentrations. Am J Physiol 143: 53–66
4. Somerville ER (1984) Orthostatic transient ischemic attacks: A symptom of large vessel occlusion. Stroke 15: 1066–1067
5. Kendall RE, Marshall J (1963) Role of hypotension in the genesis of transient focal cerebral ischemic attacks. Br Med J 2: 344–348 reprint (1976) Br Med J51: 577–692
6. Heiss W-D, Prosenz P, Tschbitscher H (1972) Effect of low molecular dextran on total cerebral blood flow within ischemic brain lesions. Eur Neurol 8: 129–133
7. Wood JH, Fleischer AS (1982) Observations during hypervolemic hemodilution of patients with acute focal cerebral ischemia. JAMA 248: 2999–3004
8. Strandgaard S (1976) Autoregulation of cerebral blood flow in hypertensive patients. The modifying influence of prolonged hypertensive treatment on the tolerance to acute, drug induced hypotension. Circulation 53: 720–727
9. Jones JV, Fitch W, Mackenzie ET (1976) Lower limit of cerebral blood flow autoregulation in the baboon. Circ Res 39: 555–557
10. Pistolese GR, Agnoli A, Prencipe M (1977) CBF studies in hypertensive patients during acute controlled hypotension and after a period of medical treatment. Pathophysiological and clinical correlations. Acta Neurol Scand 56 (Suppl LXIV): 72–73
11. Gilliksen G, Hòjer-Pedersen E, Moller M (1983) Autoregulation of cerebral blood flow in patients with malignant hypertension and hypertensive encephalopathy. In: Strandgaad S, Barry DI (eds) Cerebral blood flow, hypertension and antihypertensive treatment. Acta Med Scand 678: (Suppl I) 43–49

Discussion

Kuramoto (Tokyo): You showed the lower limit of autoregulation is about 80% or 90% of blood pressure: and I think in the study of 24-h monitoring of blood pressure, the nighttime blood pressure usually falls 30–40 mmHg compared to the daytime pressure. But, there is no ischemic syndrome shown after that. So, how do you account for this phenomenon? And second, do you recommend omitting the nighttime dose in elderly patients?

Kuriyama (Osaka): This is a study of the acute lowering of blood pressure, which I think is the initial goal in elderly hypertensive, including cases with large vessel occlusions. I emphasize that caution must be paid not to lower the blood pressure too acutely.

Marchetta (Bologna): Just a short question — maybe you mentioned it, but I did not get it — a question on the methods. Did you also study the large vessels of the neck with duplex-scanning, i.e., echodoppler techniques, in your patients? If you did, what was the correlation between the echodoppler and the angiography findings?

Kuriyama: Do you mean doppler scanning? We usually use B-mode echo of cardiography and pulse Doppler method. We do not know the exact data on the correlation between the echodoppler and angiography. All cases in this study were made by conventional angiography.

Birkenhäger (Rotterdam): Could I ask you, did the technology allow you to measure cerebral blood flow in the standing position also — not only during tilting but also during standing? That is the more usual practice in situations where there is excess risk of cerebral ischemia. Could you do that? If so, do you have any data?

Kuriyama: We usually use 35-degree head-up tilting and not standing. The aim of the study is not to induce muscle exercise, muscle contraction.

Birkenhäger Yes, I understand.

Treatment of the Hypertensive Diabetic: Focus on Calcium Channel Blockade

Peter Weidmann, Bernhard N. Trost, and Paolo Ferrari[1]

Summary. In diabetes mellitus (DM) type 1, blood pressure (BP) tends to rise in association with incipient diabetic nephropathy. In DM type 2, hypertension (HT) may develop before or during DM or nephropathy. Regardless of DM type, sodium retention and vascular hyper-reactivity seem to be important factors in the pathogenesis of HT. DM and HT may concomitantly promote cardiovascular complications and the course of diabetic nephropathy and retinopathy.

Considering the high risk of early cardiovascular and renal disability or death, dietary and, if necessary, drug treatment in diabetic patients aims at normalizing metabolic risk correlates as well as BP. Thiazide diuretics are not ideal for initial antihypertensive therapy; although they may simultaneously improve BP, body sodium, and vascular hyperreactivity, they as well as loop diuretics can impair glucose tolerance further, promote hypokalemia with its arrythmogenic potential, and increase potentially atherogenic serum cholesterol and triglyceride fractions. β_1-blockers have fewer, although still some unwanted metabolic or cardiovascular side effects. Calcium channel blockers or angiotensin-converting enzyme (ACE) inhibitors may often improve hypertension without causing relevant metabolic impairment or modifying hypoglycemic symptoms. Treatment with nitrendipine in hypertensive type 2 diabetics lowered not only BP and vascular reactivity, but also serum uric acid, while carbohydrate and lipid metabolism were unchanged. Differential effects of antihypertensive drugs on the progression of human diabetic nephropathy and long-term prognosis in diabetics remain to be determined. In the meantime, calcium channel blockers offer a potentially useful alternative for first-line treatment of HT in diabetic patients.

Key words: Hypertension accompanying diabetes mellitus — Pathogenesis — Antihypertensive treatment — Calcium channel blockers — Angiotensin-converting enzyme inhibitors — Glucose metabolism — Lipids

Pathogenetic Aspects

Hypertension (HT) and diabetes mellitus (DM) occur commonly together. In *DM type 1*, blood pressure (BP) tends to rise slightly in association with incipient diabetic nephropathy, i.e., microalbuminuria of 30–300 mg/24 h, normal serum creatinine, and a tendency for high glomerular filtration rate (GFR) [1]. The prevalence of HT increases progressively in the presence of clinical nephropathy (proteinuria >

---

[1] Medizinische Poliklinik, University of Berne, CH-3010 Berne, Switzerland

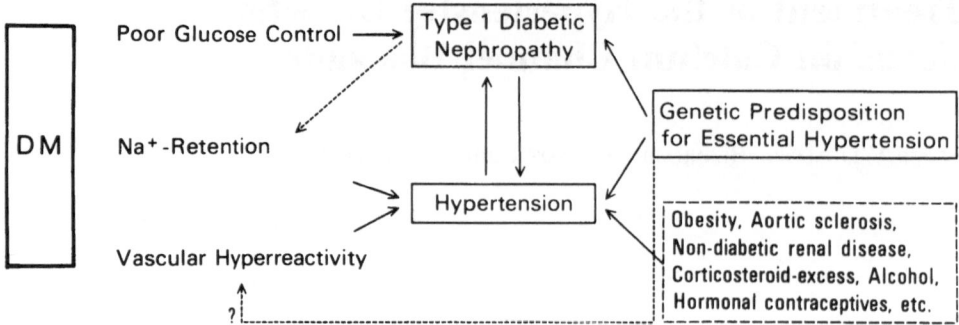

Fig. 1. Diabetes mellitus (*DM*), hypertension, and nephropathy: some possible pathogenetic interactions

300 mg/24 h) and with advancing renal failure [2, 3]. In *DM type 2*, HT may develop before or during DM or nephropathy. HT preceeding the onset of DM presents itself most often as essential and/or obesity-associated HT. In elderly patients, advanced aortic sclerosis may promote systolic HT.

Regardless of DM type, sodium (Na$^+$) retention [4, 5] vascular hyperreactivity to norepinephrine, and probably angiotensin II as well [5–8] tend to occur early (before clinical diabetic nephropathy, retinopathy, or neuropath) and seem to be important factors in the pathogenesis of HT [5, 9] (Fig. 1). The excess body Na$^+$ differentiates DM-associated HT from essential HT, where body Na$^+$ is, on the average, normal [10]. Thus, *diabetic HT* represents a pathogenetically distinct form of HT [5]. Pathogenetic mechanisms characteristic for DM may, (a) alone or together with a predisposition for essential HT, *contribute to the development of de novo HT*, or (b) complement pre-existing forms of HT (essential, obesity-associated, aortic sclerosis-induced, etc.) (Fig. 1).

The combined presence of HT and DM further increases the risk of cardio-vascular and renal complications. The tendency of HT to promote retinopathy, stroke, coronary heart disease, heart failure, nephrosclerosis and additional athero-sclerotic damage may be complemented by DM-induced micro- and macroangio-pathy and, at least in DM type 1, also by an adverse influence of HT on the course of diabetic nephropathy [3, 11].

In *DM type 1*, a poor glycemic control and a presumably genetic pre disposition for HT seem to be concomitant risk factors for the development of diabetic nephro-pathy [12, 13] (Fig. 1); glomerular capillary HT may play an important patho-genetic role [14]. Once systemic HT develops, it can aggravate albuminuria, pro-mote the progression from incipient to clinical nephropathy and, at the latter stage, accelerate the rate of decline in GFR [3, 11]. On the other hand, antihypertensive treatment may, in type 1 diabetics with incipient nephropathy, reduce micro-albuminuria and inhibit the progression to clinical nephropathy, and, in patients with clinical nephropathy, decrease proteinuria and the rate of decline in GFR [11, 15]. In *DM type 2*, relationships between HT and nephropathy are unclear, although a high BP may possibly also promote the development of renal failure [16].

Cardiovascular problems and renal failure lead to early disability or death in the majority of diabetics. It follows that in the long-term care for diabetic patients, treatment of hyperglycemia and associated metabolic disturbances favoring atherosclerosis must be combined with careful monitoring of BP and therapy of co-existing HT.

Antihypertensive Treatment

Occasionally, diabetic patients have secondary HT due to excessive alcohol consumption, hormonal contraceptives, renal artery stenosis, non-diabetic renal disease, primary hyperaldosteronism, glucocorticoid excess, acromegaly, or additional rare causes. These possibilities must be considered in the diagnostic work-up. A reduced alcohol intake, replacement of hormonal by another form of contraception, or operative correction of potentially curable lesions can improve BP in some diabetics.

Antihypertensive long-term treatment in DM is based on 3 legs [17]. These include (a) a careful diabetes therapy, (b) general measures, as in essential HT, aimed at reducing BP and/or associated risk factors, such as reduction of overweight, treatment of hyperlipidemia (both primarily by diet), restriction of salt intake to an amount which is acceptable to the patient under ambulatory conditions (if possible, about 3–5 g NaCl/day), no smoking, no oral contraceptives, appropriate physical exercise, and (c) antihypertensive drugs. It has been suggested that a diet low in Na^+ combined with a low fat and high fiber one exerts an antihypertensive effect and, thus, may be a useful non-pharmacologic baseline approach [18].

The exact level of BP at which antihypertensive pharmacotherapy becomes necessary and may improve the cardiovascular prognosis in diabetic patients is unknown. Considering the established beneficial effects of drug treatment in moderate to severe HT without associated DM [19], a lowering of BP would seem to be at least as warranted as when similar degrees of HT are further complicated by DM. In mild HT (90–105 mmHg diastolic) without DM, a conventional pharmacotherapy based on diuretics distinctly reduced the incidence of strokes, but not coronary complications [20, 21]. An adverse influence of thiazide-type diuretics given in high dosage is suspected. β-blockers slightly decreased cerebral and coronary complications in non-smokers only [21]. In patients with DM type 1 and mild HT, arguments in favor of antihypertensive pharmoacotherapy are complemented by a possible beneficial effect of a maintained normal BP as regards the progression of nephropathy [11, 15] and diabetic retinopathy [22].

It seems reasonable to conclude that in DM, HT of either mild or more severe degree should always be treated with general measures (as mentioned) as the basic approach. Considering the probable additional risk when mild HT is complemented by DM, we favor the institution of pharmacotherapy when BP remains > 140/90 mmHg despite appropriate diabetes therapy and general measures. Nevertheless, when antihypertensive drugs are prescribed in DM-associated mild HT, it would appear particularly important that they are subjectively well tolerated and do not adversely affect the glucose, potassium, or lipid metabolism or other potential

Conventional, metabolic problems   Alternative, less metabolic problems

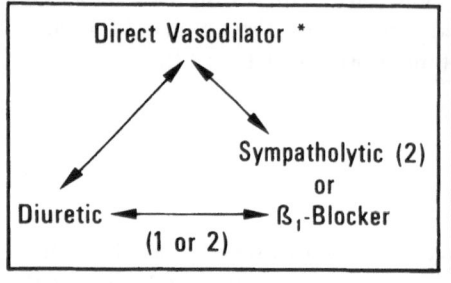
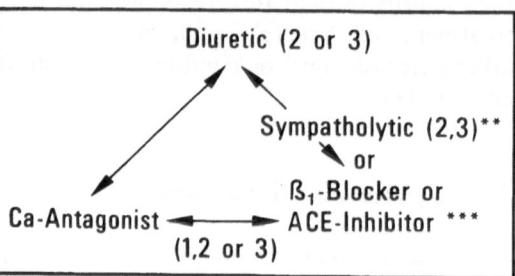

* (Di) hydralazine,   ** Prazosin, Guanfacin
   in men if necessary minoxidil   *** With normal S-creatinine or on dialysis

Fig. 2. Antihypertensive pharmacotherapy in diabetes mellitus: the "conventional" approach as compared with an alternative approach utilizing CA^{++} channel blockers and/or angiotensin-converting enzyme (ACE) inhibitors. Numbers in parentheses indicate treatment steps

cardiovascular risk correlates, thus, potentially offsetting a beneficial effect of lowered BP on cardiovascular prognosis. Apart from metabolic "neutrality" or even an ameliorating influence, the desired profile of antihypertensive drugs in DM should, if possible, be devoid of a tendency to promote orthostatic hypotension, sexual dysfunction, or functional aggravation of peripheral and coronary vessel disease in patients whose primary disease makes them already prone to these complications.

The undesirable effects of antihypertensive drugs on metabolic, autonomic, and cardiovascular functions in DM have been reviewed in detail elsewhere [17, 23] and are summarized in Table 1.

It is obvious that the conventional approach with diuretics or β-blockers as first-line drugs (Fig. 2), an approach which imitates the empirical stepped-care plan used widely in essential HT, is more problematic in DM. Although *thiazide diuretics* could represent a rational antihypertensive therapy which simultaneously improves BP, excess body Na^+, and the exaggerated cardiovascular reactivity to norepinephrine in DM [6], they as well as loop diuretics, are not ideal step 1 drugs; both tend to impair the glucose tolerance further [17, 23], may promote hypokalemia with its possible arrhythmogenic potential [24, 25], and can increase the ratio between the potentially atherogenic serum LDL-cholesterol and antiatherogenic HDL-cholesterol as well as the levels of serum triglycerides [26] (Table 1). Nevertheless, it is not excluded that, as in essential HT, low thiazide doses (25 mg hydrochlorothiazide or chlorthalidone) could provide a full antihypertensive effect with much more discrete metabolic actions [27] at least in some non-azotemic diabetic patients. Before these aspects and possible unwanted interactions between medium to high dose thiazide therapy and coronary heart disease are clarified, diuretics will be hotly debated as first-line choice, and care to use their lowest BP-effective dose and to avoid hypokalemia, hyperglycemia, and hyperlipidemia seems particularly warranted. Con-

Table 1. Undesirable effects of antihypertensive drugs in diabetes

Problem	Drugs
Metabolic	
Hyperkalemia	When renal function is impaired and/or insulin deficiency exists: K^+ – sparing diuretics, ACE inhibitors, ß-blockers[a]
Hypokalemia	Thiazide and loop diuretics
Hyperglycemia	Diuretics, particularly K^+ – loosing; $ß_{1+2}$-blockers[a] or their combination
Hypoglycemia	Recovery delayed by $ß_{1+2}$-blockers or ß-blockers with MSA
Dyslipoproteinemia	Most diuretics; ß-blockers without pronounced ISA
Hyperuricemia	Diuretics
Autonomic function	
Masking of hypoglycemia symptoms	Less palpitation, tachycardia (but more sweating) on ß-blockers
Catecholamine-induced hypertension during hypoglycemia	$ß_{1+2}$-blockers
Orthostatic hypotension	Diuretics, sympatholytics including α-blockers; less on ß-blockers, Ca-antagonists, ACE inhibitors[a]
Sexual dysfunction	Sympatholytics, diuretics (thiazides?)
Functional aggravation of angiopathy	
Coronary heart disease	Direct vasodilators
Raynaud, claudication	ß-blockers

[a]Very mild effect.
ACE, angiotensin-converting enzyme; MSA, membrane stabilizing activity; ISA, instrinsic sympathomimetic activity; CHD, coronary heart disease

sidering *β-blockers*, those with highly selective $β_1$-antagonism and without membrane-stabilizing activity, such as atenolol or metoprolol, are interfering less with glucose homeostasis and are quite valuable in the treatment of hypertensive diabetics [17, 23]. However, some potential metabolic or cardiovascular problems remain (Table 1), and many practicing physicians feel uncomfortable about the partial blunting of hypoglycemic symptoms. The use of *sympatholytic agents*, such as post-synaptic α_1-blockers (prazosin, etc.), methyldopa, urapidil, clonidine, or reserpin, seems to carry no relevant metabolic disadvantage [17, 23]; and post-synaptic α_1-blockers in particular may even slightly decrease serum low and very-low density lipoprotein cholesterol (LDL + VLDL-C) and triglyceride levels [28]. However, sympatholytics may promote orthostatic hypotension and, at least some of them, also sexual dysfunction (Table 1).

The need for more ideal antihypertensive drugs to treat the diabetic patient is obvious. *Calcium (Ca⁺⁺) channel blockers* and *angiotensin II-converting enzyme (ACE) inhibitors* are 2 classes of agents, which alone or in combination effectively

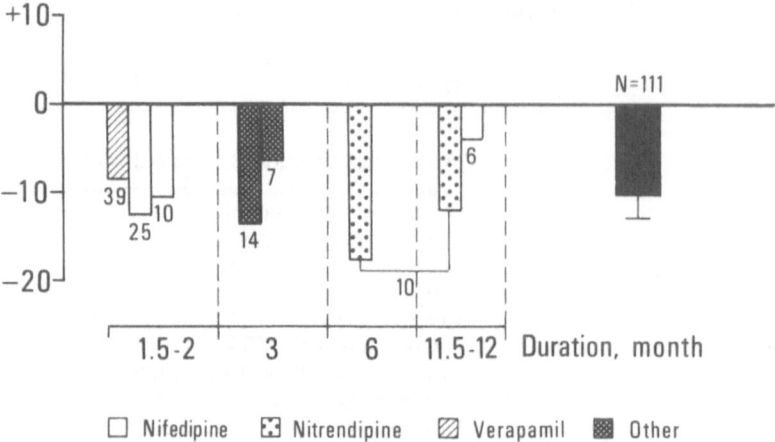

Fig. 3. Percentage responses of mean blood pressure to monotherapy with Ca^{++} channel blockers in hypertension associated with diabetes mellitus. Each column represents the average percentage change in a report based on a minimum number of 6 subjects. *Column to the right* is mean of all studies. *Nifedepine added to bendrofluazide

reduce BP in most patients with essential HT without relevant effects on plasma glucose, potassium, uric acid, and lipids [28–31]. These drugs also cause peripheral vasodilatation (rather than constriction as some β-blockers do), and no marked tendency for orthostatic hypotension has been noted [29, 30]. Thus, they deserve consideration as step 1, 2, or 3 drugs in the treatment of diabetes-associated HT (Fig. 2).

Focus on Calcium Antagonists in Hypertensive Diabetics

Trost and Weidmann [32] evaluated, in 10 type 2 diabetics with mild HT (mean age 57 years), the short-term and long-term effects of a monotherapy with the Ca^{++} channel blocker nitrendipine. Supine BP (after 1 h of bedrest) averaged 151/88 mmHg and standing BP, 151/97 mmHg (after 1 month of placebo). These values were lowered to, respectively, 128/72 and 113/69 mmHg ($P < 0.005$ and < 0.001) after 6 weeks, 128/71 and 115/71 mmHg ($P < 0.005$ and < 0.001) after 6 months, and 138/76 and 120/71 mmHg ($P < 0.5$ and < 0.005) after 12 months of nitrendipine treatment (average dose 30 mg/day).

The potency of a chronic monotherapy with Ca^{++} channel blockers in hypertensive diabetics was assessed further by an analysis of published reports with a minimal number of 6 patients per study (Fig. 3). Ca^{++} channel blockers and doses used in these studies included: nifedipine retard, 40–60 mg/day [33, 34]; nitrendipine, 20–40 mg/day [32]; verapamil, 240–480 mg/day [35]; diltiazem, 180 mg/day [36]; and nisoldipine, 10–20 mg/day [37]. One study in which nifedipine was added to a previous bendrofluazide therapy [38] is also included in Fig. 3. Although the available data do not yet allow a comparative assessment of different agents, it is evident

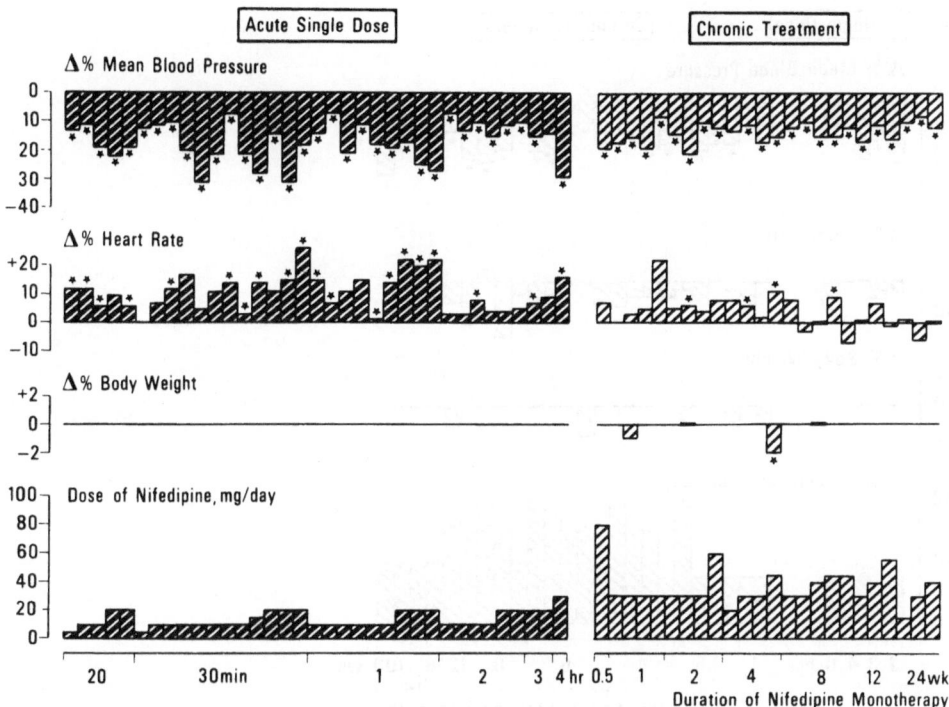

Fig. 4. Percentage responses of *mean blood pressure*, *heart rate*, and *body weight* to an acute single dose or monotherapy with nifedipine (dosage shown at *bottom*) in essential hypertension. Each column represents the average percentage change in a report based on a minimal number of 6 subjects. From Weidmann et al. [30]

that chronic Ca^{++} channel blocker therapy administered to a total of 111 hypertensive diabetics (10 insulin-treated, 101 non insulin-dependent) lowered mean BP on average by 10%, and this effect did not appear to dissipate with progressive duration of treatment. Nevertheless, the comparative efficacy of different Ca^{++} channel blockers and their long-term BP-lowering effect in hypertensive diabetics require further evaluation.

The antihypertensive effect of Ca^{++} channel blockers in patients with DM may well resemble their efficacy in non-diabetic patients with essential HT [30] (Fig. 4, 5). In the latter, Ca^{++} channel blockers can be usefully combined with ACE inhibitors or β-blockers. β-blockers are suitable companions for nifedipine or nitrendipine, while a combination of β-blockers with oral verapamil or diltiazem warrants precaution and is contraindicated with regard to i.v. verapamil or diltiazem. Whether the addition of a diuretic to a Ca^{++} channel blocker can distinctly enhance the antihypertensive action obtained with the Ca^{++} channel blockers alone is questionable [30, 39]. Considering the therapeutic profile in essential HT [30], it is probable that Ca^{++} channel blockers may, in addition to monotherapy (Fig. 3), be useful as step 2 or 3 drugs in hypertensive diabetics.

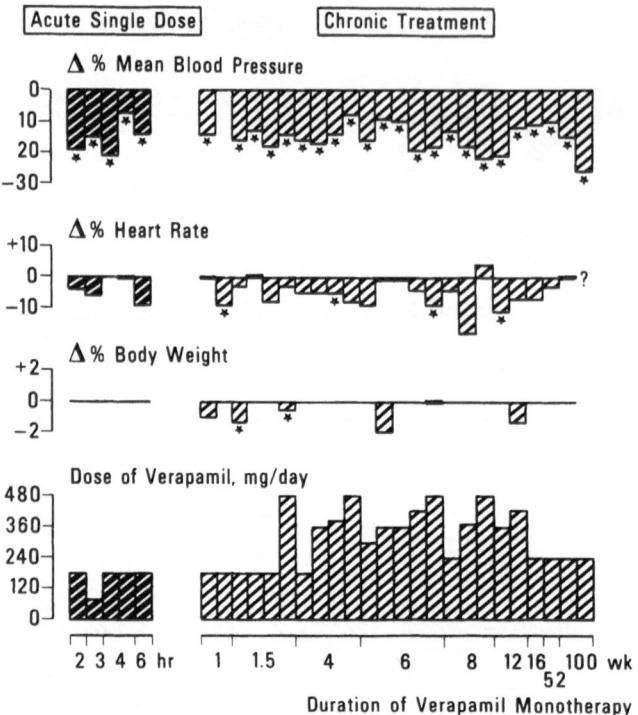

Fig. 5. Percentage responses of *mean blood pressure*, *heart rate*, and *body weight* to an acute single dose or monotherapy with verapamil (dosage shown at *bottom*) in essential hypertension. Each column represents the average percentage change in a report based on a minimal number of 6 subjects. From Weidmann et al. [30]

Ca^{++} channel blockers seem to lower BP in hypertensive diabetics at least in part by improving their vascular hyperreactivity to norepinephrine and angiotensin II. In the study by Trost and Weidmann [17], 6 weeks of nitrendipine monotherapy reduced, in 10 hypertensive type 2 diabetics, the supine and upright BPs by 16% and 25%, respectively; normalized the pressor dose of norepinephrine, i.e., the infusion rate necessary to increase mean BP 20 mmHg, from the initially diminished value of 77 ± 28 ($\pm$ Standard error of mean) ng/kg per min to 178 ± 44 ng/kg per min ($P < 0.005$); and also blunted the pressor effect of angiotensin II. This improvement could not be explained by extracellular Na$^+$-fluid volume depletion, since the existing increase in exchangeable Na$^+$ (113% of normal on placebo, 111% after Ca^{++} channel blockade) and whole blood volume (100% of normal on placebo, 97% after Ca^{++} channel blockade) were largely unchanged by nitrendipine [17].

Since the 2nd phase of insulin release depends on increased transmembranous influx of Ca^{++} into pancreatic β-cells, Ca^{++} channel blockers could potentially impair insulin secretion. However, a recent review of the available information suggests that Ca^{++} channel blockers probably do not produce clinically relevant alterations in glucose homeostasis in the large majority of patients with or without DM, although

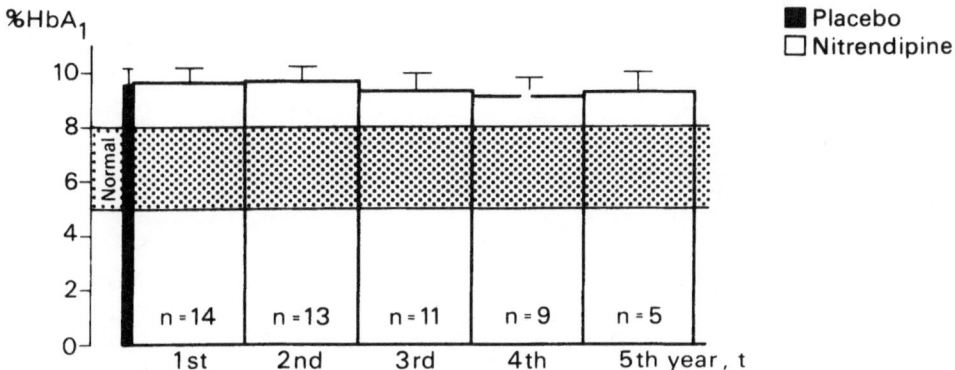

Fig. 6. *Hb A₁* (major component of adult hemoglobin) on *placebo* ($n = 14$; 1 month) and during long-term monotherapy with *nitrendipine* in hypertensive type 2 diabetics. Mean ± standard error of mean; paired *t*-tests. From Trost et al. [33]

minor influences, especially of higher doses, cannot be excluded [31]. In the 14 hypertensive type 2 diabetics followed by Trost and Weidmann [32, 40], monotherapy with nitrendipine did not modify Hb A₁ (gpycosylated component of adult hemoglobin) (Fig. 6) in up to 5 years of treatment. Assessment of published reports with a minimum of 6 hypertensive diabetics receiving a chronic Ca^{++} channel blockers therapy also reveals no consistent modification of plasma glucose, Hb A₁ or insulin levels [32, 33–38, 40–44] (Fig. 7). Nevertheless, isolated cases with suspected Ca^{++} channel blocker-induced hyperglycemia have been reported [45]. Considering that regular glucose monitoring is an integral part of care for every diabetic patient, deterioration of glucose metabolism should, if it ever occurs during chronic Ca^{++} channel blockade, be easily detected and corrected.

Ca^{++} channel blockers also do not seem to unfavorably affect other metabolic correlates of cardiovascular risk such as serum lipoproteins and potassium [28, 31]. Most available observations relate to non-diabetic patients with essential HT (Fig. 8). Nevertheless, serum lipids and/or lipoprotein fractions were unaltered in several groups of diabetics receiving Ca^{++} channel blockers [17, 31, 37, 38]. In the study of hypertensive type 2 diabetics by Trost and Weidmann [17], total cholesterol, low-density lipoprotein (LDL) and high-density lipoprotein (HDL) cholesterol, apoproteins A1, A2, and B, as well as total and very low-density lipoprotein (VLDL) triglycerides were stable after 6 weeks of nitrendipine montherapy. Moreover, serum uric acid, a risk correlate rather than risk factor per se, was significantly lowered.

Angiotensin-Converting Enzyme Inhibitors

The BP-lowering potency of a chronic monotherapy with ACE inhibitors in hypertensive diabetics was assessed by an analysis of published reports with a minimum of 8 patients [46–53] (Fig. 9). It is evident that ACE inhibitors can distinctly improve HT in diabetics; a BP-lowering effect was similarly apparent between 1 month and 1 year of monotherapy and averaged -12.5%.

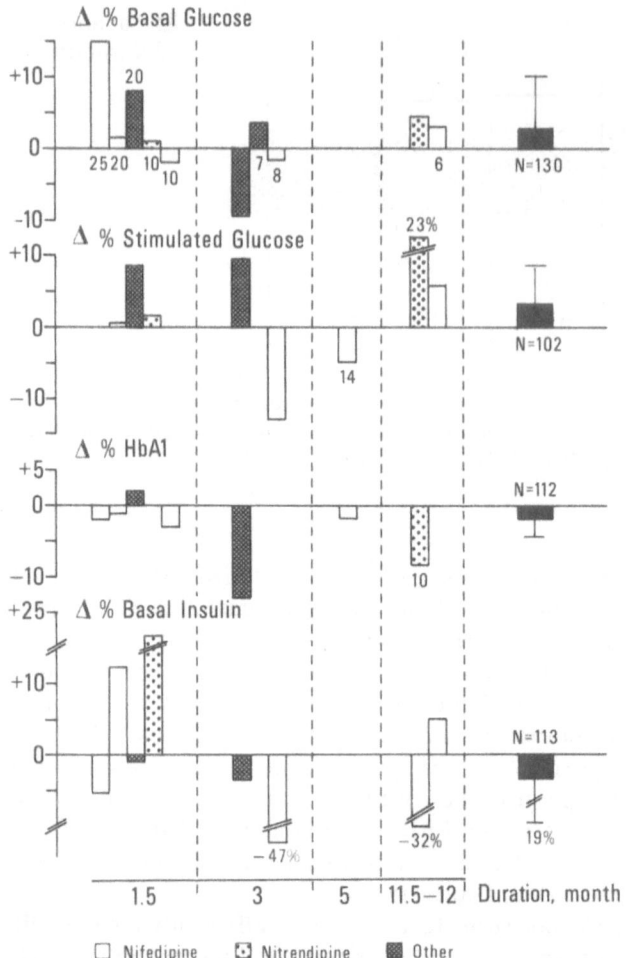

Fig. 7. Percentage changes in indices of carbohydrate metabolism during monotherapy with Ca^{++} channel blockers in hypertension associated with diabetes mellitus. Each column represents the average percentage change in a report based on a minimum number of 6 subjects. *Right column* is mean of all studies. *Niifedipine added to bendrofluazide

The neutrality of ACE inhibitors with regard to glucose and lipoprotein metabolism in non-diabetic patients with essential HT [28, 29] probably applies also for hypertensive patients with DM [46–53]. Potassium deserves particular consideration. Some diabetic patients develop hyporeninemic hypoaldosteronism [54, 55]. ACE inhibitors may promote hypoaldosteronism [56]. When hypoaldosteronism coexists with impaired kidney function and/or insulin deficiency [54, 57], serum potassium homeostasis by renal and/or extrarenal disposition of potassium [57, 58] is critically reduced and hyperkalemia may occur. It follows that ACE inhibitors should produce no relevant serum potassium changes in metabolically stable dis-

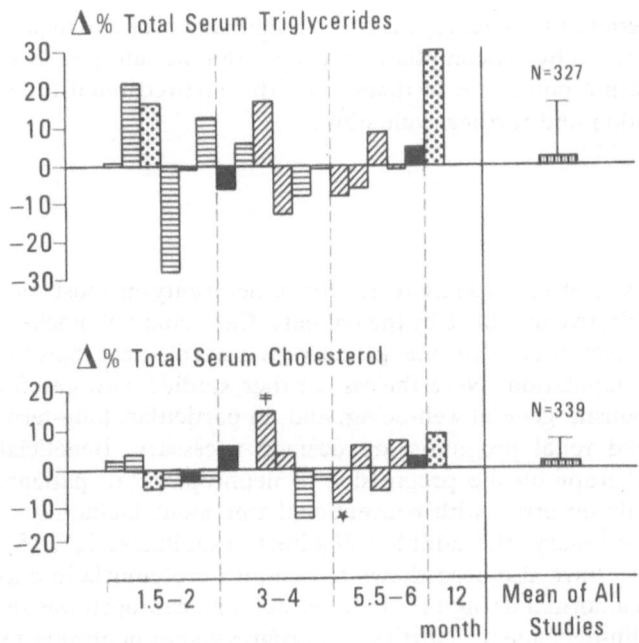

Fig. 8. Percentage responses of serum total lipids to a monotherapy with Ca^{++} channel blockers. Each column represents the average percentage change in a report based on a minimum number of 10 subjects. From Weidmann et al. [28]

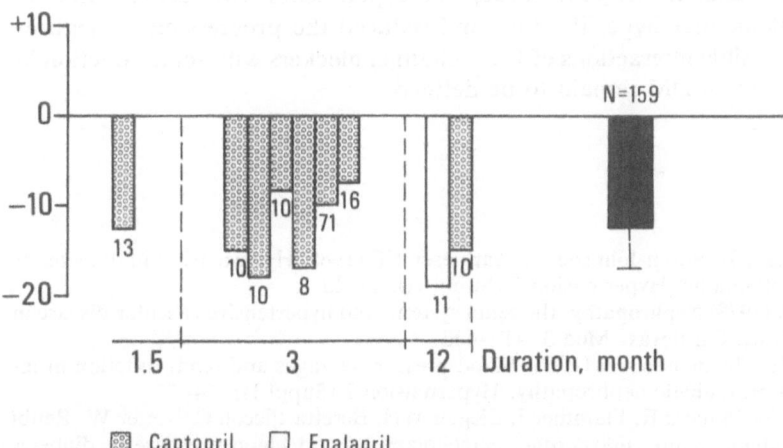

Fig. 9. Percentage responses of mean blood pressure to a monotheraphy with angiotensin-converting enzyme (ACE) inhibitors in hypertension associated with diabetes mellitus. Each column represents the average percentage change in a report based on a minimum number of 8 subjects. *Right column* is mean of all studies

betics with normal renal function, but these agents could potentially promote hyperkalemia during insulin withdrawal by noncompliant diabetics, and the safety of ACE inhibitors with regard to plasma potassium in diabetics with impaired renal functions warrants close observation and further evaluation.

Outlook

Based on their antihypertensive effect, apparent metabolic neutrality in most diabetics, and an acceptable subjective tolerance by the patients, Ca^{++} channel blockers and ACE inhibitors have the potential to become primary pharmacological tools for HT control in the diabetic population. Nevertheless, further studies with careful monitoring of glucose metabolism, general well-being, and, in particular, long-term effects on cardiovascular and renal prognosis are deemed necessary. Beneficial effects of antihypertensive therapy on the progression of nephropathy in patients with DM type 1 were initially observed with conventional treatment including β-blockers, diuretics and, if necessary, the addition of direct vasodilators [11, 15]. More recently, ACE inhibitors have also been shown to diminish proteinuria in diabetics with nephropathy and a normal or high BP [50, 59, 60]; and captopril was reported to slow, in some insulin-dependent diabetics, the progression of nephropathy [61]. In non-diabetic rats with 5/6 nephrectomy, a conventional triple therapy with hydrochlorothiazide, reserpine, and hydralazine, or a monotherapy with enalapril were similarly effective in controlling systemic hypertension; however, the ACE inhibitor only controlled glomerular hypertension and limited the development of proteinuria and glomerular lesions [62]. In rats with experimental DM, ACE inhibitors also prevented glomerular hyperfiltration and reduced the progression of nephropathy [14]. The possible interactions of Ca^{++} channel blockers with renal function in experimental or human DM remain to be defined.

References

1. Feldt-Rasmussen B, Borch-Johnsen K, Mathiesen ER (1985) Hypertension in diabetes as related to nephropathy. Hypertension 7 (Suppl II): 18–20
2. Christlieb AR (1978) Nephropathy, the renin system, and hypertensive vascular disease in diabetes mellitus. Cardiovasc Med 3: 417–432
3. Mogensen CE, Christensen CK (1985) Blood pressure changes and renal function in incipient and overt diabetic nephropathy. Hypertension 7 (Suppl II): 64–73
4. De Chatel R, Weidmann R, Flammer J, Ziegler WH, Beretta-Piccoli C, Vetter W, Reubi FC (1977) Sodium, renin, aldosterone, catecholamines and blood pressure in diabetes mellitus. Kidney Int 12: 412–421
5. Weidmann P, Beretta-Piccoli C, Trost BN (1985) Pressor factors and responsiveness in hypertension accompanying diabetes mellitus. Hypertension 7 (Suppl II): 33–42
6. Weidmann P, Beretta-Piccoli C, Keusch G, Glück Z, Mujagic M, Grimm M, Meier A, Ziegler WH (1979) Sodium-volume factor, cardiovascular reactivity and hypotensive mechanisms of diuretic therapy in hypertension associated with diabetes mellitus. Am J Med 67: 779–784
7. Beretta-Piccoli C, Weidmann P (1981) Exaggerated pressor responsiveness to norepine-

phrine in non-azotemic diabetes mellitus. Am J Med 71: 829–835
8. Drury PL, Smith GM, Ferriss JB (1984) Increased vasopressor responsiveness to angiotensin II in uncomplicated type I (insulin-dependent) diabetes. Diabetologia 27: 174–179
9. Weidmann P (1988) Pathogenesis of hypertension accompanying diabetes mellitus. In: Heidland A, Koch K(eds) Contributions to Nephrology. Karger, Basel (in press)
10. Beretta-Piccoli C, Weidmann P (1984) Circulatory volume in essential hypertension. Relationships with age, blood pressure, exchangeable sodium, renin, aldosterone and catecholamines. Miner Electrolyte Metab 10: 292–300
11. Parving HH, Andersen AR, Hommel E, Schmidt U (1985) Effects of long-term antihypertensive treatment on kidney function in diabetic nephropathy. Hypertension 7 (Suppl II): 114–117
12. Krolewski AS, Canessa M, Warram JH, Laffel LMB, Christlieb AR, Knowler WC, Rand LI (1988) Predisposition to hypertension and susceptibility to renal disease in insulin-dependent diabetes mellitus. N Engl J Med 318: 140–145
13. Mangili R, Bending JJ, Scott G, Li LK, Gupta A, Viberti GC (1988) Increased sodium-lithium countertransport activity in red cells of patients with insulin-dependent diabetes and nephropathy. N Engl J Med 318: 146–150
14. Zatz R, Dunn BR, Meyer TW, Anderson S, Rennke HG, Brenner BM (1986) Prevention of diabetic glomerulopathy by pharmacological amelioration of glomerular capillary hypertension. J Clin Invest 77: 1925–1930
15. Christensen CK, Mogensen CE (1985) Effect of antihypertensive treatment on progression of incipient diabetic nephropathy. Hypertension 7 (Suppl II): 109–113
16. Hasslacher Ch, Wolfrum M, Stech G, Wahl P, Ritz E (1987) Diabetische Nephropathie bei Typ II diabetes. Dtsch Med Wochenschr 112: 1445–1449
17. Trost BN, Weidmann P (1985) Antihypertensive therapy in diabetic patients. Hypertension 7 (Suppl II): 102–108
18. Pacy PJ, Dodson PM, Kubicki AJ, Fletcher RF, Taylor KG (1984) Comparison of the hypotensive and metabolic effects of bendrofluazide therapy and a high fibre, low fat, low sodium diet in diabetic subjects with mild hypertension. J Hypertens 2: 215–220
19. Veterans Administration Cooperative Study Group on Antihypertensive Agents (1970) Effects of treatment on morbidity in hypertension. II. Results in patients with diastolic blood pressure averaging 90 through 114 mmHg. JAMA 213: 1134–1152
20. Multiple Risk Factor Intervention Trial Research Group (1982) Multiple risk factor intervention trial: risk factor changes and mortality results. JAMA 248: 1465–1477
21. Medical Research Council Working Party (1985) MRC trial of treatment of mild hypertension: principal results. Br Med J 291: 97–104
22. Chahal P, Inglesby DV, Sleightholm M, Kohner EM (1985) Blood pressure and the progression of mild background diabetic retinopathy. Hypertension 7 (Suppl II): 79–83
23. Struthers AD, Murphy MB, Dollery CT (1985) Glucose tolerance during antihypertensive therapy in patients with diabetes mellitus. Hypertension 7 (Suppl II): 95–101
24. Holland OB, Nixon JV, Kuhnert L (1981) Diuretic-induced vertricular ectopic activity. Am J Med 70: 762–768
25. Solomon JR, Cole AG (1981) Importance of potassium in patients with acute myocardial infarction. Acta Med Scand 859: S87–S93
26. Weidmann P, Gerber A, Mordasini R (1983) Effects of antihypertensive therapy on serum lipoproteins. Hypertension 5 (Suppl III): 120–131
27. Materson BJ, Oster JR, Michael UF, Bolton SM, Burton ZC, Stambaugh JE, Morledge J (1978) Dose response to chlorthalidone in patients with mild hypertension. Clin Pharmacol Ther 24: 192–198
28. Weidmann P, Ferrier C, Saxenhofer H, Uehlinger DE, Trost BN (1988) Serum lipoproteins during treatment with antihypertensive drugs. Drugs 35 (Suppl 6): 118–134
29. Weinberger MH (1983) Influence of an angiotensin converting-enzyme inhibitor on diuretic-induced metabolic effects in hypertension. Hypertension 5 (Suppl III): 132–138
30. Weidmann P, Gnaedinger MP, Uehlinger DE (1986) Calcium channel blockers in the treatment of hypertension. In: Kaufmann W, Bönner G, Lang R, Meurer KA (eds)

Primary hypertension — Basic mechanisms and therapeutic implications. Springer, Heidelberg, pp 170-200

31. Trost BN, Weidmann P (1988) Metabolic effects of calcium antagonists in humans, with emphasis on carbohydrate, lipid, potassium and uric acid homeostases. Cardiovasc Pharmacol 12 (Suppl 6): S86-S92
mellitus. J Cardiovasc Pharmacol 9 (Suppl IV): IV-S280-S285

33. Winocour PH, Barnes PC, Anderson DC (1986) The effect of nifedipine on blood pressure and exercise tolerance in insulin-treated diabetics with hypertension. Eur J Clin Invest 16:A23

34. Gill JS, Al-Hussary N, Zezulka AV, Pasi KJ, Atkin TW, Beevers DG (1987) Effect of nifedipine on glucose tolerance, serum insulin, and serum fructosamine in diabetic and nondiabetic patients. Clin Ther 9 (Suppl III): 304-310

35. Cruickshank JK, Anderson NMcF (1987) Treating hypertensive diabetics: a comparison of verapamil and metoprolol in black and white patients. In: Fleckenstein A, Laragh JH (eds) Hypertension — the next decade: verapamil in focus. Churchill Livingstone, New York, pp 208-211

36. Wada S, Nakayama M, Masaki K (1982) Effects of diltiazem on serum lipids: comparison with beta-blockers. Clin Ther 5: 163-173

37. Odigwe Co, McCulloch AJ, Williams DO, Tunbridge WMG (1986) A trial of the calcium antagonist nisoldipine in hypertensive non-insulin-dependent diabetic patients. Diabetic Med 3: 463-467

38. Corcoran JS, Perkins JE, Hoffbrand BI, Yudkin JS (1987) Treating hypertension in non-insulin-dependent diabetes: a comparison of atenolol, nifedipine, and captopril combined with benrofluazide. Diabetic Med 4:164-168

39. MacGregor GA, Pevahouse JB, Cappuccio FP, Markandu ND (1987) Nifedipine, sodium intake, diuretics and sodium balance. Am J Nephrol 7 (Suppl I): 44-48

40. Trost BN, Weidmann P (1988) Five years of antihypertensive monotherapy with nitrendipine do not alter carbohydrate homeostasis in diabetic patients. J Cardiovasc Pharmacol S184 (Abstr)

41. Abadie E, Villette JM, Gauville C, Tabuteau F, Fiet J, Passa Ph (1985) Effets de la nifédipine sur le métabolisme hydrocarboné chez le diabétique non insulino-dépendent. Diabete Metab 11: 141-146

42. Kanatsuna T, Nakano K, Mori H, Kano Y, Nishioka H, Kajiyama S, Kitagawa Y, Yoshida T, Kondo M, Nakamura N, Aochi O (1985) Effects of nifedipine on insulin secretion and glucose metabolism in rats and in hypertensive type 2 (non-insulin dependent) diabetics. Arzneimittelforschung 35 (Suppl II): 514-517

43. Collins WCJ, Cullen MJ, Feely J (1986) The effect of therapy with dihydropyridine calcium channel blockers on glucose tolerance in non-insulin dependent diabetes. Br J Clin Pharmacol 21: P568

44. Fagan TC, Nelson EB, Lasseter KC, Crook J, Morledge J, Conrad KA (1985) Once- and twice-daily nitrendipine in patients with hypertension and noninsulin-dependent diabetes. Pharmacotherapy 6: 128-136

45. Bhatnagar SK, Amin MAA, Al-Yusuf AR (1984) Diabetogenic effects of nifedipine. Br Med J 289: 19

46. Gambaro G, Morbiato F, Cicerello E, Del Turco M, Sartori L, D'Angelo A, Crepaldi G (1985) Captopril in the treatment of hypertension in type I and type II diabetic patients. J Hypertens 3 (Suppl II): S149-S151

47. Ricci PD, Fazzi L, Ricci F (1985) Il captopril nel controllo dell'ipertensione arteriosa essenziale del soggetto diabetico. Clin Ter 113 (Suppl I): 33-38

48. Sullivan PA, Kelleher M, Twomey M, Dineen M (1985): Effects of converting enzyme inhibition on blood pressure, plasma renin activity (PRA) and plasma aldosterone in hypertensive diabetics compared to patients with essential hypertension. J Hypertens 3 (Suppl IV): 359-363

49. Dominguez JR, de la Calle H, Hurtado A, Robles RG, Sancho-Rof J (1986) Effect of converting enzyme inhibitors in hypertensive patients with non-insulin-dependent diabetes

mellitus. Postgrad Med J 62 (Suppl I): 66–68

50. Hommel E, Parving HH, Mathiesen E, Edsberg B, Nielsen MD, Giese J (1986) Effect of captopril on kidney function in insulin-dependent diabetic patients with nephropathy. Br Med J 293: 467–470

51. Matthews DW, Wathen CG, Bell D, Collier A, Muir AL, Clarke BF (1986) The effect of captopril on blood pressure and glucose tolerance in hypertensive non-insulin dependent diabetics. Postgrad Med J 62 (Suppl I): 73–75

52. Passa Ph, LeBlanc H, Marre M (1987) Effects of enalapril in insulin-dependent diabetic subjects with mild to moderate uncomplicated hypertension. Diabetes Care 10 (Suppl II): 200–204

53. Shionori H, Iino S, Inoue S (1987) Glucose metabolism during mono- and combination therapy in diabetic hypertensive patients: a multiclinic trial. Clin Exp Hypertens 9: A671–A674

54. Weidmann P, Reinhart R, Maxwell MH, Massry SG, Lupu AN, Coburn JW, Kleeman CR (1973) Syndrome of hyporeninemic hypoaldosteronism and hyperkalemia in renal disease. J Clin Endocrinol Metab 36: 965–977

55. Weidmann P, Beretta-Piccoli C, Glück Z, Keusch G, Reubi FC, de Châtel R, Cottier C (1980) Hypoaldosteronism without hyperkalemia. Klin Wochenschr 58: 185–194

56. Rimmer JM, Horn JF, Gennari FJ (1987) Hyperkalemia as a complication of drug therapy. Arch Intern Med 147: 867–869

57. Cox M, Sterns RH, Singer I (1978) The defense against hyperkalemia: the roles of insulin and aldosterone. N Engl J Med 299: 525–532

58. Van Ypersele de Strihou C (1977) Potassium homeostasis in renal failure. Kidney Int 11: 491–504

59. Taguma Y, Kitamoto Y, Futaki G, Ueda H, Monma H, Ishizaki M, Takahashi H, Sekino H, Sasaki Y (1985) N Engl J Med 313: 1617–1620

60. Marre M, Leblanc, H, Suarez L, Guyenne TT, Ménard J, Passa P (1987) Converting enzyme inhibition and kidney function in normotensive diabetic patients with persistent microalbuminuria. Br Med J 294: 1448–1452

61. Björck S, Nyberg G, Mulec H, Granerus G, Herlitz H, Aurell M (1986) Beneficial effects of angiotensin converting enzyme inhibition on renal function in patients with diabetic nephropathy. Br Med J 293: 471–474

62. Anderson S, Rennke HG, Brenner BM (1986) Therapeutic advantage of converting enzyme inhibitors in arresting progressive renal disease associated with systemic hypertension. J Clin Invest 77: 1993–2000

Discussion

Leonetti (Milan): The metabolic side effects that you have shown, are they observed with all doses, or do you advise employing small doses? Second, you have shown that the total body sodium was not decreased during treatment with a calcium antagonist. Did you observe the acute nondiuretic and diuretic effect in diabetic patients?

Weidmann (Bern): To the first, I think there is no doubt (as pointed out the day before) that in essential hypertension, and particularly in the elderly, we should use the lowest possible dosage of diuretics and other agents. There is no doubt about that. The side effects, as you all know, are dose related except for the lipoproteins. There are no data on their relationships to low doses and lipoproteins. Now, in diabetes, unfortunately, I cannot tell you that low doses of diuretics in the range of 12.5 or 25 mg hydrochlorothiazide are very effective. The data is limited even with regard to diuretics. It is possible that if one used a very low diuretic dose in a diabetic one might achieve a good clinical effect. It also did not mean to condemn the diuretics in diabetics; since, as all clinicians know, sometimes we do need the diuretics, because they tend to retain sodium. With regard to exchangeable body sodium, undoubtedly in these studies and with any other calcium antagonist, one sees an acute diuresis. The diuresis (or natriuresis, as I should say, because that is the initiating event) goes away or disappears — dissipates — within one or a very few days, and after about 1 week of treatment sodium balance is achieved. In the long range, there might be mild sodium retention. Now, with the calcium antagonist, as I showed, we do not modify the retention. This might be a disadvantage, I do not know; we haven't seen it as a disadvantage so far.

Other questions? Please, Dr. Takeda.

Takeda (Osaka): Concerning the glomerular fraction in diabetic patients with hypertension, you mentioned that the high blood pressure per se causes the degradation of the glomerular function. In our analysis of the renal function in diabetic patients, some patients have hyperfiltration per glomeruli. It is usually unfavorable to produce the glomerular damage. What is your opinion about the drug to be used to keep the glomerular function, especially in the afferent and efferent arterioles?

Weidmann: I think it is an important question. As I mentioned, there is no doubt that glomerular hyperfiltration is a very important pathogenic event in diabetic kidney disease. Also, I must tell you that (you probably are aware of the data) in type 2 in elderly or insulin-independent diabetes, the kidney disease does not start with hyperfiltration. It starts in type 1. This is one pathogenetic factor. With regard to all the drugs that differ in prevention of this nephropathy, the early data I showed by Parving are based on conventional therapy — beta-blockers, metoprolol, together with diuretics and vasodilators. So, even conventional therapy may have some effect in humans when it is not apparent in the rat, as in the studies from Brenner. Humans differ anyway.

Now, we would like to know whether calcium antagonists are beneficial. We know that converting enzyme inhibitors can prevent it experimentally, and a whole series very recently (British medical journal from Scandinavia) suggests that they might also be effective in humans with this calcium antagonist, I think that so far there is very little data on proteinuria or kidney function in the diabetic. I think it is an important field to study. We cannot at the present time say that one drug or another may be better in preventing this type of nephropathy.

Calcium Antagonists in Combination Therapy

Gastone Leonetti and Alberto Zanchetti[1]

Summary. In "non-responders" to monotherapy with calcium antagonists, the combination of dihydropyridine derivatives with beta-blockers appears very rational: indeed, the two classes have different mechanisms of actions and each can counteract side effects caused by the other. Clinical experience has confirmed the validity of this combination, which is particularly useful in hypertensive patients with ischemic heart disease. More attention must be used in the combination of calcium antagonists of the papaverine and benzothiazepine groups with beta-blockers. Another useful combination of calcium antagonists is that with converting enzyme inhibitors. In spite of the fact that both types of drugs are vasodilators, clinical experience has shown their combination induces a more powerful antihypertensive effect and can also prevent the modest rise in heart rate caused by dihydropyridine derivatives. An intriguing problem is the combination of calcium antagonists with diuretics. Contrasting results are available in the literature: according to some authors the combination of a calcium antagonist diuretic is more effective than monotherapy with either compound; for other authors, the combination is useless. Undoubtedly, the combination of diuretics and calcium antagnosts does not prevent the hormonal and metabolic effects of diuretics. According to our experience, diuretics were equally effective as beta-blockers or converting enzyme inhibitors in potentiating the antihypertensive action of nicardipine in partial-responders. A low-sodium diet reduced the acute antihypertensive action of nifedipine, but the blood pressure level reached was nevertheless lower than that induced by nifedipine during normal sodium intake. In our hands, the percentage of patients treated with calcium antagonists and requiring a combination treatment was similar in young, adult, and elderly hypertensives.

Key words: Calcium antagonists Hypertension — Combination treatment

Introduction

Antihypertensive monotherapy is effective in only 40%–60% of hypertensive patients, irrespective of the class of drugs being used. Therefore, there is frequently a need for combination therapy in the management of hypertension. The following aspects are commonly considered as rational requirements for combination treatment: 1) the different drugs should have different and therefore additive pharmaco-

[1] Istituto di Clinica Medica Generale e Terapia Medica, Università di Milano, Centro di Fisiologia Clinica e Ipertensione, Ospedale Maggiore, Milano, Italy

dynamic mechanisms; 2) the drug to be added should counteract pressor compensatory mechanisms activated by the first drug; and finally, 3) the drug to be added should oppose the unfavorable metabolic changes or side effects of the initial drug. Furthermore, the addition of a second antihypertensive agent frequently allows a reduction in the dose of the initial drug with a consequent improvement in side effects.

In this paper we discuss only the rational for combination of calcium antagonists of the dihydropyridine group with diuretics, converting enzyme inhibitors, and beta-adrenergic blocking agents and the influence of the sodium state on the antihypertensive efficacy of this group of calcium antagonists.

Dihydropyridine Derivatives and Diuretics

A survey of available information on the antihypertensive efficacy of the combination of dihydropyridine derivatives and thiazide diuretics provides contradictory results. Indeed, in 4 out of 8 studies [1–4], no additive antihypertensive effect was found when a dihydropyridine derivative and a diuretic were combined, whereas in the other 4 studies [5–8], an additive effect from the combination was found. However, independently of the variable effects on blood pressure, the combination of calcium antagonists and diuretics caused, in all studies, the expected rise in serum uric acid and plasma renin activity and the expected decrease in serum potassium.

According to Sever and Poulter [7], the conflicting results so far obtained could largely be due to the inappropriate design of several studies. For instance, the number of patients investigated was too low and the studies did not have the power to detect statistically significant differences. Other authors [4] have suggested that the limited usefulness of the combination between the dihydropyridine derivatives and diuretics might result from pharmacodynamic interferences. For instance, the natriuretic and diuretic actions of calcium antagonists might blunt the natriuretic and perhaps the vascular action of thiazides; although the natriuretic action of the dihydropyridine derivatives seems to be on distal convoluted tubules and collecting ducts [9], therefore distal to that of thiazide diuretics. Moreover, since it is by no means clear which basic mechanisms are involved in the vasorelaxant properties of thiazides, it would be premature to propose that such an unknown action might be antagonized by calcium entry blockers.

Dihydropyridine Derivatives and Converting Enzyme Inhibitors

There is an almost complete agreement among the available studies [10–17] on the usefulness of the combination between calcium antagonists and converting enzyme inhibitors. Indeed, in 7 [10–16] of 8 studies an additive antihypertensive effect of this combination was found. As shown by Guazzi et al. [11] and by Salvetti et al. [16], when captopril and nifedipine are combined for the treatment of arterial hypertension, there is not only a greater reduction in blood pressure, but also less ankle edema than during nifedipine monotherapy. The reduction in ankle edema may be explained by the vasodilating effect of captopril on the venous side of the circulation, counterbalancing the increase in capillary pressure induced by the arterial vaso-dilating effect of nifedipine.

The additive antihypertensive efficacy and good tolerance of the combination between dihydropyridine derivative calcium antagonists and converting enzyme inhibitors can be explained by the fact that the vasodilatating mechanisms of these drugs are different. Furthermore, converting enzyme inhibitors can reduce sympathetic nervous system activity and may in this way blunt the reflex activation induced by dihydropyridines [18]. Finally, nifedipine has been shown to activate the renin-angiotensin system [19, 20], and angiotensin II generation is blocked by the converting enzyme inhibitors.

Another potential benefit of this association results from the observation that neither of these 2 classes of drugs affects lipid, carbohydrate, and electrolyte metabolism [21]. It is therefore unlikely that their combination will induce the negative metabolic changes described for other antihypertensive compounds.

Dihydropyridine Derivates and Beta-Blockers

There are numerous reports in the literature on the useful association of beta-blockers and dihydropyridine derivatives in the treatment of arterial hypertension [22–29]. This combination is effective not only in inducing a further reduction in blood pressure, but also in reducing incidence of adverse effects and metabolic changes, in improving renal function, and in the well-being of the patient. Kirkendall et al. [28] and De Divitiis et al. [24] have shown that the incidence of dropouts is very low in patients treated with this combination, and the incidence of adverse effects is lower during the combination treatment than during monotherapy with either drug. According to the review by Brouwer et al. [30], the dihydropyridine/beta-blocker combination does not appear to carry out a significant risk of cardiac conduction disturbances and heart failure; on the other hand, the combination of verapamil and beta-blockers can give rise to such complications more frequently [31]. Jennings et al. [32] have shown that nifedipine can safely and effectively be given to severe hypertensive patients in the presence of previous treatment with beta-blockers, even when the left ventricular ejection fraction is relatively low. In spite of all these encouraging data, there have been occasional reports of bradyarrhythmias and heart failure with this combination [33–35].

The combination of dihydropyridine derivatives and beta-blockers may also have a favorable effect on renal circulation. Indeed, Christensen et al. [36] have reported a reduction in renal vascular resistances with a trend toward an increase in glomerular filtration rate and renal plasma flow when nifedipine was acutely added to hypertensive patients under beta-blockade in spite of the further and significant blood pressure reduction. Finally, the combination of dihydropyridine derivatives and beta-blockers has been found to cause minimal changes in laboratory tests of serum uric acid, calcium, potassium, blood sugar, and serum cholesterol.

Dihydropyridine Derivatives in Different Combinations: Evidence from Uncontrolled Studies

In a multicentric study, Kirkendall et al. [28] compared the effectiveness of the associations between nitrendipine and a diuretic or a beta-blocker and that between a beta-blocker and a diuretic. All 3 pharmacological combinations caused similar blood pressure reductions without significant difference among them. According to Mroczec et al. [37], diuretics and beta-blockers caused similar percentages of blood pressure normalization when added to non-responders to nitrendipine monotherapy. Finally, in a multicentric study [38], we have found differences (not significant) in blood pressure reduction when diuretics, beta-blockers, or converting enzyme inhibitors were added to nicardipine monotherapy. Therefore, all 3 multicentric studies suggest that the associations of dihydropyridine derivatives with diuretics, beta-blockers, or converting enzyme inhibitors are equally potent.

Dihydropyridine Derivatives and Sodium Intake

It has been claimed [39–40] that sodium intake can influence calcium ion transport at the cell membrane level and consequently the antihypertensive efficacy of calcium antagonists. The influence of sodium intake on the antihypertensive response to calcium antagonists has been investigated in an acute study by our group [14] and in an acute and short-term study by Cappuccio et al. [42]. In our study, the administration of a single dose of nifedipine after adequate periods of normal- (100 mEq/day) and low- (10 mEq/day) sodium intake caused similar diastolic blood pressure reductions (–7 and –5 mmHg respectively), while systolic blood pressure fell to a greater (not significant) extent during normal sodium intake (–17 mmHg) than in the depleted state (–10 mmHg). However, in spite of the slightly greater blood pressure reduction during normal-sodium intake, the blood pressure values attained after acute nifedipine administration were lower during sodium depletion than during normal-sodium intake, because of the blood pressure reduction caused by the low-sodium diet. Cappuccio et al. [42] have found that a single dose of nifedipine caused smaller percentage reductions in mean arterial pressure during low- and normal-sodium diets than during high-sodium intake. However, the average blood pressure after nifedipine was lowest during low-sodium intake, due to the blood pressure reduction caused by the low-sodium diet. Similar results were found by these authors during short-term (5 days) repeated administration of nifedipine. Therefore, all these studies suggest that nifedipine can lower the blood pressure of hypertensive patients independently of their sodium intake, and that nifedipine can cause a further blood pressure reduction in patients whose blood pressure has been partially reduced by a low-sodium diet.

Conclusions

The following conclusions can be drawn from available studies:

1. The combination of calcium antagonists of the dihydropyridine series with beta-adrenergic blocking agents and converting enzyme inhibitors has an additive anti-hypertensive effect, while some of the side effects due to each class of drugs are partly reduced or prevented.
2. The antihypertensive efficacy of the combination of dihydropyridine derivatives and thiazide diuretics is controversial, and further studies are necessary in order to reach a definite conclusion.
3. Nifedipine caused a significant blood pressure reduction independently of the state of sodium intake and can further exaggerate the blood pressure reduction induced by a low-sodium diet.

Although there are no studies specifically designed to assess the antihypertensive efficacy of calcium antagonists in combination with other antihypertensive drugs in the elderly, we have found no evidence in published studies to suggest that efficacy and/or tolerability of the various combinations may be related to the patient's age in an age range of up to 79 years. Therefore, we can tentatively conclude that the combination of calcium antagonists with other drugs is equally effective and tolerated in old and young people, although this tentative conclusion needs to be confirmed in adequately controlled studies.

References

1. Rosenthal J (1982) Antihypertensive effects of nifedipine, mefruside and a combination of both substances in patients with essential hypertension. In: Kaltenbach M, Neufeld HN (ed) New therapy of ischemic heart disease and hypertension. Excerpta Medica Amsterdam, pp 175–181.
2. Mimran A, Ribstein J (1986) Effect of nifedipine in hypertension not controlled by converting enzyme inhibitors and diuretic. Postgrad Med J 62 (Suppl I): I-135–138.
3. Magagna A, Abdel-Haq B, Pedrinelli R, Salvetti A (1986) Does chlorthalidone increase the hypotensive effects of nifedipine? J Hypertens 4 (Suppl V): V-S519–S521
4. MacGregor GA, Pevahouse JB, Cappuccio FP, Markandu ND (1987) Nifedipine, diuretics and sodium balance. J Hypertens 5 (Suppl IV): IV-S127–S131
5. Hedner T, Samuelsson O, Sjogren E, Elmfeldt D (1986) Treatment of essential hypertension with felodipine in combination with diuretics. Eur J Clin Pharmacol 30: 133–139
6. Massie BM, Tubau JF, Szlachcic J, Vollmer C (1986) Comparison and additivity of nitrendipine and hychochlorothiazide in systemic hypertension. Am J Cardiol 58: D16–D19
7. Sever PS, Poulter NR (1987) Calcium antagonists and diuretics as combined therapy. J Hypertens 5 (Suppl IV): IV-S123–S126
8. Ferrara AL, Pasanisi F, Marotta T, Rubba P, Mancini M (1986) Calcium antagonists and thiazide diuretics in the treatment of hypertension. J Cardiovasc Pharmacol 10 (Suppl X): X-S136–S137
9. Di Bona GF (1985) Effects of felodipine on renal function in animals. Drugs 29 (Suppl II): II-168–175
10. Stornello M, Di Rao G, Iachello M, Pisani R, Scapellato L, Pedrinelli R, Salvetti A (1983) Haemodynamic and humoral interactions between captopril and nifedipine. Hypertension 5 (Suppl II): II-154–156
11. Guazzi MD, De Cesare N, Galli C, Salvioni A, Tramontana C, Tamborini G, Bartorelli A (1984) Calcium-channel blockade with nifedipine and angiotensin converting-enzyme inhibition with captopril in therapy of patients with severe primary hypertension. Circulation 70: 279–284

12. MacGregor GA, Markandu ND, Smith SJ, Sagnella GA (1985) Captopril: contrasting effects of adding hydrochlorotiazide, propranolol or nifedipine. J Cardiovasc Pharmacol 7: S82–S87
13. Brouwer RML, Bolli P, Erne P, Lonen D, Kiowski W, Buhler FR (1985) Antihypertensive treatment using calcium antagonists in combination with captopril rather than diuretics. J Cardiovasc Pharmacol 7: S88–S91
14. White WB, Viadero JJ, Lane TJ, Podesla S (1986) Effects of combination therapy with captopril and nifedipine in severe or resistant hypertension. Clin Pharmacol Ther 39: 43–48
15. Mimram A Ribstein J (1985) Effects of chronic nifedipine in patients inadequately controlled by converting enzyme inhibitor and a diuretic. J Cardiovasc Pharmacol 7 (Suppl I) I-S92–S95
16. Salvetti A, Innocent PF, Iardella M, Pambianco F, Saba GC, Rossetti M, Botta GF (1987) Captopril and nifedipine in the treatment of essential hypertension: a crossover study. J Hypertens 5 (Suppl IV): IV-S139–S142
17. Klein WW, Stuhlinger W, Mahr G (1986) Crossover comparison between captopril and nifedipine. Postgrad Med J 62 (Suppl I): I-108–110
18. Zanchetti A (1988) Nitrendipine and ACE inhibitors. (in press) J Cardiovasc Pharmacol 12 (Suppl IV)
19. Leonetti G, Cuspidi C, Sampieri L, Terzoli L, Zanchetti A (1982) A comparison of cardiovascular, renal and humoral effects of acute administration of two calcium-channels blockers in normotensive and hypertensive subjects. J Cardiovasc Pharmacol 4: 319–324
20. Lederballe-Pedersen O, Mikkelsen E, Christensen NJ, Kornerup HJ, Pederson EB (1979) Effects of nifedipine on plasma renin, aldosterone and catecholamines in arterial hypertension. Eur J Clin Pharmacol 15: 235–240
21. Weidmann P, Ferrier C, Saxenhofer H, Vehlinger DE, Trost BN (1988) Serum lipoprotein during treatment with antihypertensive drugs. Drugs 35 (Suppl VI) VI-118–134
22 Ekelund LG, Ekelund C, Rossner S (1982) Antihypertensive effects at rest and during exercise of a calcium blocker nifedipine, alone and in combination with metoprolol. Acta Med Scand 212: 71–75
23. Eggersten R, Hansson L (1981) Effect of treatment with nifedipine and metoprolol in essential hypertension. Eur J Clin Pharmacol 21: 389–390
24. De Divitiis O, Petito M, Di Somma S, Fazio S, Galderisi M, Villari B, Liguori U, Santomauro M (1984) Acebutolol and nifedipine in the treatment of arterial hypertension: efficacy and acceptability. Arzneimittel forschung 34: 710–715
25. Maltz MB, Davies DW, Lau CP, Creamer JE, Banim SO, Camm AJ (1986) The effects of oral nitrendipine and propranolol, alone and in combination, on hypertensive patients with special reference to AV conduction Br J Clin Pharmacol 22: 463–467
26. Dekoch M, Melin JA, Nannan ME, Robert A, Beckers C, Lavenne F, Detry JMR (1986) Alternation of left ventricular diastolic filling in hypertensive patients: effects of nitrendipine and atenolol. Eur Heart J 7: 792–799
27. Daniels AR, Opie LH (1986) Atenolol plus nifedipine for mild to moderate systemic hypertension after fixed doses of either agent alone. Am J Cardiol 57: 965–970
28. Kirkendall WM, Adlin V, Canzanello V, Cubberley R, Haider B, MacCarthy P, Mroizek W, Nelson E, Schoenberger J, Solomon R (1987) Comparative study of safety and effectiveness of nitrendipine, atenolol and hydrochlorothiazide in combination in the treatment of hypertension. J Cardiovasc Pharmacol 9 (Suppl IV): IV-S232–S237
29. Singer DRJ, Markandu ND, Shore AC, Mac Gregor GA (1987) Nifedipine and acebutolol in combination for the treatment of moderate to severe essential hypertension. J Hypertens 1: 31–37
30. Brouwer RML, Follath F, Buhler FR (1985) Review of the cardiovascular adversity of the calcium antagonist beta-blocker combination: implications for antihypertensive therapy. J Cardiovasc Pharmacol 7 (Suppl IV): IV-S38–S44
31. Hutchison SJ, Lorimer AR, Lakhdar A, McAlpine SG (1984) Beta-blockers and verapamil:

a cautionary tale. Br Med J 289: 659–660
32. Jennings AA, Jee LD, Smith JJ, Commerford PJ, Opie LH (1986) Acute effects of nifedipine on blood pressure and left ventricular ejection fraction in severely hypertensive outpatients: predictive effects of acute therapy and prolonged efficacy when added to existing therapy. Am Heart J 111: 557–563
33. Anastassiades CJ (1980) Nifedipine and beta-blocking drugs. Br Med J 281: 1251–1252
34. Opie EH, White DA (1980) Adverse interactions between nifedipine and beta-blockers. Br Med J 281: 1462
35. Robson RH, Viswanath MC (1982) Nifedipine and beta-blockade as a cause of cardiac failure. Br Med J 284: 104
36. Christensen CK, Pedersen OL, Mikkelsen E (1982) Renal effects of acute calcium blokade with nifedipine in hypertensive patients receiving beta-adrenoceptor-blocking drugs. Clin Pharmacol Ther 32: 572–576
37. Mroczek WJ, Burris JF, Allenby KS (1988) Nitrendipine in severe hypertension. Hypertension 11 (Suppl I): I-225–228
38. Leonetti G (on behalf of the participants) (1987) Antihypertensive efficacy of nicardipine, in monotherapy and association, in mild or moderate hypertensives with and without concomitant disease: interim report of Italian multicenter studies. J Hypertens 5 (Suppl V): V-S575–S577
39. Blaustein MP (1977) Sodium ions, calcium ions, blood pressure regulation and hypertension: a reassessment and a hypothesis. Am J Physiol 232: C165–C173
40. Resnick LM, Nicholson JP, Laragh JH (1985) Calcium metabolism and the renin angiotensin system in essential hypertension. J Cardiovasc Pharmacol 7: S187–S193
41. Leonetti G, Rupoli L., Sangiorgio P, Grandik R, Cuspidi C, Bolla G, Zanchetti A (1987) Effects of different sodium intakes on the antihypertensive and renal effects of single oral doses of nifedipine in hypertensive patients. J Cardiovasc Pharmacol 10 (Suppl X): X-S138–S139
42. Cappuccio EP, Markandu N, MacGregor GA (1987) Calcium antagonists and sodium balance: effects of changes in sodium intake and of the addition of a thiazide diuretic on the blood pressure lowering effect of nifedipine. J Cardiovasc Pharmacol 10 (Suppl X): X-S57–S60

Discussion

Omae (Osaka): What is your explanation for sodium restrictions having an additive effect to the antihypertensive effect of nifedipine, but diuretics not necessarily doing so. It is controversial. What is your explanation for that?

Leonetti (Milan): I think the explanation is that the antihypertensive effects of nifedipine and all the other dihydropyridine derivatives are not mediated through any effect on the sodium balance. It is an effect independent from the sodium balance. This may explain why we still had a reduction when the sodium state was really reduced.

Omae: I see. Frequently we use some thiazide diuretics plus calcium antagonists, but we thought that diuretics were more important in losing sodium than that. The calcium antagonists also show some diuretic action, but thiazide has a stronger diuretic action. So, we not infrequently combine both, thinking we can expect some additive effect.

Leonetti: Well, as I have shown, when you go through the literature and look at the effect of the studies which were specifically designed to investigate if there was an additive effect from this combination, I have found 4 positive and 4 negative results. What I am suggesting is that, in connection with what I have told you before, the antihypertensive effect, either of a calcium antagonist or the long-term effect of a diuretic, is independent from the effect on the sodium balance. You know we have shown many years ago, when I was still a medical student, that the total body sodium reduction caused by diuretics is limited in time. If you check either plasma volume and total body sodium after 4–8 weeks of diuretic treatment, you do not see any reduction in total body sodium and plasma volume. So, it is just a short-term effect.

Omae: Thank you.

Leonetti: You're welcome.

Ogihara (Osaka): Any questions?

Ogihara: Dr. Leonetti, what do you think are the most useful combination drugs with a calcium antagonist in treating elderly hypertension in general?

Leonetti: Well, as I said, there was no specific study which was concerned with the effect of the combination of a calcium antagonist with other drugs in the elderly. But, because I believe that there is an additive effect between calcium antagonists and diuretics, I think that may be a good association. At the same time, I do not have anything against the combination of a converting enzyme inhibitor and a calcium antagonist; because as we have just heard, they are both indicated in the elderly patient. So, from the pharmaco-dynamic and pharmacokinetic point of view, I think that the calcium antagonist and a converting enzyme inhibitor or the calcium antagonist and a diuretic would be a good combination for the treatment of hypertension in the elderly.

Marchetta (Bologna): What do you think about the possible improvement of the cardioprotective effect of beta-blocker therapy by combination with nifedipine or calcium antagonist? Beta-blockers, of course, are not contraindicated in low doses in the elderly.

Leonetti: Well, unfortunately, at present we know nothing about the cardio-protective effect of both a calcium antagonist and a converting enzyme inhibitor. So, if we can guess from what we have found up to now concerning the regression of left ventricle hypertrophy, the metabolic effects, I think that we could hopes; but hope is not enough for scientific research. Any comments from the audience? Well, I do not have any public opinion; I call tell you in private.

Onrot (Vancouver): I would suggest from your last slide that the addition of nife-dipine to salt restriction is not of benefit. It seemed to me that the benefit was derived in 2 patients whose blood pressure remained high after salt restriction and then had a lowering after the nifedipine. In the 4 patients whose blood pressure was somewhat lower during the salt restriction, there was no additional benefit from the nifedipine. So, I think it would only follow if you had a benefit from salt restriction. There is not much more to be expected from nifedipine. If you have no benefit from salt restriction, then there is not much point in continuing on with salt restriction.

Leonetti: Well, I think it is a general assumption, and I agree completely — when you have a lowered blood pressure, at a certain level, it is almost impossible to further reduce blood pressure, because the counteracting mechanisms are very effective. The last slide, unfortunately, was not mine but was MacGregor's slide, So, I get your point and I agree with you.

Ogirhara: OK, last question, please.

Jannetti (Genova): What about the combination of 2 calcium antagonists in treatment of hypertension — 2 different kinds of calcium antagonists? I usually treat angina with 2 calcium antagonists, for example diltiazem and nifedipine, to counteract the sympathetic activity provoked by nifedipine. What do you think about this possibility?

Leonetti: Well, I do not have any personal experience with the combination of 2 calcium antagonists, and from what I know from the literature, I have found no study on this combination. Perhaps, Dr. Lund-Johansen, can you help me? No, he could not. Well, I think there might perhaps be, in some patients, an additive effect This is just a hypothetical point. Certainly before claiming that 2 different calcium antagonists can be additive in antihypertensive treatment, we should make a very complex Latin square, double-blind, and long-term study. Certainly they have something different at the cellular level. If this is also reflected in the hemodynamic effect, I cannot say. Perhaps angina patients are different from hypertensive patients.

Posters

Prevalence, Treatment, and Control of Hypertension in the Elderly: Study on Blood Pressure in Elderly Outpatients (SPAA)

Emanuela Taioli[1], Claudio Alli[1], Fausto Avanzini[1], Giuseppe Bettelli[1], Fabio Colombo[1], Rocco Corso[1], Maria Angelica Devoto[1], Marco Di Tullio[1], Roberto Marchioli[1], Giancarlo Mariotti[2], Maria Radice[2], Gianni Tognoni[1], Massimo Villella[1], Alessandro Zussino[1], and the participating doctors of the "Gruppo di studio sulla pressione arteriosa nell' anziano"*

Summary. The prevalence, quality of care, and degree of control of arterial hypertension have been studied in 3858 elderly outpatients (mean age 72.7 ± 4.9 years) randomly recruited from the practice of 444 general practitioners. Hypertension (defined either as blood pressure [BP] ≥ 160 and/or 90 mmHg and/or the presence of antihypertensive treatment) was found in 67.8% of the screened cohort, with a higher prevalence in females than males (73.1% vs 61.0%) and in the older age group (71.1% in those over 80 years vs 64.8% in the 65–69-year group). The hypertensive status was unknown to both the doctors and the patients in 21.4% of cases. Over 90% of the known hypertensives were on treatment with no age-or sex-related differences, but less than 30% of them had BP $< 160/90$ mmHg. One drug was prescribed to 50.2% of treated patients, only 5.5% were receiving three or more drugs. Low-dosage treatment schedules were frequently used, often associated with non-daily drug administration. Despite the high proportion of subjects on treatment, hypertension in the elderly we studied seemed to be poorly controlled. The study also documents the need for a more rational approach to detection and control of hypertension in this age group, for whom clearly defined recommendations or criteria are lacking.

Key words: Elderly — Blood pressure — Hypertension — Treatment status — Control of blood pressure

Introduction

People over 65 years are an increasing proportion of the population in Western countries; this undoubtly amplifies the need for health care, resulting in an ever increasing expense. Although hypertension is common in the elderly, a lot of problems remain. For example, the influence of BP on survival and quality of life in this age group is still uncertain [2, 3], leading to a lack of clear guidelines for drug treatment [4, 5]. Data are scant and have usually been derived from studies not specifically designed to assess the prevalence and prognostic significance of hypertension or the benefit/risk profile for pharmacological treatment in elderly patients, who are usually only a subgroup of the studied population.

---

[1] Istituto di Ricerche Farmacologiche "Mario Negri", Milano, Italy
[2] Istituto di Scienze Biomediche Bassini, Università di Milano, Italy
* The names of the 444 participating doctors were published in [1]

The aim of our study was to evaluate the prevalence and natural history of hypertension in an elderly population, selected a group of Italian general practitioners (GP), in order to highlight the main problems arising in relation to hypertension in general practice. This could provide useful information for planning further ad hoc studies.

Patients and Methods

The study protocol and organization have been described elsewhere [6]. A total of 444 self-selected GP from all over Italy each agreed to recruit a random sample of 10 patients aged 65 years or more from their practice. The resulting population consisted of 3858 subjects (1678 males, 2180 females), mean age 72.7 ± 4.9 years (range 65–91 years). The baseline clinical assessment was the result of two visits, one week apart, in 1983. At each visit blood pressure was recorded after 5 min in supine position. Details of antihypertensive treatment were taken. Subjects were defined as hypertensive if they had systolic blood pressure (SBP) ≥ 160 mmHg and/or diastolic blood pressure (DBP) ≥ 90 mmHg (average of the measurements at the two first visits) or if they were receiving antihypertensive therapy.

Results

Prevalence, Treatment, and Control of Hypertension

Hypertension was found in 67.8% of the screened cohort, with a higher prevalence in females than males (73.1% vs 61.0%) and rising with age (from 64.8% in the 65–69-year group to 71.1% in those over 80 years). Figure 1 illustrates the frequency distribution of the whole study population according to BP categories, awareness of hypertension, and treatment status. In 557 patients (21.3% of the 2616 hypertensives), the hypertension was unknown to the patient and GP. Regardless of medication status, almost half of the hypertensive cases (46.1%) were mild, 6.7% were moderate or severe, and 26.6% had an isolated systolic hypertension.

More than 90% of known hypertensives were on treatment, but less than one third of the treated subjects (28.9%) had their blood pressure well controlled.

Characteristics of Antihypertensive Treatment

Among the 2059 treated subjects, 50.2% were taking one drug, 44.3% were taking two, and 5.5% more than two drugs. Diuretics were the most frequent single-drug therapy (Table 1) and the main drugs of multi-drug therapies. The most widely prescribed association of two substances was a diuretic plus a centrally acting agent; three active substances were mostly: a diuretic, an adrenergic neuron blocker, and a direct arteriolar vasodilator. Low-dosage treatment schedules were frequently used, especially for diuretics, often in association with non-daily drug administration.

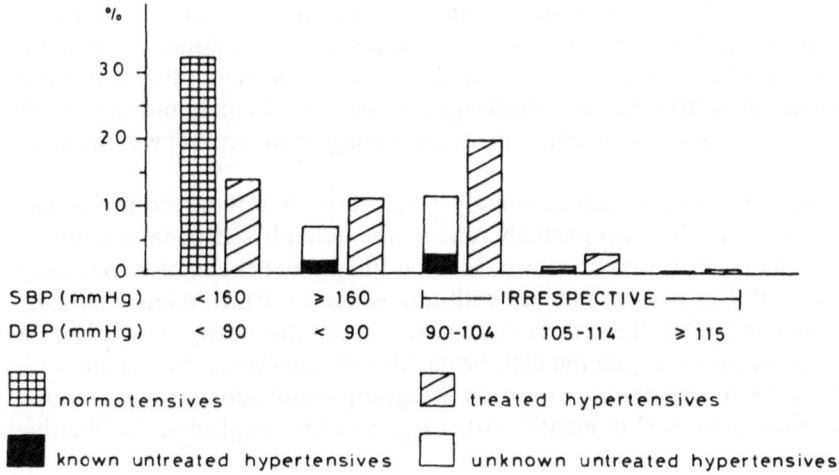

Fig. 1. Distribution of whole population in relation to systolic (*SBP*) and diastolic (*L'BP*) blood pressures, awareness of hypertension, and treatment status

Table 1. Distribution of drugs taken by treated hypertensives

Therapeutic classes	Treated patients (%) ($n = 1865$)
Diuretics	85.5
Centrally acting agents	32.0
Adrenergic neuron blockers	19.5
Beta-blockers	10.5
Direct arteriolar vasodilators	3.4
Alpha-blockers	2.1
ACE inhibitors	1.8
Ca channel blockers	1.5

Discussion

The prevalence of hypertension observed in the SPAA is higher than in other studies [7-11], even after adjustment for diagnostic criteria used. One possible explanation of this excess prevalence is that our cases were elderly outpatients, which probably resulted in subjects being specifically selected, as some of them would have contacted their physician because of their high blood pressure.

A particularly high proportion of subjects were known hypertensives, and a high percentage were already receiving antihypertensive treatment, in accordance with other recent studies [10, 11]. This tendency to treat geriatric hypertension is typical of the industrialized countries. It is also a clear example of how clinical practice does not always apply research findings, as we still lack definite proof of the utility of treating mild diastolic and isolated systolic hypertension in the elderly.

The type and distribution frequency of drugs included in treatment schedules needs some comment. It is likely that the qualification of hypertension as a chronic and unchangeable condition is the basis for the wide use of "old" drugs: present treatments reflect the carry-over from prescriptions issued in the past and continued without readjustment or reassessment – the drugs having proved free of troublesome side effects.

Furthermore, there is a tendency to employ lower doses than those recommended in the early 1980's [12, 13]. This partially reflects the care physicians take to minimize iatrogenic damage. It may, however, also be the manifestation of uncertainty and of a passive attitude of doctors faced with a question for which there is no concrete answer. In conclusion, the control of hypertension in the elderly population we studied seems to be poor, despite the high proportion of subjects on treatment. The lack of clear guidelines for treatment in this age group could substantially account for this, underlining the need to identify criteria particularly applied to the elderly.

Acknowledgements. The work was supported by a grant from the National Council of Research (CNR) for the development of Clinical Pharmacology and the generous contributions of the Italian Federation of Physicians (FNOM) and of the Fondazione Angelo and Angela Valenti, Milan, Italy. We warmly thank Miss Angela Palumbo for data input and management and Mrs. Teresa Nigro and Mrs. Lorena Guzzetti for secretarial assistance. Language-editing was kindly done by J. Baggot. Dr. Roberto Marchioli was the recipient of a fellowship from the Centro di Formazione e Studi per il Mezzogiorno-Formez (Progetto Speciale "Ricerca Scientifica Applicata nel Mezzogiorno").

References

1. Avanzini F, Alli C, Andreani A, Colombo F, Conforti L, Di Tullio M, Mariotti G, Pirone F, Radice M, Spagnoli A, Taioli E, Tognoni G, Tundo G, Villella M, Zussino A (1984) SPAA: studio sulla pressione arteriosa in pazienti anziani ambulatoriali. The Practitioner (Edizione Italiana) 75: 74-83
2. Kannel WB, Gordon T (1978) Evaluation of cardiovascular risk in the elderly: the Framingham Study. Bull, NY Acad Med 54: 573-91
3. Mattila K, Haavisto M, Rajala S, Heikinheimo R (1988) Blood pressure and five year survival in the very old. Br Med J 296: 887-9
4. The Joint National Committee on Detection, Evaluation, and Treatment of High Blood Pressure (1984) The 1984 Report of the Joint National Committee on Detection, Evaluation, and Treatment of High Blood Pressure. Arch Intern Med 144: 1045-57
5. Larochelle P, Bass MJ, Birkett NJ, De Champlain J, Myers MG (1986) Recommendations from the Consensus Conference on Hypertension in the Elderly. CMAJ 135: 741-5
6. Avanzini F, Alli C, Bettelli G, Colombo F, Conforti L, Di Tullio M, Mariotti G, Pirone F, Radice M, Spagnoli A, Taioli E, Tognoni G, Villella M, Zussino A (1987) Feasibility of a large prospective study in general practice: an Italian experience. Br Med J 294: 157-60
7. Garland C, Barrett-Connor E, Suarez L, Criqui MH (1983) Isolated systolic hypertension and mortality after age 60 years. Am J Epidemiol 118: 365-76
8. Curb JD, Borhani NO, Schnaper H, Kass E, Entwisle G, Williams W, Berman R (1985) Detection and treatment of hypertension in older individuals. Am J Epidemiol 121: 371-6
9. Stamler J, Stamler R, Riedlinger WF, Algera G, Roberts RH (1976) Hypertension

screening of 1 million Americans. Community hypertension evaluation clinic (CHEC) program, 1973 through 1975 JAMA 235: 2299-306

10. Hale WE, Marks RG, Stewart RB (1981) Screening for hypertension in an elderly population: report from the Dunedin program. J Am Geriatr Soc 29: 123-5

11. Subcommittee on definition and prevalence of the 1984 Joint National Committee (1985) Hypertension prevalence and the status of awareness, treatment, and control in the United States. Final report. Hypertension 7: 457-68

12. Williams SH, Jagger Pl, Braunwald E (1980) Hypertensive vascular disease. In: Isselbacher KJ, Adams RD, Braunwald E, Petersdorf RG, Wilson JD (eds) 9 Edition McGraw Hill, New York, pp 1167-1178

13. The Joint National Committee on Detection, Evaluation, and Treatment of High Blood Pressure (1980) The 1980 report of the The Joint National Committee on Detection, Evaluation, and Treatment of High Blood Pressure. Arch Intern Med 140: 1280-5

Comparison of Cardiovascular Regulatory Functions in Elderly Hypertensive Patients and Normal Elderly Subjects

Akiko Kawamoto[1], Kazuyuki Shimada[1], Kozo Matsubayashi[1], Taishiro Chikamori[1], Osamu Kuzume[1], Hiroshi Ishida[1], Hisakazu Ogura[2], and Toshio Ozawa[1]

Summary. In order to dissociate the effects of an elevated blood pressure on cardiovascular regulatory functions from those of aging in elderly hypertension, resting hemodynamic and circulatory autonomic functions of 30 elderly hypertensive patients were compared with those of 30 healthy, age-matched, normotensive volunteers with mean age of 65 years. The hypertensives showed significantly lower cardiac index and higher total peripheral resistance. β-receptor and baroreflex sensitivity indices were only marginally reduced in hypertensives as compared to normotensives, while the variability of the resting heart rate as an index of cardiac parasympathetic control did not differ between the two groups. Plasma renin activity, but not plasma aldosterone, was significantly decreased in the hypertensives. Group results showed plasma norepinephrine level inversely related to resting mean blood pressure ($r = -0.31$, $P < 0.05$). Thus, it is unlikely that either sympathetic nervous system or renin-angiotensin system is responsible for the increase in peripheral resistance in elderly hypertension. Furthermore, high blood pressure has a very limited influence on circulatory regulatory functions, which in the older subjects have already been substantially altered by age.

Key words: Elderly hypertension — Autonomic nervous system — Hemodynamics — Aging — Blood pressure

Introduction

There is relatively little information about the pathophysiologic state of the cardiovascular system in hypertension of the elderly, whose cardiovascular autonomic regulatory functions have been altered by both advancing age and high arterial blood pressure [1]. Age is well known to be associated with a progressive reduction in β-adrenoceptor responsiveness [2], baroreflex sensitivity [3], and parasympathetic control of heart rate [4] in normotensive subjects. The inhibitory effects of hypertension on these autonomic functions have also been well described, mainly in middle-aged or younger patients [2-4]. Still, little is known about how an elevated blood pressure per se affects the cardiovascular system in the elderly, which has already been altered by another important modulating factor — age. The present study,

Department of Medicine and Geriatrics[1] and Department of Medical Information[2], Kochi Medical School, Kochi, Japan

undertaken to answer this question, compares hemodynamic and cardiovascular autonomic parameters in elderly hypertensive patients with those in elderly normotensive controls who had undergone extensive health-screening tests.

Methods

Subjects

The study population consisted of 30 hypertensive patients (21 men and 9 women) aged 56–76 years, and 30 male normotensive subjects aged 58–77 years. All hypertensive patients had diastolic pressure ≥ 90 mmHg and/or systolic pressure ≥ 160 mmHg on two separate visits to the clinic (without medication) and were at WHO stages I or II. All normotensive subjects were volunteers recruited from the community and maintained moderate levels of daily physical activity. The results of physical and laboratory examinations, including maximal exercise tests, were normal.

Study Protocol

Twenty-four hour blood pressure monitoring: Indirect ambulatory blood pressure was recorded at 10 min intervals by using a finger volume-oscillometric device BP-100 (ME-Commercial, Tokyo, Japan) [5].

Hemodynamics and autonomic function tests: Following 30 min supine rest in the morning after an overnight fast, blood was sampled to determine plasma norepinephrine level [6], plasma renin activity, and plasma aldosterone. Cardiac index was measured by cuvette dye dilution methods. As an index of parasympathetic heart rate control, coefficient variation of RR intervals (CV) was obtained from 100 heart beats at rest with Autonomic R100 (ME-Commercial) [7]. Baroreflex sensitivity was measured by the change in RR intervals per unit change in systolic blood pressure during phases II and IV of the Valsalva maneuver [6,8]. Isoproterenol hydrochloride sensitivity was measured from dose/response curves to rapid intravenous injection as the dose required to increase the heart rate by 25 beats/min [9].

Results

Clinical Findings

Age, body height, weight, and body surface area were similar in both elderly groups. The hypertensive group showed significantly higher blood pressure levels than the normotensive group, not only at the clinic ($162 \pm 3/96 \pm 1$ vs $126 \pm 2/80 \pm 1$ mmHg, $P < 0.001$), but also in the mean of blood pressure measurments taken at 10 min intervals during 24 h ambulatory monitoring ($143 \pm 4/91 \pm 3$ vs $116 \pm 2/75 \pm 2$ mmHg, $P < 0.001$). Heart rate and the standard deviations of blood pressure and heart rate in the ambulatory recording were similar.

Table 1. Comparison of hemodynamics and cardiovascular regulatory functions

	Normotensives (n = 30)	Hypertensives (n = 30)	Unit
Cardiac index	2.8 ± 0.1	2.4 ± 0.1*	liters per min/M^2
TPRI	2716.5 ± 131.8	3793.2 ± 198.0***	dynes · sec · cm^{-5} · M^2
CD$_{25}$/BS	1.5 ± 0.2	1.9 ± 0.2$^+$	μg/M^2
BRSI-II	2.8 ± 0.6	1.5 ± 0.3**	ms/mmHg
BRSI-IV	2.1 ± 0.3	2.7 ± 0.4	ms/mmHg
CV	2.8 ± 0.2	2.7 ± 0.2	%
PNE	219.8 ± 15.9	186.6 ± 13.5	pg/ml
PRA	1.00 ± 0.17	0.56 ± 0.10*	ng/ml per hour
ALD	72.0 ± 4.1	67.8 ± 7.2	pg/ml
UNa	8.6 ± 0.6	8.4 ± 0.8	g/day

TPRI, total peripheral resistance index; CD$_{25}$/BS, chronotropic dose of isoproterenol to increase heart rate by 25 beats/min, corrected by body surface area; BRSI-II and –IV, baroreflex sensitivity index during phase II and IV of the Valsalva maneuver; CV, coefficient variation of resting heart rate; PNE, plasma norepinephrine; PRA, plasma renin activity; ALD, plasma aldosterone; UNa, urinary sodium
$^+P = 0.055$, $*P < 0.05$, $**P < 0.01$, $***P < 0.001$ (by Mann-Whitney test)

Hemodynamic Findings

Results are summarized in Table 1. Cardiac index was significantly lower by approximately 15% in hypertensives than in normotensives, while total peripheral resistance index (TPRI) was significantly higher (approximately 40%) in the hypertensive group.

Autonomic Functions

Chronotropic dose of isoproterenol corrected for body surface area (CD$_{25}$/BS) was slightly, but significantly larger, and baroreflex sensitivity index derived from phase II of the Valsalva maneuver (BRSI-II) also slightly, but significantly less, in the hypertensive group than each in the normotensive group. These statistical significances were apparent in the nonparametric Mann-Whitney test but not evident in the less sensitive Student's t-test. Neither variability of resting heart rate (CV), baroreflex sensitivity index from phase IV of the Valsalva maneuver (BRSI-IV), nor plasma norepinephrine level (PNE) were significantly different between the two groups. However, group analysis showed a significant inverse relationship of plasma norepinephrine level to resting mean blood pressure ($r = -0.31$, $P < 0.05$).

Renin-Aldosterone System

Plasma renin activity (PRA) was significantly lower in the hypertensive group, while plasma aldosterone (ALD) was similar in the two groups. Both groups excreted a similar amount of urinary sodium (UNa) during a 24-h period.

Discussion

Our hemodynamic data are consistent with the previous findings of Terasawa et al. [10], who reported that the hemodynamic pattern of elderly hypertension is of the low output and high peripheral resistance type. The exact mechanisms contributing to these hemodynamic characteristics are currently unknown. Plasma norepinephrine and renin activity tended to be depressed in hypertensives in comparison with normotensives under similar sodium intakes, indicating that neither sympathetic nervous system nor renin-angiotensin system is likely responsible for the increased peripheral resistence in elderly hypertension.

Our study emphasized the subtlety of changes in cardiovascular autonomic functions in the elderly patients with mild essential hypertension in comparison with the elderly normotensives. Thus, β-receptor and baroreceptor reflex sensitivities were only marginally depressed in the hypertensive patients, and the variability of resting heart rate did not differ between hypertensive and normotensive groups. These results suggest that high blood pressure, though an important modulating factor in the younger subjects [2-4], has a very limited, if any, influence on the cardiovascular regulatory functions in the older subjects whose autonomic functions have already been substantially altered by advancing age.

References

1. Franklin SS (1983) Geriatric hypertension. Med Clin North Am 67: 395-417
2. Bertel O, Buhler FR, Kiowski W, Lutold BE (1980) Decreased beta-adrenoceptor responsiveness as related to age, blood pressure, and plasma catecholamines in patients with essential hypertension. Hypertension 2: 130-138
3. Gribbin B, Pickering G, Sleight P, Peto R (1971) Effect of age and high blood pressure on baroreflex sensitivity in man. Circ Res 29: 424-431
4. Alicandri C, Boni E, Fariello R, Zanielli A, Minotti F, Cantalamessa A, Muiesan G(1987) Parasympathetic control of heart rate and age in essential hypertensive patients. J Hypertens 5 (Suppl V): 345-347
5. Imai Y, Nihei M, Abe K, Sasaki S, Minami N, Munakata M, Yumita S, Onoda Y, Sekino H, Yamakoshi K, Yoshinaga K (1987) A finger volume-oscillometric device for monitoring ambulatory blood pressure: Laboratory and clinical evaluations. Clin Exper Hypertens 9: A2001-A2025
6. Shimada K, Kitazumi T, Sadakane N, Ogura H, Ozawa T (1985) Age-related changes of baroreflex function, plasma norepinephrine, and blood pressure. Hypertension 7: 113-117
7. Kageyama S, Mochio S, Taniguchi I, Abe M (1981) A proposal of a quantitative autonomic function test. Jikeikai Med J 28: 81-85
8. Goldstein DS, Horwitz D, Keiser HR (1982) Comparison of techniques for measuring baroreflex sensitivity in man. Circulation 66: 432-439
9. Cleaveland CR, Rangno RE, Shand DG (1972) A standardized isoproterenol sensitivity test; The effects of sinus arrhythmia, atropin, and propranolol. Arch Intern Med 130: 47-52
10. Terasawa F, Kuramoto K, Hon Ying L, Suzuki T, Kuramochi M (1972) The study on the hemodynamics in old hypertensive subjects. Acta Gerontol Jpn 56: 47-55

Role of Dipyridamole-Echocardiography Tests in the Diagnosis of Coronary Artery Disease in Hypertensives

Fabio Lattanzi[1], Alessandra Renata Lucarini[2], Eugenio Picano[1], Silva Severi[1], Enrico Orsini[1], Alessandro Distante[1], Antonio Salvetti[2], and Antonio L'Abbate[1]

Summary. In hypertensive patients, the exercise-electrocardiography test shows limited feasibility and diagnostic accuracy for the noninvasive detection of coronary artery disease (CAD). Recently, the dipyridamole-echocardiograpy test (2-dimensional echo monitoring with a dipyridamole infusion of up to 0.84 mg/kg over 10 min) has been proposed as an exercise independent method for the diagnosis of CAD. In order to establish the relative diagnostic usefulness of the exercise-electrocardiography test (EET) and the dipyridamole-echocardiography test (DET) in the detection of CAD, the 2 tests were performed consecutively in 114 inpatients with a chest-pain syndrome and essential hypertension. Forty patients had previous myocardial infarction. Criteria of positivity were: for EET, a horizontal or downsloping ST segment shift > 0.1 mV; and for DET, a transient dyssynergy of contraction.
  Coronary angiography showed significant CAD ($> 70\%$ lumen reduction of at least 1 major coronary vessel) in 84 patients. Sensitivity was 68% for EET and 77% for DET ($P = $ ns); specificity was 52% for EET and 90% for DET ($P < 0.05$). Thus, DET test appears to be of greater diagnostic value than EET in the noninvasive detection of CAD in hypertensives with a chest-pain syndrome.

Key words: Coronary artery disease (CAD) — Hypertension — Dipyridamole — Echocardiography

Introduction

As an exercise independent method of detecting coronary artery disease (CAD), dipyridamole stress is gaining popularity [1–4].

In particular, with the high dose dipyridamole-echocardiography test (DET) [2], the diagnostic end point is represented by a transient dyssynergy of contraction, a marker of myocardial ischemia much more specific than ST segment changes on ECG. This mechanical market of ischemia is not affected by factors like arterial hypertension and/or left ventricular hypertrophy and old myocardial infarction, which reduce the diagnostic usefulness of the exercise-electrocardiography stress test (EET) and the dipyridamole-electrocardiography test [5]. Furthermore, DET does not require the ability to exercise and does not induce a significant hypertensive reaction (but rather a mild hypotension).

Istituto di Fisiologia Clinica del C.N.R. and Patologia Medica[1] and Clinica Medica I[2], Universita' di Pisa, Pisa, Italy

The aim of this study was therefore to evaluate the relative diagnostic accuracy of DET vs EET in the diagnosis of angiographically assessed CAD in essential hypertensives with a chest-pain syndrome and/or previous myocardial infarction.

Materials and Methods

Selection of Patients

From August 1985 to April 1988, 114 patients (79 male, 35 female, mean age 54 ± 10) with essential arterial hypertension (diastolic blood pressre > 95 mmHg) and chest-pain syndrome were referred to our institution. We excluded patients with: (1) cardiac failure; (2) congenital or valvular heart disease; (3) documented cardiomyopathy; (4) bundle-branch blocks; (5) poor acoustic window; or (6) inability to exercise. All patients performed EET and DET on different days and in random order.

Exercise-Electrocardiography Test

All patients performed a multistage, upright bicycle ergometer test, with an initial load of 25 W and subsequent increments of 25 W every 2 min. A 12 lead electrocardiogram and blood pressure determination were performed at baseline and thereafter every min. Criteria for interrupting the test were severe chest pain, diagnostic ST segment shift, fatigue, excessive blood pressure rise (systolic blood pressure greater than 280 mmHg, diastolic blood pressure greater than 140 mmHg), limiting dyspnea, or maximal predicted heart rate in absence of ischemia.

Electrocardiographic tracing was considered diagnostic for myocardial ischemia when there was an ST segment shift of at least 0.10 mV, 0.08 after the J point compared with the baseline.

Dipyridamole-Echocardiography Test

Two-dimensional echocardiographic and 12-lead electrocardiographic monitoring were performed in combination with a dipyridamole infusion [2]: 0.56 mg/kg over 4 min followed by 4 min of no dose and then 0.28 mg/kg in 2 min. The cumulative dose was therefore 0.84 mg/kg over 10 min. Aminophylline (240 mg), which promptly reverses the effects of dipyridamole, was readily at hand (Fig. 1).

During the procedure, the blood pressure and the electrocardiogram were recorded each min. The electrocardiographic criteria for ischemia during this test were the same as during the exercise stress test. Two-dimensional echocardiograms were continuously recorded during and up to 20 min after dipyridamole administration. A commercially available wide-angle, phased-array imaging system (Hewlett Packard Mod. 77020, 2.5 and 3.5 MHz transducers) was used. In the baseline studies, all standard echocardiographic views were obtained when possible. During the test, new areas of abnormal wall motion were identified on multiple views of rapidly moving

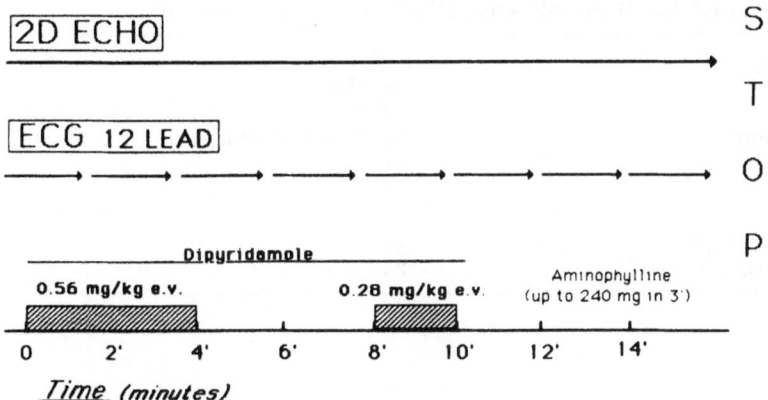

Fig. 1. Schematic representation of the study protocol of high-dose dipyridamole-echocardiography test

the ultrasound transducer through various positions. After an optimal position for the observation of abnormal wall motion was established, the transducer was held stationary throughout the remainder of the study and the recovery period.

Segmental anatomy and wall motion were assessed in a qualitative manner as previouly reported [1, 2]. Wall motion was graded as hyperkinetic, normal, hypokinetic, akinetic or dyskinetic. The grading of the dyssynergy as well as the regional localization of the dyssynergy were reached by consensus between the 2 observers. Positivity of the test was linked to detection of a transient dyssynergy of contraction or worsening of baseline dyssynergy.

Angiographic Study

Patients underwent biplanar left ventriculography and selective right and left coronary arteriography, using either the Judkins or the Sones technique. Multiple views of each coronary artery were obtained, including craniocaudal views. A vessel was considered to have significant obstruction if its diameter was narrowed by 70% or more with respect to the pre-stenotic tract. Two independent observers, blind to the results of both EET and DET, analyzed the coronary angiograms.

Statistical Analysis

Differences between the results of EET and DET were compared using the chi-squared test; a Fisher exact test was utilized when appropriate. A P value < 0.05 was considered statistically significant. For both tests; sensitivity, specificity, accuracy, and predictive value of positive and negative tests in detecting angiographically assessed CAD were calculated according to standard definitions.

Table 1. Clinical characteristics of patients who performed both provocative tests

Number of patients	114
Mean age (years)	54 ± 10
Sex (M/F)	79/35
Arterial blood pressure	Diastolic > 95 mmHg
Diabetics	11
Smokers	82
Hyperlipemia	32
Left ventricular hypertrophy	41
Coronary artery disease	84

Results

Clinical Characteristics

Forty-one patients had echocardiographic evidence of left ventricular hypertrophy; 22 of them had electrocardiographic left ventricular hypertrophy, and 8 also had resting ST and T wave repolarization changes. Other clinical characteristics of the study patients are shown in Table 1. Twenty-nine patients performed the tests under antihypertensive therapy (angiotensin-converting enzyme-inhibitors, diuretics, beta-blockers, and/or calcium-antagonists).

Comparison with Angiographic Findings

At coronary angiography, 30 patients had nonsignificant and 84 significant CAD: 31 of these had single, 33 had double, 20 had triple vessel disease. In the subgroup of 74 patients without previous myocardial infarction, significant CAD was present in 45. DET showed a specificity of 27/30, EET of 16/30 (90% vs 52%, $P < 0.05$) (Fig. 2). The sensitivity was 65/84 for DET, and 57/84 for EET (77% vs 68%, $P =$ ns) (Fig. 2).

Of the 68 patients with positive DET, 28 has regional hypokinesia, 32 akinesia, and 8 dyskinesia after dipyridamole administration. The transient dyssynergy mainly involved the septum in 27, anterolateral wall in 13, inferoposterior wall in 15, and apex in 13 patients. Of the 36 patients with previous myocardial infarction and baseline ventricular dyssynergy, 22 showed a worsening of the basal dyssynergy, and 14 developed a new dyssynergy. All the patients of this last group had a multi-vessel coronary disease. Except for the 3 false-positives, in all cases there was a good correspondence between the location of the transiently dyssynergic region and the presence of significant stenosis in the coronary artery feeding that region. In all cases, the dyssynergy was promptly reversed (usually within 2 min) by aminophylline infusion.

The accuracy was 79% for DEET and 60% for EET ($P < 0.05$); the predictive value of a positive test was 96% for DET and 79% for EET ($P < 0.05$); and the predictive value of a negative test was 58% for DET and 34% for EET ($P < 0.05$) (Fig. 2).

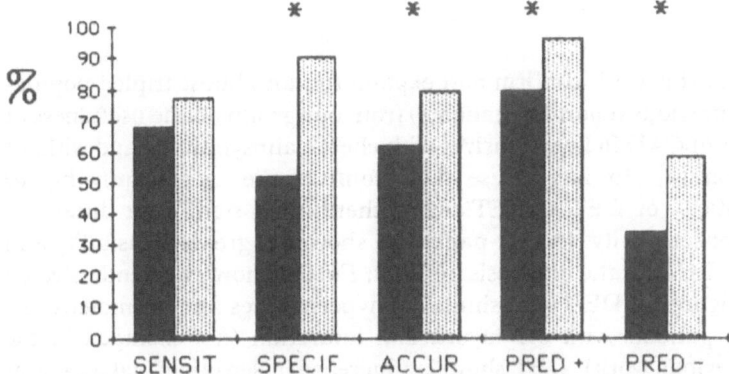

Fig. 2. Histograms representing the relative sensitivity (*SENSIT*), specificity (*SPECIF*), accuracy (*ACCUR*), and the predictive value of positive (*PRED +*) and of negative (*PRED −*) tests of EET (dark columns) and of DET (light columns) for the diagnosis of CAD in hypertensives (* *P* < 0.05)

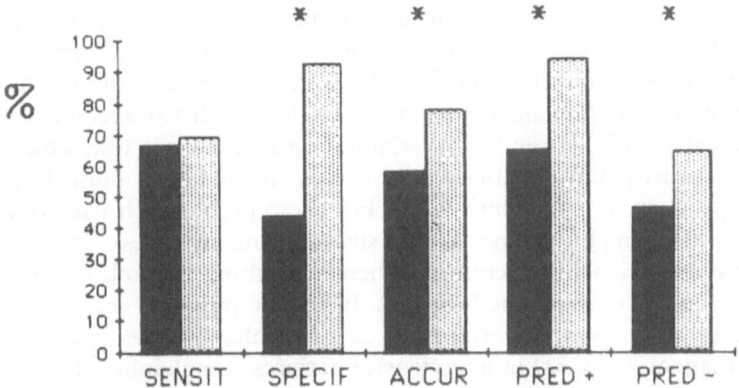

Fig. 3. Histograms representing results of tests in hypertensive patients without previous myocardial infarction (compare Fig. 2).

Chest pain during dipyridamole test occurred in 52 patients: 30 had CAD, 22 had no CAD. Of these 22 patients without CAD, 15 also had ECG evidence of ischemia during dipyridamole. Of these last 15 patients, 8 had echocardiographic evidence of left ventricular hypertrophy.

Considering only the 74 patients without previous myocardial infarction, the sensitivity for DET and EET was 31/45 and 30/45, (69 vs 67%, *P* = ns), respectively while specificity was 27/29 and 13/29 (93% vs 44%, *P* < 0.05). The accuracy was 78% and 58% (*P* < 0.05); the predictive value of positive tests was 94% and 65% (*P* < 0.05); and the predictive value of negative tests was 64% and 46% (*P* < 0.05) for DET and EET, respectively (Fig. 3).

Discussion

The data presented in this work confirm and expand (on an almost tripled population) the results of a previous report (43 patients) from our group on the usefulness of DET in the diagnosis of CAD in hypertensives with chest-pain syndrome and without myocardial infarction [4]. In fact, these data confirm the significantly higher feasibility and specificity of DET vs EET, while there is no significant difference between the values of sensitivity. In that paper, we showed a greater feasibility and specificity of DET vs EET for the diagnosis of CAD. Furthermore, we demonstrated that the diagnostic figures of DET were similar in hypertensives and normotensives. Indeed, considering patients with old myocardial infarction (not included in the population of the previous work), DET shows an increase in sensitivity value, maintaining the same specificity. On the contrary, EET values of specificity and sensitivity are similar considering patients with previous myocardial infarction as well (Figs. 2 and 3). The diagnostic value of DET is even more clinically appealing if one considers that other tests are also much more sophisticated and expensive than EET and not reliable for the diagnosis of CAD in hypertensives.

In a recent review of this argument, Prisant et al, stated that "no noninvasive screening test has been found to adequately discriminate between hypertensive patients with and without associated coronary atherosclerosis" [6]. For example, it has been demonstrated that radionuclide angiography, although an excellent indicator of myocardial ischemia in normotensive patients, has a low predictive accuracy in hypertensives with chest pain [7]. Even the 201-thallium exercise stress test, which shows a very good sensitivity and specificity in normotensive patients, presents a significant drop in specificity in hypertensives [8]. For these problems, it has been stated that "noninvasive testing by routine exercise stress testing and stress radionuclide angiography are not reliably predictive of ischemia resulting from obstructive epicardial CAD and should be abandoned for that diagnostic purpose" [6].

In this context, DET assumes an important role as a feasible, reliable, and inexpensive tool for the diagnosis of CAD in hypertensive patients complaining of chest pain.

Acknowledgment. We are indebted to Ms. Antonella Distante for secretarial assistance.

References

1. Picano E, Distante A, Masini M, Morales AM, Lattanzi F, L'Abbate A (1985) Dipyridamole-echocardiography test in effort angina pectoris. Am J Cardiol 56: 452–456
2. Picano E, Lattanzi F, Masini M, Distante A, L'Abbate A (1986) High dose dipyridamole-echocardiography test in effort angina pectoris. J Am Coll Cardiol 8: 848–854
3. Picano E, Lattanzi F, Masini M, Distante A, L'Abbate A (1987) Different degrees of ischemic threshold stratified by the dipyridamole-echocardiography test. Am J Cardiol 59: 71–73
4. Picano E, Lucarini AR, Lattanzi F, Distante A, Di Legge V, Salvetti A, L'Abbate A (1988) Dipyridamole-echocardiography test in essential hypertensives with chest pain. Hypertension 12: 238–243

5. Picano E, Lucarini AR, Lattanzi F, De Prisco F, Masini M, Del Prato C, Salvetti A, Distante A (1987) Dipyridamole-echocardiography test in essential hypertensives. (abstract) Circulation 76: 4
6. Prisant LM, Frank MJ, Carr AA, von Dohlen TW, Abdulla AM (1987) How can we diagnose coronary artery disease in hypertensive patients? Hypertension 10: 467–72
7. Wasserman AG, Katz RJ, Varghese PJ, (1984) Exercise radionuclide ventriculographic response in hypertensive patients with chest pain. N Engl J Med 311: 1276–1280
8. Schulman DS, Francis CK, Black HR, Wackers FJT (1986) Thallium-201 stress imaging in hypertensive patients. Hypertension 10: 16–21

The Systolic Hypertension in the Elderly Program (SHEP): Rationale, Design, Recruitment, and Baseline Data

Jeffrey L. Probstfield[1], William B. Applegate[2], J. David Curb[3], Nemat O. Borhani[4], C Morton Hawkins[5], Jeffrey A. Cutler[6], Barry R. Davis[5], Curt D. Furberg[7] Edward Lakatos[8], Lot B Page[3], H. Mitchell Perry, Jr.[9], and W. McFate Smith[10] for the SHEP Cooperative Research Group*

Summary. The Systolic Hypertension in the Elderly Program (SHEP) is a randomized, double-blind, placebo-controlled trail to determine if antihypertensive treatment of isolated systolic hypertension (ISH) (systolic blood pressure [SBP] $\geq$ 160 mmHg, diastolic blood pressure [DBP] < 90 mmHg) reduces the 5-year incidence of fatal and nonfatal stroke. Recruitment was demanding; however, 4736 persons (target 4800) with ISH, age 60 years and over, were enrolled (1% of those initially contacted) between March 1, 1985 and January 15, 1988. Potential participants were those who met blood pressure criteria or those on antihypertensive medication and without documented diastolic hypertension who had their medication tapered and discontinued (consent obtained from participant and primary care physician) and then met blood pressure criteria.

Eligible participants were randomized to stepped-care therapy with chlorthalidone and atenolol (alternative, reserpine) or matching placebos as first and second steps. Sixty-six percent of participants were not on antihypertensive medication prior to randomization. The group is 38.6% nonblack male, 47.5% nonblack female, 4.5% black male, and 9.3% black female. At baseline the age-range distribution was 41%, 60–69; 45%, 70–79; and 14%, 80 and over (mean 71.6). The cohort's SBP distribution was 57%, 160–169 mmHg; 27%, 170–179 mmHg; and 16%, 180 mmHg and over, (mean 170.3). The mean DBP was 76.6 mmHg; and 59.8% had codeable baseline electrocardiographic abnormalities. The trial is now in follow-up phase with scheduled termination in 1991.

Key words: Systolic hypertension — Prevention — Stroke — Drug treatment — Total mortality — Quality of life

[1] Clinical Trials Branch, National Heart Lung and Blood Institute, Bethesda, MD, USA
[2] University of Tennessee School of Medicine, Memphis, TN, USA
[3] National Institute on Aging, Bethesda, MD, USA
[4] University of California School of Medicine at Davis, Davis, CA, USA
[5] University of Texas at Houston School of Public Health, Houston, TX, USA
[6] Prevention and Demonstration Research Branch, National Heart, Lung, and Blood Institute, Bethesda, MD, USA
[7] Bowman-Gray School of Medicine, Winston Salem, NC, USA
[8] Biostatistics Research Branch, National Heart, Lung, and Blood Institute, Bethesda, MD, USA
[9] Washington University School of Medicine, St. Louis, MO, USA
[10] Medical Research Institute of San Francisco, Pacific Medical Center, San Francisco, CA, USA
* See footnote on page 142.

Rationale and Background

Isolated Systolic Hypertension (ISH) is an important unresolved clinical and public health problem; data on large-scale long-term clinical trials are not available on the treatment of this condition. The Systolic Hypertension in the Elderly Program (SHEP) is a current investigation in the United States sponsored by the National Heart, Lung, and Blood Institute (NHLBI) and the National Institute on Aging (NIA). This multicenter, randomized, placebo-controlled trial has as its main objective to answer the question: will antihypertensive drug treatment in men and women age 60 and over with sustained isolated systolic hypertension, i.e., elevated systolic blood pressure (SBP) (160–219 mmHg) and nonhypertensive diastolic blood pressure (DBP) (< 90 mmHg) reduce the number of strokes (fatal and nonfatal) compared with participants on placebo? Ascertainment of whether or not antihypertensive drug therapy reduces total or other cause specific mortality in this group is considered an important secondary objective.

In previous randomized, controlled trials on efficacy of antihypertensive drug treatment, including the few that had older people, the focus has been on the problem of elevated DBP (≥ 90 mmHg) and that has been used as the sole or main blood pressure entry criterion [1–10].

Epidemiologic studies have shown that ISH is associated with an increased risk of stroke, coronary heart disease, all-cardiovascular and all-cause mortality in both middle-aged and older people [11–18]. Although the prevalence of ISH in the general population may be declining [19], it is progressively and markedly higher within certain age groups, particularly among persons age 60 and older, in both men and women, black and white [20]. In the SHEP Pilot Study (SHEP-PS), the prevalence of ISH in those screened was 6% in the age group 60–69 years, 11% in the 70–79 age group, and 18% in those 80 years and over [21].

In 1980 the United States census data showed that there were 35.6 million people 60 years and older in the country. Based on a prevalence rate for ISH, i.e., $SBP \geq 160$ mmHg and $DBP < 90$ mmHg, in this age group of about 8%–11% [20] at any given time, there could be more than 3 million people with ISH in the U.S. ISH is a public health problem, and there is a lack of knowledge on efficacy and safety of drug treatment of ISH, a strong justification is in evidence for the SHEP trial.

The feasibility of SHEP was demonstrated by the results of the SHEP-PS [22]. This double-blind, randomized, placebo-controlled trial was conducted in 5 clinical centers and had as its main objectives testing methods of recruitment, success of enrollment, and adherence to, efficacy of, and frequency of side effects from antihypertensive medication for lowering blood pressure in an older population with sustained ISH.

Further, the pilot study was designed to develop and test methods of ascertaining stroke and other disease end points. An additional objective was to evaluate the potential impact of the intervention regimen on mood and cognitive states with periodic behavioral assessment. The 5 centers recruited 551 eligible participants (2% of those screened). Adherence to the intervention regimen was excellent, dropout and drop-in rates were acceptable and goal blood pessure was reached by

75% of the drug-treated group at 3 months. Troublesome symptoms in about 50% of participants at 1 year were reported equally in the actively treated and placebo groups. Based on the drugs used in the SHEP-PS, low-dose chlorthalidone and a beta-blocker were seleted as the most appropriate medications for the full-scale study. NHLBI and NIA, after selection of 17 participating institutions, constituted a steering committee to develop the SHEP protocol.

Design

General

The SHEP design, including information on study sizing and subgroup hypotheses, has been more fully reported elsewhere [23]. Briefly, this is a double-blind, placebo-controlled, randomized clinical trial of 4736 (target 4800) [24] participants stratified within centers according to their previous use of antihypertensive medication. Men and women aged 60 years or older were enrolled who had sustained $SBP \geq 160$ mmHg and DBP of < 90 mmHg according to a specific set of criteria for measurements and visits. A stepped-care drug treatment regimen with chlorthalidone and atenolol, each at 2 doses (Fig. 1), is employed as necessary to reduce blood pressure to goal within 6 months of enrollment. A reduction in SBP

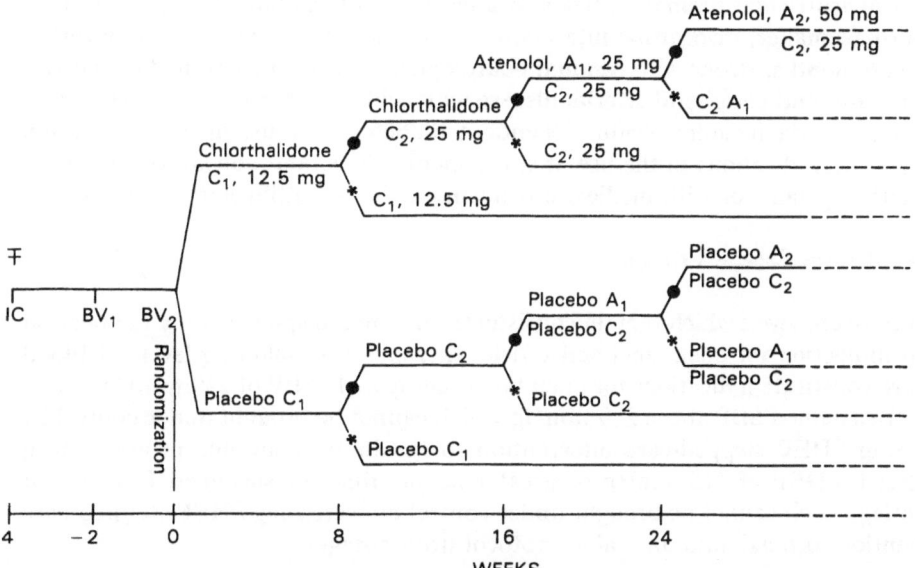

Fig. 1. SHEP clinic visit and treatment schedule. ‡All those first seen while on antihypertensives must have these drugs discontinued through an additional series of visits. ● Indicates those with blood pressure not reduced to or below goal. ● Indicates those with blood pressure reduced to or below goal. *IC*, initial contact; BV_1 and BV_2, baseline visits 1 and 2, respectively. Drug dosages are per day. Reprinted from [23], p 1200, with permission

of at least 20 mmHg or to below 160 mmHg, depending upon entry level, is the treatment goal. Reserpine can be used as an alternative step 2 drug for those who are intolerant of atenolol.

Follow-up

Participants are being followed quarterly for an average of 5 years from randomization. Measurements include: interval history and physical examination, blood pressure, ECGs, hematologic and biochemical parameters, and urinalysis. Potassium supplementation is indicated if on 2 consecutive visits the level of serum potassium is less than 3.5 mEq/l. Specific step-down procedures are described for those whose SBP falls below 110 mmHg. Specific guidelines for the institution of "open label" medication have been defined for those whose blood pressure cannot be satisfactorily reduced or controlled. Although stroke (fatal and nonfatal) is the primary end point, the detection of adverse effects from the interventions, various morbid and fatal cardiovascular events, and specific behavioral variables, e.g., depression and dementia, are considered important and are defined as end points in the study.

Inclusion and Exclusion Criteria

The 2 main inclusion criteria are age (≥ 60 years) and the level of SBP (160–219 mmHg, with DBP < 90 mmHg). The cardiovascular exclusion criteria include: atrial fibrillation or flutter, 2nd or 3rd degree atrioventricular (AV) block, multifocal ventricular premature beats, bradycardia of less than 50 beats/min, permanent pacemaker, myocardial infarction or coronary artery bypass surgery within the past 6 months, stroke with residual neurological deficit, uncontrolled congestive heart failure, and peripheral arterial disease with evidence of ischemic injury. Other exclusion criteria include: insulin-dependent diabetes mellitus, history of alcohol abuse, contraindications to the use of study medications, and obligatory treatment with anticoagulants or with medications having a known antihypertensive effect.

Blood Pressure Escape Criteria

Blood pressure levels which remain consistently elevated in spite of study medication are an indication for open-label active drug therapy. The following levels of blood pressure constitute indications for open label therapy: (1) SBP of 240 mmHg at any time, or sustained SBP above 220 mmHg which cannot be brought under control by increasing SHEP stepped-care intervention to maximum allowable protocol drug dosages; (2) DBP of 115 mmHg or greater at any time, or sustained DBP about 90 mmHg which cannot be brought under control by increasing SHEP stepped-care intervention to maximum allowable protocol drug dosages.

Study End Points

Combined fatal and nonfatal strokes are the focus of the primary end point analysis. One event per patient is permitted for analytic purposes and all events are analyzed dichotomously. There is a hierarchy of 3 levels of events described below. All events have been defined a priori for study purposes.

1. Stroke (fatal and nonfatal)
2. Non-stroke cardiovascular events and other conditions including: total mortality, sudden death, other cardiovascular death, acute myocardial infarction (fatal and nonfatal), coronary artery bypass surgery, carotid surgery, other arterial surgery, peripheral vascular disease, renal dysfunction, transient ischemic attack, angina, left ventricular hypertrophy, significant ventricular arrhythmia, and aortic aneurysm
3. Other events including: noncardiovascular death, fractures, depression, dementia (multi infarct and other), hospitalizations, and nursing home admissions.

Stroke is defined as the abrupt onset of a new neurological deficit lasting at least 24 h, with specific localizing findings confirmed by unequivical physical examination or laboratory data (computerized tomography [CT] scan) and without evidence for an underlying nonvascular cause.

Behavioral Evaluation

The assessment of the quality of life of participants who are in the 2 treatment groups is seen as an important aspect of SHEP. The objectives of the behavioral evaluation component of SHEP are: (1) to define the level of cognitive functioning and affective functioning, the activities of daily living, and the nature of social supports at baseline; and (2) to measure changes in these variables over time in relation to treatment assignment and blood pressure levels. There are 2 parts to the evaluation. Part I, given to all participants, includes: the SHORT CARE questionnaire (reduced to those items required for detecting clinically significant depression and dementia) [25], the Center for Epidemiologic Studies-Depression Scale (CES-D) [26], Activities of Daily Living (ADL) [27] and Social Network Questionnaire (social support) [28]. Behavioral part II is being done at 6 clinical centers and is a more in-depth evaluation of cognitive function. The behavioral evaluation is being administered at baseline and semiannually.

Quality Control and Monitoring

Monthly reports are distributed from the Data Coordinating Center (some by the distributed data entry system) to the clinics on a regular basis. During recruitment, this was an essential aspect of monitoring and the basis for further planning. During the follow-up phase, information regarding adherence to study medications, visit attendance, and forms completion are valued feedback to the clinics. Quality control site visits are done at the clinical centers on a regular basis by·program office and coordinating center personnel. A standard protocol has been developed. The progress of the study and the safety of the participants is reviewed on a regular basis by an independent data and safety monitoring board.

Recruitment

The recruitment phase of SHEP began in March 1985 and was scheduled for completion on March 31, 1987. Although the pilot study had successfully enrolled about 2% of those initially screened, recruitment was about twice as difficult for the full-scale study. Over 80% of initial contacts were excluded for failing to meet blood pressure criteria, chiefly because of low SBP. Nearly 450,000 age-eligible candidates had blood pressures taken to find the 4736 that were finally enrolled. A recent study suggests that ISH may be decreasing in its prevalence [19]. Active recruitment was extended 7 months with an additional 2½ months for processing all potential participants. A full description of the SHEP recruitment is in preparation. Briefly, while multiple recruitment strategies were employed, mass mailing and community screening were the most useful. Where mass mailing was coordinated with targeted advertising and community screening, the combined strategy was particularly successful.

Baseline Data

An overview of the SHEP participant baseline characteristics is given in Table 1. The 2 randomized groups are comparable (data not shown) including the number who were originally on antihypertensive medication when first contacted, the number with codeable ECG abnormalities, and those with cognitive impairment or depressive symptoms. It has been noted that information is lacking on the effect of treatment for those over age 80. Approximately 650 participants for the full-scale SHEP above age 80 will provide information on this group.

Conclusion

Previous and ongoing trials in elderly populations have focused on the efficacy of treatment of DBP or a combination of DBP and SBP elevations [3, 5–8]. Isolated systolic hypertension is a prevalent problem in the elderly. Whether or not efficacy of treatment can be demonstrated to confer benefit by prevention of stroke or other mortal or morbid events, remains open to question. Further, the quality of life for those in this age group being treated with antihypertensive medications has yet to be evaluated fully. SHEP aims to obtain information on these issues. The follow-up phase of the trial is planned for completion in the early 1990s.

References

1. Veterans Administration Cooperative Study Group on Antihypertensive Agents (1970) Effects of treatment on mobility in hypertension. II. Results in patients with diastolic blood pressure averaging 90 through 114 mmHg. JAMA: 1143–1152
2. Management Committee of the Australian Therapeutic Trial in Mild Hypertension (1980) The Australian Therapeutic Trial in Milo Hypertension. Lancet 1: 1261–1267

Table 1. Baseline characteristics of SHEP participants

Characteristics	Mean (SD) or percent total
Number	4736
Age (years) (%)	
60–69	41.4
70–79	44.8
80 +	13.7
Mean (SD)	71.6 (6.7)
Race and sex (%)	
Black male	4.5
Black female	9.3
Non black male	38.6
Non black female	47.5
Education (years) (%)	
0–7	10.0
8–11	26.1
12	33.2
13–15	14.7
16 +	16.0
Baseline systolic blood pressure (mmHg)	170.3 (9.4)
Baseline diastolic blood pressure (mmHg)	76.6 (9.7)
Depressive symptoms (%)[a]	11.0
Evidence of cognitive impairment (%)[b]	0.4
Medications at initial contact (%)	33.2
Codeable ECG abnormalities (%)	59.7

[a] SHORTCARE depression score 7 + .
[b] SHORTCARE dementia score 4 + .

3. Blaufox MD (guest ed) The Hypertension Detection and Follow-up Program Cooperative Group Editorial Board (1986) Results and implications of the hypertension detection and follow-up program. Prog Cardiovasc Dis 29 (Suppl I): 1–124
4. Medical Research Council Working Party (1985) MRC trial of treatment of mild hypertension: Principal results. Br Med J 291: 97–104
5. Amery A, Birkenhager W, Brixko P, Bulpitt C, Clement B, Deruyttere M, DeSchaepdryver A, Dollery C, Fagard R, Forette F, Forte J, Hamdy R, Henry JF, Joossens JV, Leonetti G, Lund-Johansen P, O'Malley K, Petrie J, Strasser T, Tuomilehto J, Williams B (1985) Mortality and mobility results from the European working party on high blood pressure in the elderly trial. Lancet 1: 1349–1354
6. Amery A, Birkenhager W, Brixko P, Bulpitt C, Clement D, Deruyttere M, Deschaepdryver A, Dollery C, Fagard R, Forette F, Forte J, Hamdy R, Henry JF, Joossens JV, Leonetti G, Lund-Johansen P, O'Malley K, Petrie JC, Strasser T, Tuomilehto J, Williams B (1986) Efficacy of antihypertensive drug treatment according to age, sex, blood pressure, and previous cardiovascular disease in patients over the age of 60. Lancet 2: 589–592
7. Coope J, Warrender TS (1986) Randomized trial of treatment of hypertension in elderly patients in primary care. Br Med J 293: 1145–1151
8. Dahlof B, Hansson L, Lindholm L, Rastam L, Schersten B, Wester PO (1986) STOP Hypertension: Swedish trial in old patients with hypertension. J Hypertens 4: 511–513
9. MacMahon SW, Cutler JA, Furberg CD, Payne GH (1986) The effects of drug treatment for hypertension on morbidity and mortality from cardiovascular disease: A review of randomized controlled trials. Prog Cardiovasc Dis 29 (Suppl I): 99–118
10. Hebert PR, Fiebach NH, Eberlein KA, Taylor JO, Hennekens CH (1988) The community-

based randomized trials of pharmacologic treatment of mild-to-moderate hyptension. Am J Epidemiol 127: 581–590

11. Society of Actuaries (1959) Building and blood pressure study (vol 1). Chicago
12. Shekelle R, Ostfeld A, Klawans HL Jr (1974) Hypertension and risk of stroke in an elderly population. Stroke 5: 71–75
13. Kannel WB, Dawber TR, Sorlie P, Wolf B (1976) Components of blood pressure and risk of atherothrombotic brain infarction: The Framingham study. Stroke 7: 327–331
14. Dyer AR, Stamler J, Shekelle RB, Schoenberger JA, Farinaro E (1977) Hypertension in the elderly. Med Clin North Am 61: 513–529
15. Colandrea MA, Friedman GD, Nichaman MZ, Lynd CN (1970) Systolic hypertension in the elderly. An epidemiologic assessment. Circulation 41: 239–245
16. Garland C, Barrett-Conner E, Suarez L, Criqui MH (1983) Isolated systolic hypertension and mortality after age 60 years. A prospective population-based study. Am J Epidemiol 118: 365–376
17. Curb JD, Borhani NO, Entwisle G, Tung B, Kass E, Schnaper H, Williams W, Berman R (1985) Isolated systolic hypertension in 14 communities. Am J Epidemiol 121: 362–370
18. Stamler J (1989) Blood pressure (systolic and diastolic) and risk of fatal coronary heart disease. J Hypertens (in press)
19. McClellan W, Hall WD, Broga D, MartinezB, Wilber JA (1987) Isolated systolic hypertension: Declining prevalence in the elderly. Prev Med 16: 686–695
20. (1986) Blood pressure of adults by race and area: United States, 1976–1980. National Center for Health Statistics, Series II, No. 234
21. Vogt TM, Ireland CC, Black D, Camel G, Hughes G (1986) Recruitment of elderly volunteers for multi-center clinical trial; the SHEP pilot study. Controlled Clin Trials 7: 113–118
22. Hulley SB, Furberg CD, Gurland B, McDonald R, Perry M, Schnaper HW, Schoenberger JA, Smith WM, Vogt TM, For the SHEP Research Group (1985) Systolic hypertension in the elderly program (SHEP): Antihypertensive efficacy of chlorthalidone. Am J Cardiol 56: 913–920
23. The Systolic Hypertension in the Elderly Program (SHEP) Cooperative Research Group (1988) Rational and design of a randomized clinical trial on prevention of stroke in isolated systolic hypertension Clin Epideiol 41: 1197–1208
24. Lakatos E (1986) Sample size determination in clinical trials with time-dependent rates of losses and non-compliance. Controlled Clin Trials 7: 189–199
25. Gurland B, Golden RR, Teresi JA, Challop (1984) The short care: An efficient instrument for the assessment of depression, dementia, and disability. J Gerontol 39: 166–169
26. Radloff LS (1977) The CES-D scale: A self-report depression scale for research in the general population. Appl Psychol Meas 1: 385–401
27. Branch LG, Katz S, Kniepmann K (1984) A prospective study of functional status among community elders. Am J Public Health 74: 266–268
28. Branch LG, Berkman LF, Brock DB, Cosmatos D, Keough ME, Lemke H, McGloin J, Morris MC (1986) Social functioning. In: Coroni-Huntley J, Brock DB, Ostfeld AM, Taylor DO, Wallace RB (eds) Established populations for eppidemiologic studies of the elderly. Resource data book. NIH publication no 86-2443. National Institutes of Health, Bethesda MD, pp 33–55

* SHEP Investigators in addition to authors so noted; *M. Donald Balufox* Albert Einstein College of Medicine; *W. Dallas Hall* Emory University School of Medicine; *Thomas Vogt* Kaiser Permanent Center for Health Research; *Jeffrey Raines* Miami Heart Institute; *David Berkson* Northwestern University Medical School; *Helen Petrovitch* Pacific Health Research Institute; *John B. Kostis* Robert Wood Johnson Medical School; *Harold W. Schnaper* University of Alabama, Birmingham; *Gordon Guthrie* University of Kentucky Medical Center; *Richard H. Grimm, Jr.* University of Minnesota; *Robert McDonald* University of Pittsburgh; *Henry Black* Yale University; *Kenneth G. Berge* Mayo Clinic (Steering Committee Chairman); *Eleanor Schron* National Heart, Lung, Blood Institute

Antihypertensive Therapy with Uncontrolled Systolic Pressure and Increased Aortic Rigidity

M.E. Safar, Ph.L. Soubies, A.M. Safavian, R.G. Asmar, and St. Laurent[1]

Summary. Sixty patients with sustained essential systolo-diastolic hypertension were submitted to a stepped-care approach in order to obtain an adequate control of blood pressure with antihypertensive drugs. After a 24-month follow-up survey, 30 patients (group I) had adequate control of both systolic and diastolic pressures; while, in another 30 patients (group II), diastolic pressure was controlled and systolic pressure remained elevated. Compared to patients in group I with the same age and mean arterial pressure, patients in group II exhibited higher values in carotido-femoral pulse wave velocity ($P < 0.001$). The higher values of pulse wave velocity could not be explained on the basis of differences in therapeutic regimen or associated clinical atherosclerotic diseases. The Sokolow Lyon index was significantly higher in group II than in group I. The study provided evidence that, in patients treated for systolo-diastolic hypertension: (1) an adequate control of diastolic pressure may be obtained while systolic pressure remains elevated; and (2) the increased systolic pressure indicates an enhanced rigidity of the arterial wall with possible consequence to cardiac structure and function.

Key words: Essential hypertension — Antihypertensive therapy — Pulse wave velocity — Arterial compliance

Introduction

In clinical treatment of patients with hypertension, guidelines and long-term follow-up of antihypertensive treatment are based on diastolic blood pressure measurement [1, 2]. Systolic pressure is rarely taken into consideration. However, the usual management of patients indicates that an adequate control of diastolic pressure is often associated with a systolic pressure which remains elevated.

While diastolic pressure is mainly determined by the degree of dilatation of the small arteries, systolic pressure is influenced by other hemodynamic mechanisms such as the level of ventricular ejection and the rigidity of the arterial wall [3, 4]. Consideration of the latter mechanism may be important in hypertension, since the decrease in blood pressure due to antihypertensive treatment is expected to cause per se an improvement in arterial distensibility and compliance through the simple reduction of distending pressure [4].

---

[1] Hypertension Research Center, Broussais Hospital, Paris, France

In the present study, a long-term follow-up of patients treated for systolo-diastolic hypertension is presented. Patients are classified as those with an adequate control of both systolic and diastolic pressures and those with an adequate control of diastolic pressure while systolic pressure remains elevated. This particular hemodynamic pattern is related to the most widely used clinical index of arterial distensibility, pulse wave velocity [3-7].

Material and Methods

Patients

The study was performed in 60 men with sustained essential hypertension. Ages ranged between 45 and 59 years (mean: 51 years). Body weight was between 59 and 130 kg (mean: 80 kg). Mean height was 170 ± 1 cm (± 1 standard error of the mean).

Selection of patients was based on the following criteria. First, sustained hypertension was diagnosed when, during a 1-month untreated, ambulatory period, at least three diastolic blood pressure measurements (determined as indicated below) were equal or superior to 100 mmHg. Second, essential hypertension was ascertained by thorough investigation including plasma and urinary electrolytes, plasma creatinine, urinary catecholamine determination, and timed intravenous pyelography, as described previously [4]. Third, antihypertensive therapy (started in all cases), caused a significant decrease in blood pressure with a diastolic blood pressure equal or below 95 mmHg (60 patients).

In the 60 subjects, antihypertensive therapy was performed using the classic stepped-care approach [2]. In 41 patients, diuretics (hydrochlorothiazide: 50 mg/day), beta-blocking drugs (acebutolol: 600 mg/day), or both were sufficient to obtain a diastolic blood pressure equal to or below 95 mmHg. In 12 patients, dihydrallazine (50-75 mg/day), alpha-methyldopa (500 mg/day), or both were added in order to obtain the same blood pressure reduction. In the 7 remaining, resistant, hypertensive patients, normalization of diastolic pressure was achieved with nifedipine (30 mg/day) associated with acebutolol, methyldopa, or a combination of these different drugs. All drugs were administered orally, b.i.d. In all cases, follow-up lasted more than 12 months with a mean survey duration of 24 ± 1 months.

At the end of the follow-up period, the 60 patients were divided into two groups. In group I, diastolic pressure was equal to or below 95 mmHg and systolic pressure was equal to or below 145 mmHg. In group II, diastolic pressure was equal to or below 95 mmHg while systolic pressure was consistantly above 150 mmHg.

Procedure

At the end of the follow-up survey, the 60 patients were submitted to a day of hospitalization while continuing antihypertensive treatment. Tests were performed in the following order: biological investigations; blood pressure measurements and determination of pulse wave velocity after 30 min rest in supine position; and non invasive hemodynamics including continuous Doppler measurements. Arterial pressure was measured according to the American Heart Association Recommendation [8] with a standard mercury sphygmomanometer. The auscultatory method used followed Korotkoff's phases: phase I for the systolic arterial pressure (SAP), and phase V for the diastolic arterial pressure (DAP). Mean arterial pressure (MAP) was calculated in mmHg as the diastolic pressure plus ⅓ pulse pressure. Heart rate (b/min) was measured on the basis of the ECG recording immediately after the blood pressure determination.

For the evaluation of pulse wave velocity [6, 7], two pulse transducer probes (Electronics for Medicine) were fixed to the skin over the most prominent parts of the brachial and radial arteries of the right arm. The foot-to-foot wave velocity, which contains the high frequency information [9], was measured as the interval between the foot of the brachial and the radial waves, using a recorder with paper speed of 150 mm/s. The foot, identified as the point where the sharp systolic upstroke commenced, was defined by extrapolating the wave front downwards to the intersection of this line with a straight-line extrapolation of the last part of the diastolic curve. The time delay was measured between the feet of simulateneously recorded waves. This was averaged over at least 1 respiratory cycle of about 10 beats. Measurement of the distance between transducers was then used to calculate pulse wave velocity. The duplication of estimates by the same observer was $8 \pm 5\%$. Reproductivity and normal values have been published else where [10].

Since no patient had clinical symptoms suggesting arteriosclerosis obliterans of the lower limbs or ischemic cerebrovascular disease, continuous Doppler examination was used to detect stenosis of the large arteries in the carotid and iliofemoral circulations. For the lower limbs, the ratio between brachial and ankle systolic arterial pressure was evaluated using the method of Yao et al. [11]. Normal laboratory values for those between 40 and 60 years are $126\% \pm 4\%$. For the carotid circulation, standard methods were used [12]; only stenosis of the internal carotid artery above 80% was considered as significant [12]. Coronary insufficiency was assessed on the basis of characteristic symptoms and/or well-established electrocardiographic findings according to the criteria detailed by Sokolow and Perloff [13]. Left ventricular hypertrophy was assessed on the basis of the Sokolow-Lyon index. Classic methods previously published [4, 10, 12] were used to evaluate plasma and urinary electrolytes, plasma creatinine, cholesterol, glucose, and uricacid. For the statistical study [14], the Student's t-test was performed to compare mean values. A P value inferior to 0.05 was considered statistically significant.

Results

Table 1 shows that, for the same age and the same diastolic arterial pressure as patients in group I, patients in group II exhibited higher values in systolic and mean arterial pressures.

Figure 1 shows that pulse wave velocity was significantly higher in group II patients than in group I patients ($P < 0.01$). Figure 2 indicates that, in 10 patients from group I and 10 patients from group II selected for the same age and the same mean

Table 1. Clinical characteristics

	Group I	Group II
Number of patients	30	30
Age (years)	51 ± 1	51 ± 1
Weight (Kg)	82 ± 2	78 ± 2
Height (cm)	171 ± 1	170 ± 1
Systolic arterial pressure (mmHg)	129 ± 2	162 ± 2*
Diastolic arterial pressure (mmHg)	86 ± 1	88 ± 1
Mean arterial pressure (mmHg)	100 ± 1	113 ± 1*
Heart rate (beats/min)	69 ± 2	73 ± 3

Values given are ± 1 standard error of the mean
*$P < 0.001$

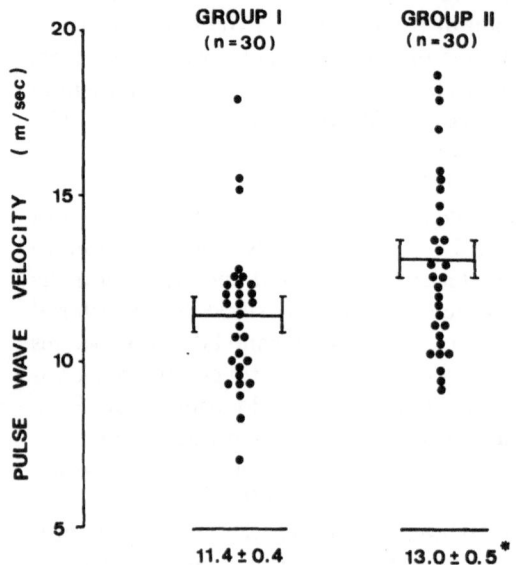

Fig. 1. Pulse wave velocity in groups I and II. *$P < 0.01$

arterial pressure, pulse wave velocity was significantly higher in patients from group II ($P < 0.001$). In addition to significantly higher values for systolic pressure ($P < 0.001$), patients from group II exhibited lower values for diastolic pressure ($P < 0.05$).

Tables 2 and 3 show that the biochemical parameters and the evaluated indices of vascular disease were similar in the two groups. However, the Sokolow-Lyon index was more elevated ($P < 0.05$) in patients in group II.

Table 4 indicates that the distribution of antihypertensive drugs was similar in groups I and II. Due to difficulties in reducing systolic pressure, a higher incidence of administration of calcium inhibitors was noticed in group II.

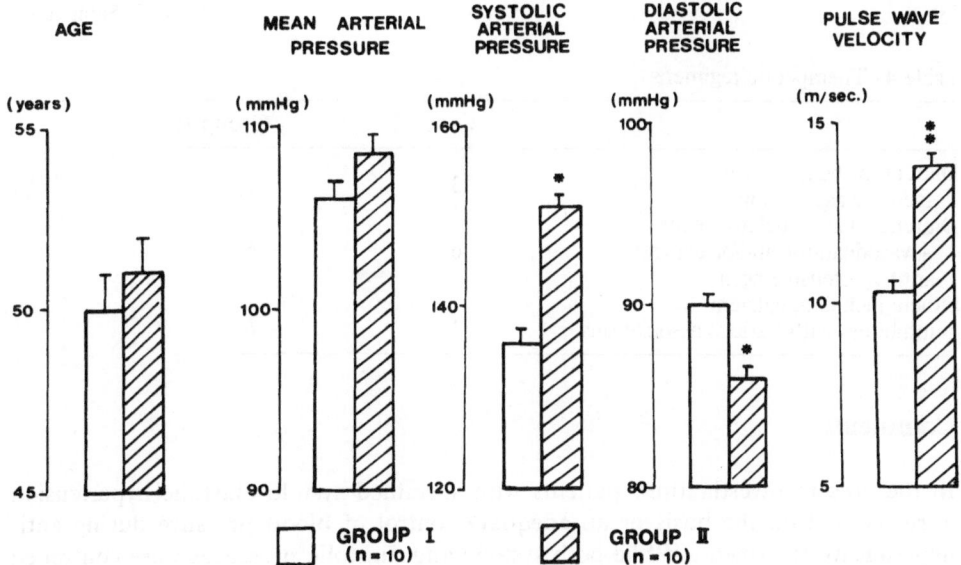

Fig. 2. Pulse wave velocity in 10 patients from group I and 10 patients from group II selected for corresponding ages and mean arterial pressures. * P<0.05; **P<0.001

Table 2. Biological parameters

	Group I	Group II
Hematocrit (%)	48 ± 1	48 ± 1
Urine		
Sodium (mmol/24 h)	156 ± 14	193 ± 19
Potassium (mmol/24 h)	65 ± 5	78 ± 10
Plasma		
Sodium (mmol/l)	143 ± 1	143 ± 1
Potassium (mmol/l)	3.8 ± 0.1	4.0 ± 0.1
Glucose (mmol/l)	6.0 ± 0.3	6.4 ± 0.3
Cholesterol (mmol/l)	6.1 ± 0.2	6.4 ± 0.2
Triglyceride (mmol/l)	2.1 ± 0.3	1.8 ± 0.2
Creatinine (μmol/l)	109 ± 4	102 ± 3
Uric Acid (μmol/l)	374 ± 17	359 ± 13

Values given are ± 1 standard error of the mean.

Table 3. Indices of vascular disease

	Group I	Group II
Sokolow Lyon (mm)	22 ± 1	26 ± 1*
Coronary insufficiency (N : T)	4 : 30	5 : 30
Brachial and ankle systolic arterial pressure ratio (%)	113 ± 2	111 ± 3
Stenosis of the internal carotid artery (N : T)	3 : 30	4 : 30

Values given are ± 1 standard error of the mean.
N, number of patients with arterial disease; T, total number of subjects
* P<0.05

Table 4. Therapeutic regimens

	Group I	Group II
Diuretic or beta-blocking agent or association	23	18
Diuretic + beta-blocking agent + vasodilatator and/or central antihypertensive agent	6	6
Others including calcium inhibitors with various associations	1	6

Comments

In the present investigation, patients with sustained systolo-diastolic hypertension were selected on the basis of an adequate control of blood pressure during anti-hypertensive treatment. While both systolic and diastolic pressures were controlled in group I patients, only diastolic pressure was within the normal range in group II patients, and systolic pressure remained elevated. Since pulse wave velocity was found significantly increased in patients in group II, the role of an increased stiffness of the arterial wall in the mechanism of elevated systolic pressure has to be reviewed at length.

The value of pulse wave velocity in interpreting arterial function and cardiac load results from its direct relationship to characteristic impedance, which is determined from the pulsatile arterial pressure/flow relationship in an artery [3-9]. Published studies of pulse wave velocity [3-7] have stressed it's value as an index of aortic rigidity: the higher the age, the higher the mean arterial pressure, and the stiffer the arterial wall. In the present investigation, patients in groups I and II had the same ages but different values for mean arterial pressure (Table 1). Thus, the possibility exists that the increased mean arterial pressure might explain the increased pulse wave velocity. For that reason, subgroups of patients were selected for matched age and arterial pressure from groups I and II (Fig. 2). Even with these conditions, pulse wave velocity remained higher in patients in group II. Moreover, in group II, not only an elevation of systolic pressure was noticed but also a decrease in diastolic pressure in comparison with group I. As demonstrated experimentally [15], such hemo-dynamic pattern clearly indicates an increased stiffness of the arterial wall in patients in group II, with a resulting increase in systolic and decrease in diastolic pressure.

Elevated pulse wave velocity may be related to functional factors acting on the arterial wall such as the amount of sodium intake [16], sympathetic stimulation [3], or the effect of pharmacological agents [4]. In older subjects, increased sodium intake has been shown to decrease arterial compliance and to increase systolic pressure predominantly [16]. Furthermore, salt restriction decreases pulse wave velocity independantly of its action on blood pressure [17]. However, sodium does not seem to influence greatly the findings of the present study: urinary sodium was similar in the two groups of patients, who were also receiving similar amounts of diuretic treatment. Among the most classic antihypertensive agents, some [4] are known to reduce pulse wave velocity pharmacologically (calcium inhibitors and converting enzyme inhibitors) while others produce no change (beta-blocking agents and hydralazine-like substances) for the same blood pressure reduction. However, in the present study, similar drugs were given to both groups of patients with calcium inhibitors even more frequently administered to patients in group II. Thus, antihypertensive agents did not seem to influence pulse wave velocity. Nevertheless, it might be that, in group II patients, sympathetic stimulation produced by dihydrallazine caused an exaggerated increase in pulse wave velocity on a previously more rigid arterial wall. Indeed, structural modifications of the aortic wall related to hypertensive vascular disease might have amplified the activation of the autonomic nervous system as a consequence of arteriolar vasodilatation caused by dihydrallazine [18]. In view of this observation, it seems possible that the elevated pulse wave velocity results directly or indirectly from the structural modification of the hypertensive arterial wall.

In agreement with experimental findings [3], our group [10, 19] has recently proposed that increased pulse wave velocity in untreated patients with essential hypertension might be the consequence of two different mechanisms. The first one, which affects most hypertensives, could be considered as an acceleration of the normal aging process. The second being that the form of the arterial disease could confer to the natural aging process the effects of other degenerative factors [3], perhaps atherosclerotic in nature. The latter changes could therefore cause more profound impairment of the arterial buffering function with an exaggerated amplitude of the arterial pulse pressure such as that observed in group II. However, in these patients, the findings of similar plasma cholesterol and indices of arterial in both groups (Table 3) did not favor the latter possibility. Nevertheless, in the present investigation, patient age was between 45 and 59 years while clinical observation of the atherosclerotic process occurs more frequently in those over 55 years.

Epidemiological studies have emphasized that systolic pressure was a higher independant cardiovascular risk factor than diastolic pressure for those over 50 years [20]. This problem is important in the consideration of the patients (group II) who had higher values in systolic pressure and pulse wave velocity. Both factors may contribute to an increase in ventricular afterload and thereby generate cardiac hypertrophy [3]. Indeed, a higher Sokolow-Lyon index was observed in group II. Moreover, in patients in group II, the tendency towards lower diastolic pressure (Fig. 2) might contribute to a decrease in the driving pressure of coronary circulation and abet cardiac ischemic disease [3, 15].

In conclusion, the present study has shown that some patients treated for sustained systolo-diastolic hypertension may have adequate control of diastolic pressure while systolic pressure remains elevated. Increased systolic pressure reflects an increased rigidity of the arterial wall (observed despite pharmacological blood pressure reduction). Whether this finding may influence cardiovascular morbidity and mortality in treated hypertensive patients remains an open question and requires further investigation.

Acknowledgements. This study was made possible by grants from the Institut National de la Santé et de la Recherche Médicale (INSERM), the Association pour l'Utilisation du Rein Artificiel (AURA), the Association Claude Bernard, and the Ministère de la Recherche, Paris. We thank Mrs. Danièle Saqué for her excellent assistance.

References

1. Freis ED (1982) The veterans trial and sequelae. Br J Clin Pharmacol 13: 67-72.
2. Simpson FO (1982) General strategy of antihypertensive treatment. In: Amery A, Fagard R, Lijnen P, Staessen J (eds) Hypertensive cardiovascular disease: pathophysiology and treatment. Martinus Nijhoff, The Hague Boston London, pp 873-886
3 O'Rourke MF (1982) Arterial function in health and disease. Longman, Harlow, pp 94-132, 210-224
4. Safar ME, Bouthier JA, Levenson JA, Simon ACh (1983) Peripheral large arteries and the response to antihypertensive treatment. Hypertension 5 (Suppl III): 63-68
5. Eliakim M, Sapoznikov D, Weisman J (1971) Pulse wave velocity in healthy subjects and in patients with various disease states. Am Heart J 82: 448-457
6. Gribbin B, Pickering TG, Sleight P (1979) Arterial distensibility in normal and hypertensive man. Clin Sci 56: 413-417
7. Avolio AP, Chen SG, Wang RP, Zhang CL, Li MF, O'Rourke MF (1983) Effects of aging on changing arterial compliance and left ventricular load in a northern Chinese urban community. Circulation 68: 50-58
8. Kirdendall WM, Feinleib MH, Freis ED, Mark AL (1981) Recommendation for human blood pressure determination by sphygmomanometers. Hypertension 3: A509-A519
9. McDonald DA (1974) Wave reflection, wave velocity and attenuation. In: Blood flow in arteries, 2nd edn. Edward Arnold, London, pp 309-350, 389-419
10. Asman RG, Pannia B, Santoni J Ph, Laurent St, London GM, Levy BI, Safar ME (1988) Revision of Cardiac hypertrophy and reduced arterial compliance after converting enzyme inhibition in essential hypertension. Circulation 78: 941-950
11. Yao VST, Hobbs JT, Irvine WI (1969) Ankle systolic pressure measurements in arterial disease affecting the lower extremities. Br J Surg 56: 676-687
12. Benetos A, Simon A, Levenson J, Lagneau P, Bouthier J, Safar M (1986) Pulsed Doppler: an evaluation of diameter, blood velocity and blood flow of the common carotid artery in patients with isolated unilateral stenosis of the internal carotid artery. Stroke 16: 696-972
13. Sokolow M, Perloff D (1961) The prognosis of essential hypertension treated conservatively. Circulation 23: 697-708
14. Draper N, Smith H (1966) Applied regression analysis. Wiley, New York, pp 10-50
15. Randall OS, Van DEN Bos GC, Westerhof N (1984) Systemic compliance: does it play a role in the genesis of essential hypertension Cardiovasc Res 18: 455-458
16. Levenson JA, Simon ACh, Maarek BE, Gitelman GJ, Fiessinger JN, Safar ME (1985) Regional compliance of brachial artery and saline infusion in patients with arteriosclerosis obliterans. Arteriosclerosis 5: 80-87
17. Avolio AP, Clyde KM, Beard TC, Cooke HM, Ho KKL, O'Rourke MF (1986) Improved arterial distensibility in normotensive subjects on a low salt diet. Arteriosclerosis 6: 166-169
18. Folkow B (1982) Physiological aspect of primary hypertension. Physiol Rev 62: 347-503
19. Simon ACh, Levenson J, Bouthier J, Safar ME, Avolio AP (1985) Evidence of early degenerative changes in large arteries in human essential hypertension. Hypertension 7: 675-680
20. Kannel WB, Castelli WP, McNamara PM, KcKee PA, Feinleb M (1972) Role of blood pressure in the development of congestive heart failure. The Framingham Study. Engl J Med 287: 781-787

Role of Intracellular Free Calcium in the Hypotensive Response to Nifedipine

Tetsuya Oshima, Hideo Matsuura, Koji Matsumoto, Koji Kido, Tomofumi Otsuki, Tetsuji Shingu, Ichiro Inoue, and Goro Kajiyama[1]

Summary. The acute antihypertensive effect of 10 mg of sublingual nifedipine was investigated in patients with essential hypertension in comparison with that in normotensive controls and in relation to intracellular free calcium concentration ($[Ca^{2+}]i$) in lymphocytes. Parameters predictive of the response to nifedipine such as age, pretreatment blood pressure, plasma norepinephrine concentration and plasma renin activity were also assessed. The fall in mean blood pressure with nifedipine was greater, and $[Ca^{2+}]i$ in lymphocytes was higher in patients with essential hypertension than in normotensive controls. In patients with essential hypertension, the hypotensive response to nifedipine was positively correlated with lymphocyte $[Ca^{2+}]i$ ($r = 0.82$) and negatively linked with plasma renin activity ($r = -0.65$), but unrelated to age, pretreatment mean blood pressure or plasma norepinephrine concentration. $[Ca^{2+}]i$ in lymphocytes was inversely correlated with plasma renin activity ($r = -0.66$). In normotensives, the mean blood pressure response to the drug had no relation to the variables studied. These results suggest that the acute hypotensive response to nifedipine may involve $[Ca^{2+}]i$ abnormalities and that calcium-influx-dependent vasoconstriction may be enhanced in essential hypertensive patients with suppressed plasma renin activity.

Key words: Intracellular calcium — Lymphocytes — Plasma renin activity — Nifedipine — Essential hypertension

Introduction

A number of investigators [1–3] have reported finding elevated $[Ca^{2+}]i$ and abnormal calcium handling at the cellular level in patients with essential hypertension. Clinical evidence that the hypotensive response to calcium channel blocking drugs is enhanced in patients with essential hypertension may be compatible with the pathogenetic importance of elevated $[Ca^{2+}]i$ in this disease. However, the response to calcium-channel-blocking drugs is variable in different individuals. Although several investigators [4–7] claim that the acute hypotensive efficacy of calcium-blocking drugs can be predicted by such factors as age [4], pretreatment blood pressure [4, 5] and plasma renin activity [6, 7], only limited information is available concerning the contribution of altered metabolism of cellular calcium to the hyotensive effects of these drugs.

---

[1] First Department of Internal Medicine, Hiroshima University School of Medicine, Hiroshima, Japan

We investigated the acute hypotensive response to sublingually administered nifedipine in patients with essential hypertension in relation to [Ca^{2+}]i in lymphocytes and predictive variables of this response from previous studies [4–7] such as age, pretreatment blood pressure, plasma renin activity, and plasma norepinephrine concentration.

Methods

Twenty-four patients with essential hypertension (12 male and 12 female; 54 ± 10 years old) and 11 normotensive subjects (6 male and 5 female; 53 ± 11 years old) were enrolled in the study. The hypertensive patients had sitting blood pressures of more than 160/95 mmHg in the outpatient clinic on at least 3 visits. The normotensive subjects had blood pressures consistently below 140/90 mmHg. Any medication was discontinued at least 4 weeks before the study. Informed consent was obtained from all subjects.

Based on previous studies in which we reported that [Ca^{2+}]i in lymphocytes and the antihypertensive response to nifedipine are affected by systemic sodium balance [8], our protocol entailed sharp, uniform control of dietary sodium chloride intake. All subjects were placed on a diet containing 8–10 g NaC1 per day for 1 week before the day of the study.

After an indwelling catheter was inserted into a forearm vein, fasting subjects were kept in the supine position for 30 min. Venous blood samples were then drawn for determination of [Ca^{2+}]i in lymphocytes, plasma renin activity, and plasma norepinephrine concentration. Blood pressure was determined with a mercury sphygmomanometer. Mean blood pressure was calculated by adding one third of the pulse pressure to the diastolic pressure. The subjects then received 10 mg of nifedipine sublingually, and blood pressure was measured every 5 min for 60 min. The hypotensive response to nifedipine was considered to be the maximal fall in mean blood pressure, regardless of the time elapsed after its administration. Lymphocyte [Ca^{2+}]i was measured with quin 2 (tetraacetoxy methyl ester [quin 2 AM]) and plasma renin activity by radioimmunoassay as previously described [9]. Plasma norepinephrine concentration was measured by an electrochemical method with high-performance liquid chromatography.

Data are expressed as mean $\pm$ SD. Statistical evaluation was performed using the Wilcoxon rank sum test. Correlation coefficients were calculated by Pearson correlation. Statistical significance was defined as a P value of less than 0.05.

Results

Pretreatment mean blood pressure ranged between 105 mmHg and 130 mmHg in patients with essential hypertension and between 60 mmHg and 90 mmHg in normotensive controls. Lymphocyte [Ca^{2+}]i was significantly higher in patients with essential hypertension than in normotensive controls (141 ± 13 vs 126 ± 13 nmol/1; $P < 0.01$). In both groups, the maximal response to nifedipine occured between 15 and 30 min after its administration. However, hypertensive patients had a greater

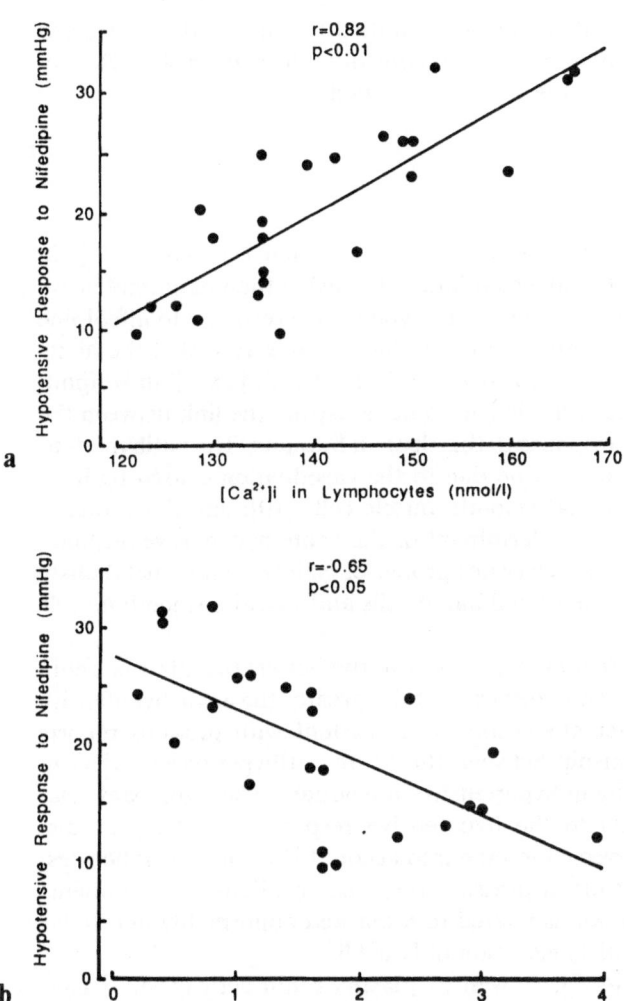

Fig. 1. The relation of [Ca^{2+}] in lymphocytes (**a**) and plasma renin activity (**b**) to the hypotensive response to nifedipine in patients with essential hypertension

fall in mean blood pressure following sublingual nifedipine, in comparison with controls (20 ± 7 vs 4 ± 3 mmHg; $P < 0.01$). Among patients with essential hypertension, [Ca^{2+}]i in lymphocytes was positively correlated with the hypotensive response to nifedipine (r = 0.82; $P < 0.01$) as shown in Fig. 1a. This response was also significantly correlated with plasma renin activity (r = −0.65; $P < 0.05$) (Fig. 1b), but not with age (r = 0.29), pretreatment mean blood pressure (r = 0.21), or plasma norepinephrine concentration (r = 0.31). A significant negative correlation was demonstrated between [Ca^{2+}]i and plasma renin activity (r = −0.66; $P < 0.01$) in hypertensive patients. The correlation between plasma renin activity and the response of mean blood pressure to nifedipine was nullified ($r = 0.12$) when corrected for $[Ca^{2+}]i$ in lymphocytes. In the normotensive controls, the hypotensive effect of nifedipine was not related to any of the variables studied.

Discussion

The results of this study confirmed our previous observation [1] that $[Ca^{2+}]i$ in lymphocytes was higher in patients with essential hypertension than in normotensive controls and the clinical report [4] that the acute hypotensive response to nifedipine was enhanced in the hypertensive patient. In addition, we observed that the acute hypotensive response to nifedipine was positively correlated with $[Ca^{2+}]i$ in lymphocytes. This study is the first, to our knowledge, to demonstrate the link between the index of cellular calcium and the response to this drug in humans. The antihypertensive effect of nifedipine is considered to be due to the vasodilation caused by inhibiting calcium inflow into the vascular smooth muscle cells [10]; and thus, altered calcium metabolism may be a major determinant of the acute hypotensive response to this drug. It seems likely that characteristics proper of cellular cation metabolism in some respects are shared by the nucleated blood cells and vascular smooth muscle cells.

We also observed that in essential hypertension the lower the plasma renin activity, the higher the $[Ca^{2+}]i$ in lymphocytes, and the greater the acute hypotensive response to nifedipine. The latter observation is consistent with previous reports [6, 7] showing a negative relationship between the acute antihypertensive effect of the drug and plasma renin activity in hypertensive individuals. The significant relationship of plasma renin activity to the hypotensive response to nifedipine disappeared when the data were corrected to take into account $[Ca^{2+}]i$ in lymphocytes. This suggests that the enhanced blood pressure response to nifedipine in patients with low-renin essential hypertension is related to a marked abnormality in cellular calcium metabolism, which results in elevation of $[Ca^{2+}]i$.

Pretreatment blood pressure [4, 5], as well as plasma renin activity [6, 7] have been reported to be clinical predictors of the acute blood pressure response to nifedipine. However, in the present study, pretreatment mean blood pressure was not significantly correlated with the hypotensive response to the drug. Our patients were relatively mild essential hypertensives with pretreatment diastolic blood pressures ranging between 90 and 110 mmHg, which were significantly lower than those of the previous reports [4, 5]. Magometshnigg [5] studied patients with a diastolic blood pressure between 120 and 160 mmHg, and MacGregor et al. [4], between 100 and 125 mmHg. It is possible that the narrow range of pretreatment blood pressure of hypertensive patients limited our ability to demonstrate the relation between pretreatment mean blood pressure and the response to nifedipine.

In summary, in patients with essential hypertension, the acute hypotensive response to nifedipine was greater than in normotensive controls, was positively linked with $[Ca^{2+}]i$ in lymphocytes, and negatively correlated with plasma renin activity. Thus, the acute fall in blood pressure after nifedipine administration may be associated with $[Ca^{2+}]i$. The link between plasma renin activity and the response to nifedipine may be mediated through modifications in $[Ca^{2+}]i$.

Acknowledgement. We are indebted to Miss Yuko Omura for her help in the preparation of this manuscript.

References

1. Oshima T, Matsuura H, Kido K, Matsumoto K, Fujii H, Masaoka S, Kajiyama G (1986) Abnormalities in intralymphocytic sodium and free calcium in essential hypertension: relation to plasma renin activity. J Hypertension 4 (Suppl VI): S334–S336
2. Erne P, Bolli P, Burgisser E, Buhler FR (1984) Correlation of platelet calcium with blood pressure: effect of antihypertensive therapy. N Engl J Med 310: 1084–1088
3. Postnov Y, Orlov SN, Shevchenko A, Adler AM (1977) Altered sodium permeability, calcium binding and Na-K ATPase activity in the red blood cell membrane in essential hypertension. Pflugers Arch 371: 263–269
4. MacGregor GA, Rotellar C, Markandu ND, Smith SJ, Sagnella GA (1982) Contrasting effects of nifedipine, captopril, and propranolol in normotensive and hypertensive subjects. J Cardiovasc Pharmacol 4 (Suppl III): 358–362   2
5. Magometshnigg D (1983) Acute hypotensive response to nifedipine. Hypertension 5 (Suppl II): II-80-84
6. Kiowski W, Bertel O, Erne P, Bolli P, Hulthen UL, Ritz R, Buhler FR (1983) Hemodynamic and reflex responses to acute and chronic antihypertensive therapy with the calcium entry blocker nifedipine. Hupertension 5 (Suppl I): 70–74
7. Resnick LM, Nicholson JP, Laragh JH (1987) Calcium, the renin-aldosterone system, and the hypotensive response to nifedipine. Hypertension 10: 254–258
8. Oshima T, Matsuura H, Matsumoto K, Kido K, Fujii H, Kajiyama G (1987) Role of cellular Ca^{2+} in salt sensitivity of patients with essential hypertension. (abstract) Hypertension 10: 367
9. Oshima T, Matsuura H, Kido K, Matsumoto K, Otsuki T, Fujii H, Masaoka S, Okamato M, Tsuchioka Y, Kajiyama G, Tsubokura T (1987) Intralymphocytic sodium and free calcium concentration in relation to salt sensitivity in patients with essential hypertension. Jpn Circ J 56: 1184–1190
10. Vanhoutte PM (1985) Calcium-entry blockers, vascular smooth muscle and systemic hypertension. Am J Cardiol 55: B17–B23

Determinants of the Hypotensive Action of Nitrendipine and Atenolol in African Black Patients

P. Lijnen[1], J.R. M'Buyamba-Kabangu[2], B. Lepira[2], R. Fagard[1], and A. Amery[1]

Summary. Thirty-five hypertensive black patients were double-blindly randomized to receive for 6 weeks either 100 mg atenolol per day ($n = 17$) or 20 mg nitrendipine daily ($n = 18$). Atenolol and nitrendipine significantly reduced blood pressure ($P < 0.05$ or less); however, the magnitude of the decrease in supine systolic (-25.0 ± 13 vs -10 ± 18 mmHg) and diastolic (-15.7 ± 8.5 vs -6.5 ± 11.2 mmHg) pressure, and in standing diastolic pressure (-17.6 ± 9.8 vs -7.8 ± 13.0 mmHg) was more pronounced ($P < 0.05$ or less) in the nitrendipine than in the atenolol group. Satisfactory control of blood pressure was obtained in 9 of the atenolol treated patients, and in 17 patients who received nitrendipine ($P = 0.016$). Pulse rate ($P < 0.05$ or less), plasma aldosterone ($P < 0.05$), and plasma renin activity ($P = 0.09$) decreased with atenolol, whereas no significant change occurred with nitrendipine. Pulse rate and plasma renin activity were lower ($P < 0.05$ or less) in the atenolol than in the nitrendipine group at the end of the study. Neither of the drugs significantly affected the red blood cell concentrations of sodium and potassium, the ouabain-sensitive efflux of sodium, or the other biochemical measurements.

In multiple regression analysis, the changes in supine systolic and diastolic pressure during nitrendipine were independently and negatively correlated with the patient's age and initial blood pressure, and positively correlated with the change in supine pulse rate. The change in supine systolic pressure was also negatively correlated with initial erythrocyte sodium concentration.

The results indicate that nitrendipine was more efficient than atenolol in the hypertensive blacks entered in this study and suggest that besides older age and higher pretreatment blood pressure level, a higher intracellular sodium concentration could predict a greater response to nitrendipine.

Key words: Atenolol — Nitrendipine — Erythrocyte sodium — Hypertension — Blacks

Introduction

In black as well as in white populations, various abnormalities of circulating blood cells sodium and potassium concentrations and transport systems have been described in patients with essential hypertension [1]. A dissociation between these

[1] Hypertension and Cardiovascular Rehabilitation Unit, University of Leuven, Leuven, Belgium
[2] Service de Endocrinology and Cardio-Renal Disease, Department of Internal Medicine, University of Kinshasa, Kinshasa, Zaïre

abnormalities and high blood pressure has been shown, however, by demonstrating similar anomalies in still normotensive subjects. Heagerty et al. [2] have therefore proposed to consider such abnormalities in hypertensive patients as simply markers of altered membrane handling of calcium. Raised intracellular-free calcium has indeed been found in various cells of hypertensive patients [3–5]. In the smooth muscle, cytosolic-free calcium appears to be the final determinant of arterial tone, hence, of blood pressure level [6, 7].

Antihypertensive treatment with calcium entry blockers [5, 8, 9] or beta-adrenoceptor blockers [8] was reported to decrease intracellular calcium in the red cells or the platelets from white hypertensive patients while lowering arterial blood pressure. The effect of these drugs on cellular sodium concentration and transport in white hypertensive patients has been controversial [10–12]. In view of the difference in cellular sodium and potassium concentration and transport between blacks and whites [13, 14], racial factors could modulate the effect of antihypertensive treatment on cellular sodium metabolism. Therefore, the present work sought to evaluate the clinical effects of atenolol and nitrendipine in hypertensive black patients, to examine the action of the two drugs on cellular sodium and potassium concentration and fluxes using the red blood cell model, and to investigate the relationship between the change in pressure with the two drugs and these red blood cell cationic variables.

Methods

Patients

Thirty-five Zairian hypertensive patients (18 men and 17 women) gave informed consent and participated in the current study. All had probable essential hypertension on the basis of history, physical examination, serum electrolytes, and urinalysis; but further specific investigations for secondary forms of hypertension were not performed. Sixteen patients had received no previous antihypertensive therapy, whereas 19 patients had been treated for an average of 3.8 years prior to entering the preliminary period in this study. None of the patients were stabilized by their previous therapy.

In all patients, serum creatinine was below 2 mg% and serum bilirubine was 1.5 mg% or less. No patient had cardiac failure, history of or impending sequelae of cerebrovascular accident, nor other significant organ damage as a result of hypertension. Other exclusion criteria included insulin-requiring diabetes mellitus, chronic obstructive respiratory disease, second and third degree atrioventricular block, and pregnancy.

Study Design

A double-blind parallel design with a double-dummy technique was used. The patients were randomized to receive for 6 weeks either atenolol (100 mg) or nitrendipine (20 mg) once a day and were seen at the outpatient clinics after 2 and 6 weeks of therapy. This active treatment period was preceded by a 6-week preliminary period during which the patients attended outpatient clinics at 3-week intervals and received, single-blindly, 2 placebo tablets each morning. At each examination, whether on placebo or active medication, 3 blood pressure readings were obtained with a standard mercury sphygmomanometer after 3 min relaxation in supine position and after 2 min standing upright. Korotkoff sounds I and V were used to characterize systolic and diastolic pressures, respectively. Pulse rate was measured under the same conditions. Body weight was measured in loose clothing without shoes, whereas height was obtained once, during the preliminary period. All measurements were performed 3–5 h after the morning dose. Compliance with therapy was assessed by tablet count and one of the investigators administered a questionnaire inquiring about complaints.

Additional Procedures

At randomization, a chest x-ray and a 12-lead ECG were obtained. A blood sample was drawn from an antecubital vein for blood cell count and determination of hemoglobin, hematocrit, serum electrolytes, creatinine, transaminases, uric acid, plasma glucose, renin activity [15], aldosterone concentration [16], the erythrocyte concentration of sodium and potassium, and the ouabain-sensitive efflux of sodium [17]. A 24-h urine collection was obtained from 17 patients (9 in the atenolol and 8 in the nitrendipine group) and was analyzed for sodium excretion.

At the end of the study, a second blood sample for the same hematological and biochemical measurements could be obtained from only 18 patients (8 on atenolol and 10 on nitrendipine) who first entered the study. These patients did not differ from the group as a whole.

Statistical Analysis

Statistic methods included paired and unpaired Student's t-tests, chi-squared test, and single and multiple regression analyses. Values are expressed as the means ± standard deviation (SD). Since the distribution of plasma renin activity and plasma aldosterone concentration were positively skewed, logarithmic transformation was applied. Therefore, geometric means and range are reported for these variables.

Individual blood pressure responses were graded in reference to predetermined, ideal response lines [18] according to initial supine diastolic pressure as follows:
1. Excelent — iDBP > 100 mmHg and final supine diastolic pressure < 90 mmHg or iDBP < 100 mmHg and a fall in supine diastolic pressure > 10 mmHg
2. Unsatisfactory — iDBP > 105 mmHg and final supine DBP > 100 mmHg or iDBP < 105 mmHg and a fall in DBP < 5 mmHg
3. Satisfactory — a response intermediate to excellent and unsatisfactory

Left ventricular hypertrophy was defined as a Romhit Estes score of 5 points or more on ECG.

Table 1. Characteristics of the patients at randomization

	Atenolol group	Nitrendipine group
Males (n)	9	9
Females (n)	8	9
Age (years)	43 ± 7	46 ± 13
Height (cm)	164 ± 13	163 ± 8
Weight (kg)	74 ± 15	69 ± 15
Supine blood pressure (mmHg)	162 ± 8	162 ± 15
	102 ± 4	103 ± 8
Standing blood pressure (mmHg)	157 ± 9	159 ± 16
	102 ± 4	102 ± 8
Supine pulse rate (beats/min)	73 ± 11	78 ± 10
Standing pulse rate (beats/min)	81 ± 13	83 ± 9
Serum creatinine (mg%)	1.03 ± 0.27	1.26 ± 0.77
Plasma renin activity (ng A_1/ml per h)[a]	0.54	0.54
	(0.14–1.49)	(0.01–2.01)
Plasma aldosterone concentration (ng%)[a]	20.0	15.5
	(11.2–40.7)	(8.9–25.1)
Urinary sodium (mmol/24 h)[b]	84 ± 29	92 ± 36
Cardiothoracic ratio	0.48 ± 0.04	0.46 ± 0.04
Left ventricular hypertrophy on ECG (n)	4	2

Values given are arithmetic mean ± SD.
[a] Geometric mean and range in parenthesis.
[b] Determined in 9 patients from atenolol group and in 8 patients from nitrendipine group.

Results

Patient Characteristics at Randomization

At randomization no significant diference was observed between the two treatment groups (Table 1).

Clinical Effects of Both Groups

All randomized patients completed the double-blind study. After 6 weeks of active therapy, supine and standing systolic and diastolic pressures were significantly reduced in the atenolol-($P < 0.05$) and in the nitrendipine-($P < 0.001$) treated patients. The hypotensive effect was more pronounced in the nitrendipine than in the atenolol group (Fig. 1), the difference being significant ($P < 0.05$ or less) for supine systolic ($-25 ± 13$ vs $-10 ± 18$ mmHg) and diastolic ($-15.7 ± 8.5$ vs $-6.5 ± 11.2$ mmHg) pressure, and for standing diastolic pressure ($-17.6 ± 9.8$ vs $-7.8 ± 13.0$ mmHg). The individual response to therapy was excellent, satisfactory, or unsatisfactory in respectively 4, 5, and 8 atenolol-treated patients and in 9, 8, and 1 patients who were given nitrendipine. The number of patients with at least a satis-

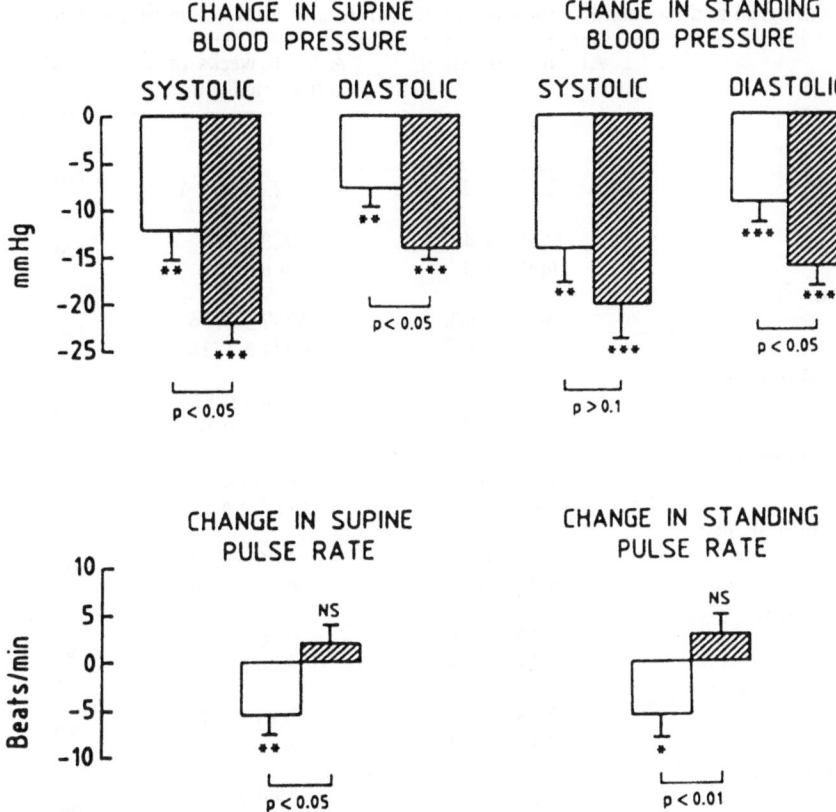

Fig. 1. Changes in blood pressure and pulse rate (means ± SE) after 6-week administration of atenolol (□) or nitrendipine (▨). The symbols * $P < 0.05$, ** $P < 0.01$, ***$P < 0.001$, and *NS* (not significant) give the significance of within group comparison; the indicated P-value compares both treatment groups

factory response to therapy was greater in the nitrendipine than in the atenolol group (17 vs 9 patients) ($X^2 = 5.86$; $P = 0.016$).

Atenolol induced a significant fall in supine (-5.6 ± 7.0 beats per min [bpm]; $P < 0.01$) and standing (-5.5 ± 9.3 bpm; $P < 0.05$) pulse rates, whereas a slight and not significant acceleration of 2.0 ± 6.0 bpm in supine and 3.0 ± 9.0 bpm in standing pulse rate occurred with nitrendipine (Fig. 1). Body weight was unchanged in the the two groups at the end of active treatment.

Effects of Therapy on Red Blood Cell, Electrolyte, and Other Laboratory Measurements

In 8 atenolol- and 10 nitrendipine-treated patients, biochemical measurements were obtained at baseline and at the end of active treatment (Table 2). The 2 subgroups were comparable for blood pressure and demographic data at baseline. After 6

Table 2. Hematological and biochemical measurements before and after active medication

	At randomization	After 6 weeks of active medication	P^b
Hemoglobin (%)			
A	12.2 ± 1.3		
N	12.7 ± 1.8	12.6 ± 1.5	NS
Hematocrit (%)			
A	36.8 ± 4.4	36.8 ± 4.3	
N	34.0 ± 1.9	34.8 ± 2.6	NS
Leucocytes (mm^{-3})			
A	6393 ± 1778	6737 ± 1756	
N	6042 ± 1472	6321 ± 1216	NS
Serum creatinine (mg%)			
A	1.03 ± 0.27	1.08 ± 0.17	
N	1.26 ± 0.77	0.88 ± 0.24	NS
Serum sodium (mmol/l)			
A	141.4 ± 3.6	140.0 ± 4.5	
N	143.5 ± 2.3	141.5 ± 4.3	NS
Serum potassium (mmol%)			
A	4.33 ± 0.36	4.06 ± 0.52	
N	4.35 ± 0.45	4.13 ± 0.28	NS
Serum calcium (mg%)			
A	9.00 ± 0.56	9.10 ± 0.64	
N	8.87 ± 1.04	9.20 ± 0.37	NS
Serum phosphorus (mg%)			
A	3.03 ± 0.13	3.15 ± 0.32	
N	3.17 ± 0.31	2.82 ± 0.75	NS
Serum protein (mEq/l)			
A	18.2 ± 1.6	18.4 ± 2.1	
N	18.4 ± 1.5	18.6 ± 1.1	NS
Serum SGOT (V/l)			
A	7.3 ± 1.1	7.9 ± 2.2	
N	15.8 ± 14.2	16.2 ± 11.8	NS
Serum SGPT (V/l)			
A	5.6 ± 1.8	5.4 ± 2.7	
N	5.8 ± 6.3	7.6 ± 3.4	NS
Plasma glucose (mg%)			
A	76.0 ± 4.8	75.1 ± 9.2	
N	86.8 ± 16.4	77.6 ± 8.7	NS
Plasma uric acid (mg%)			
A	4.45 ± 0.75	6.12 ± 1.54	
N	4.90 ± 1.19	5.32 ± 1.03	NS
Erythrocyte sodium concentration (mmol/l cells)			
A	12.70 ± 4.09	12.30 ± 4.25	
N	11.20 ± 2.64	11.02 ± 1.91	NS
Erythrocyte potassium concentration (mmol/l cells)			
A	90.82 ± 8.25	86.39 ± 3.50	
N	84.47 ± 4.18	83.94 ± 1.64	NS
Ouabain-sensitive sodium efflux (μmol/l cells per h)			
A	1.35 ± 0.43	1.40 ± 0.26	
N	1.39 ± 0.53	1.46 ± 0.69	NS

(*Table continued on the following page*)

Table 2. (*continued*)

	At randomization	After 6 weeks of active medication	P^b
Plasma renin activity (ng AI/ml per h)[a]			
A	0.54	0.49	
	(0.14–1.49)	(0.16–1.31)	
N	0.54	1.68	<0.01
	(0.01–2.01)	(0.76–7.56)	
Plasma aldosterone (ng%)			
A	21.1	14.7	
	(11.2–40.7)	(9.0–22.9)	
N	15.7	17.5	<0.01
	(8.9–25.1)	(11.0–33.9)	

A, atenolol group; N, nitrendipine group
Values given are arithmetic mean ± SD.
[a] Geometric mean and range in parentheses.
[b] *P*-value for between group comparison after 6 weeks of active medication.

weeks of administration of atenolol, plasma renin activity tended to decrease ($P = 0.09$), whereas an opposite trend was seen in the nitrendipine-treated subgroup. The difference between the two treatment groups was significant ($P < 0.01$). Plasma aldosterone concentration decreased ($P < 0.05$) in the atenolol group, whereas no change ($P < 0.10$) occurred in the nitrendipine group. Atenolol or nitrendipine did not affect serum electrolytes, creatinine, proteins, transaminases, plasma glucose, uric acid, the erythrocyte concentrations of sodium and potassium, or the ouabain-sensitive efflux of sodium. Blood hemoglobin, hematocrit, and white cell count were unchanged in both groups after active treatment.

Regression Analysis

Using single regression analysis, the nitrendipine- (but not the atenolol-) induced changes in supine systolic and diastolic ($r = -0.58$; $P < 0.05$) blood pressure (Fig. 2) were correlated negatively with age and positively with the pretreatment plasma renin activity ($r = 0.71$; $P < 0.05$) (Fig. 3). No significant relationships were observed between the nitrendipine- or the atenolol- induced changes in blood pressure and the erythrocyte concentrations of sodium or potassium.

Multiple regression analysis (Table 3) demonstrated a significant inverse relationship between the pretrial concentrations of erythrocyte sodium and the change in supine systolic pressure which was independent of age, initial supine systolic blood pressure, and change in pulse rate during nitrendipine therapy. Also, in the nitrendipine group, age and the change in supine pulse rate yielded significant partial regression coefficients with the change in supine diastolic pressure after adjusting for initial diastolic blood pressure. No combination of two or more independent variables yielded significant partial regression coefficients with the atenolol-induced changes in systolic or diastolic pressure.

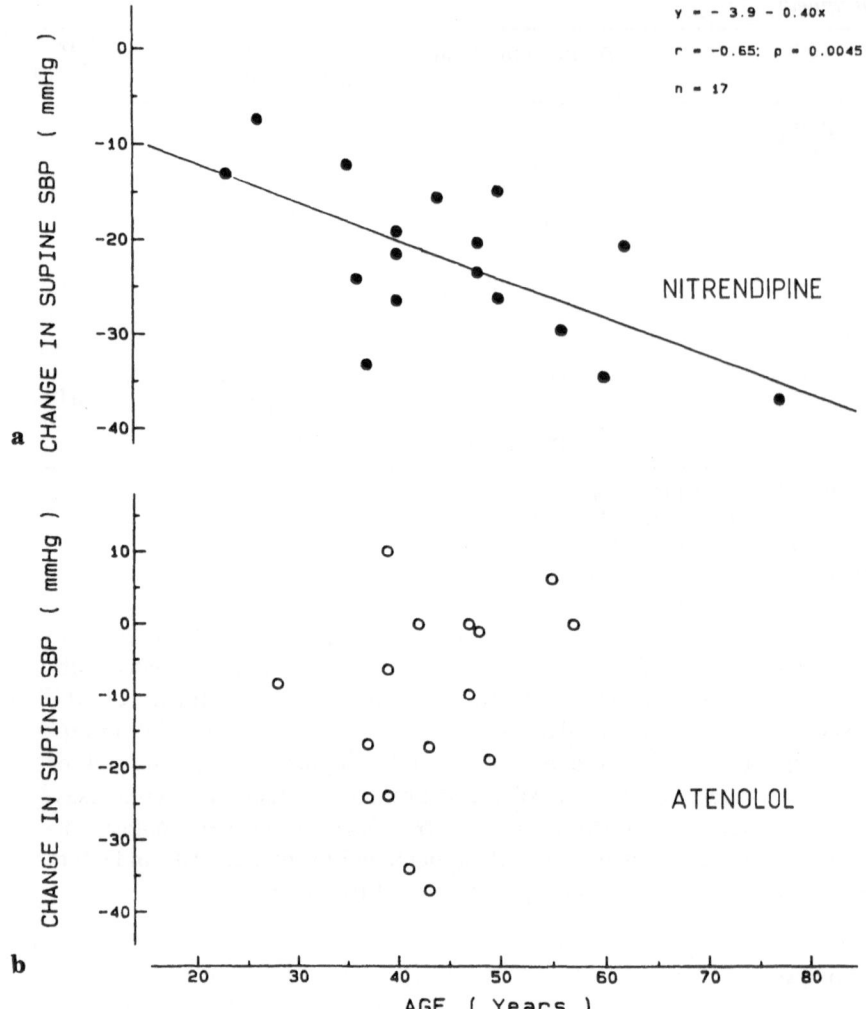

$y = -3.9 - 0.40x$

$r = -0.65; \ p = 0.0045$

$n = 17$

NITRENDIPINE

ATENOLOL

Fig. 2a, b. Relationship between the change in supine diastolic blood pressure (*DBP*) and *age* in the nitrendipine (**a**) and in the atenolol (**b**) groups

Complaints

In Table 4 the complaints at randomization and those which newly occurred or were aggravated during active treatment are listed. During the preliminary period as well as during active medication, few complaints were voiced with most complaints being as frequent in the atenolol as in the nitrendipine group. Numbness of the legs occurred only in the atenolol-treated patients, whereas palpitations were observed only in those who received nitrendipine.

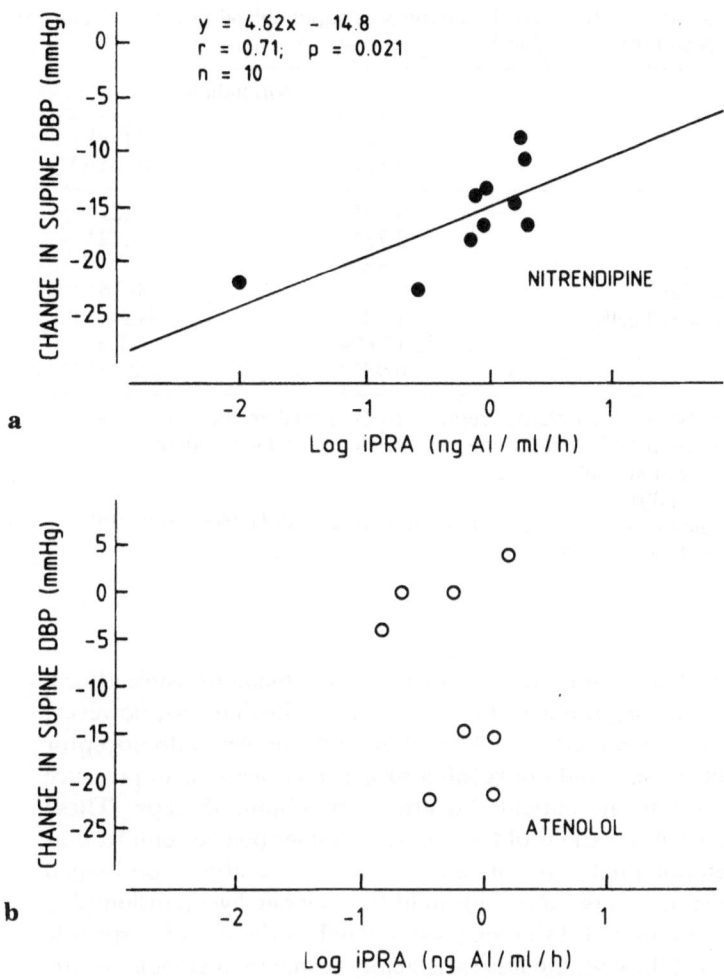

Fig. 3a, b. Relationship between the change in supine diastolic blood pressure (*DBP*) and the initial plasma renin activity (*iPRA*) in the nitrendipine (**a**) and in the atenolol (**b**) groups

Discussion

Black subjects and black hypertensive patients are characterized by low plasma renin activity and a high intracellular sodium concentration. Low plasma renin activity [19] and high intracellular sodium concentration in hypertensive patients [2] have both been proposed as reflective of increased levels of intracellular calcium. The purpose of the present study was therefore to assess and compare the hypotensive action of atenolol and nitrendipine monotherapy in hypertensive African black patients and to investigate its relationship to plasma renin activity and intracellular sodium concentration in this population. The importance of age and other variables as determinants of the anti-hypertensive effect of both drugs were also examined.

Table 3. Partial regression coefficients between the changes in supine blood pressure after 6 weeks of active medication and other variables[a]

	Nitrendipine	
	△SBP (mmHg)	△DBP (mmHg)
Age (years)	−0.18*	−0.21***
Change in pulse rate (bpm)	0.72**	0.22*
Initial systolic pressure (mmHg)	−0.82***	—
Initial diastolic pressure (mmHg)	—	−0.76***
Initial erythrocyte sodium (mmol/l cells)	−1.33	NS
Constant	129.04	71.6
r	0.98**	0.97***

[a] Besides the variables listed above, initial plasma renin activity, initial erythrocyte potassium concentration, and the change in body weight were also included as independent variables in the multiple regression analysis.
*$P < 0.05$; **$P < 0.01$; ***$P < 0.001$
—, variable not entered in the analysis; △SBP, change in supine systolic blood pressure; △DBP, change in supine diastolic pressure

Nitrendipine and atenolol both induced a significant fall in blood pressure after 6 weeks of administration. The magnitude of blood pressure reduction was, however, more pronounced with the calcium entry blocker than with the beta-adrenoceptor blocker. About half of the patients did not reach a satisfactory decrease in pressure after atenolol, whereas all but one patient did after nitrendipine therapy. These results confirm our previous observations of the relatively higher potency of nitrendipine as compared to acebutolol both after a short-term [20] and after a prolonged 40-week follow-up of black natives of Zaïre with mild to moderate hypertension [21]. It is thus unlikely that the reported difference was related to the use of a specific beta-adrenoceptor blocker. Likewise, the less satisfactory response to atenolol in the present study agrees with the well-documented, poor efficacy of various beta-adrenoceptor blocking agents in hypertensive blacks when used as monotherapy [22–26] . In contrast to the current findings, one study [27] recently reported similar blood pressure reduction after acute oral administration of atenolol (100 mg) and slow-release nifedipine in South African blacks who had malignant hypertension and high plasma renin activity which could have modulated the antihypertensive response to the administered drugs. It has certainly been shown that for beta-adrenoceptor blockers, efficiency increases the higher the renin activity, whereas the opposite is true for calcium entry-blocking agents [28]. Although no correlation was demonstrated in the present study between the change in blood pressure (after nitrendipine) and initial plasma renin activity, the latter was low given the low average urinary-sodium excretion.

In multiple regression analysis, the change in pressure after nitrendipine was independently and negatively related to age and initial erythrocyte sodium concentration, and positively correlated to changes in pulse rate. This suggests a greater fall of pres-

Table 4. Complaints during placebo and active treatment[a]

	At randomization		During active treatment	
	A	N	A	N
Total number of subjects	17	18	17	18
Patients without complaints	6	5	9	12
Patients with complaints	11	13	8	6
Patients with specific complaints				
Headache	2	1	1	3
Dizziness	3	3	2	1
Insomnia	2	6	3	1
Numbness	1	0	3	0
Palpitation	2	1	0	2
Weakness	3	2	1	1
Constipation	0	0	1	1

No significant difference was observed between the groups for any complaint.
[a] Only complaints newly occurring or aggravated during the active treatment are listed.
A, atenolol group; N, nitrendipine group

sure in older patients and those with higher intracellular sodim concentration but only a small blood pressure reduction in the patients reacting to nitrendipine with marked tachycardia. Several investigators have shown a similar relationship between the effectiveness of nitrendipine [21, 29] or other calcium entry blockers [30] and age. This relationship has been supported by the high response rate to nitrendipine among elderly patients aged 66–83 years treated for 6 months with 10–20 mg daily [31]; control of blood pressure was achieved in 89% of the series. In one study, however [32], the hypotensive effect of nitrendipine appeared to be greater in younger than in older patients. The lack of correlation between age and the atenolol-induced changes in blood pressure could be due to the narrower age-range of the patients randomized to atenolol in the present study.

It appears of particular interest that the relationship of the hypotensive response to nitrendipine with the initial erythrocyte concentration of sodium has been independent of other factors since possible interrelationships between intracellular sodium concentration, plasma renin activity, age, and pretreatment blood pressure could have been invoked.

The relationship between the hypotensive effect of a calcium entry blocker and the pretreatment level of intracellular sodium concentration can be understood on the assumption that high intracellular sodium in hypertensive patients might be linked to increased cellular-free calcium. Although intracellular calcium has not been measured in the present work, it was reported to be elevated in the red blood cells [5] and in the platelets of hypertensive patients [3 4]. A hypothesis has been put forward that elevated intracellular sodium concentration stimulates a sodium-calcium exchange across cell membrane by which the level of intracellular calcium is raised [33]. Calcium entry blockers act at least partly by inhibiting the calcium influx into the cell [34] leading to reduction in intrecellular calcium activity [5] or concentration

[3, 9]. The antihypertensive response to the calcium entry blocker, nitrendipine, was shown to parallel the decreases in cellular-free calcium concentration [8]. It appears of particular interest that the relationship of the hypotensive action of nitrendipine with the initial intracellular sodium concentration has been independent of other factors, since possible interrelationships of the erythrocyte sodium, plasma renin activity, age, and/or pretreatment blood pressure cold have been invoked.

Nonetheless, in the present study, neither atenolol nor nitrendipine affected the red blood cell sodium concentration. Likewise, in normotensive male volunteers given felodipine, the red blood cell sodium concentration remained unchanged [35]. Thus, the reduction in intracellular calcium after calcium entry blockade or beta-adrenoceptor blockade, if any, in the red blood cells, must occur through pathways not involving a change in intraerythrocyte sodium. In the current study, the ouabain-sensitive sodium efflux, an estimate of the sodium pump activity, was unaltered after nitrendipine or atenolol. Other pathways for sodium transport were not investigated however. Ambrosioni et al. [10] also found no change in intracellular sodium content of lymphocytes from hypertensive patients treated with beta-adrenoceptor blockers. However, conflicting results have been reported for the leucocyte sodium of hypertensive patients treated with calcium entry blockers. Using oral nifedipine, a significant fall in blood pressre was observed with unchanged leucocyte sodium concentration [11]. The authors concluded that treatment with calcium entry blockers does not correct a fundamental alteration of sodium-calcium exchange across the cell membrane. By contrast, a significant decrease in the leucocyte sodium concentration was seen after verapamil hydrochloride [12]; the authors could not ascertain whether this resulted from a direct effect of the drug on the cell.

A decrease in pulse rate after atenolol and no significant change after short-term and long-term dihydropyridine-derived calcium entry blocker are well-documented observations. The absence of acceleration in pulse rate by a drug with arterial vasodilator properties is suggestive of a resetting of baroreceptors. In such a context, the positive and independent correlation between the change in pressure after nitrendipine and change in pulse rate indicates that the reflex-sympathetic activation in a particular patient co-determines the degree of antihypertensive response. The reflex-sympathetic stimulation was also reflected by the observed trend of increase in plasma renin activity after nitrendipine. This did not, however, reach a statistical significance.

It was concluded that calcium entry blockade with nitrendipine was more efficient in reducing blood pressure than beta-adrenoceptor blockade with atenolol in the hypertensive blacks entered in this trial. The effectiveness of calcium entry blockade was more pronounced in older patients or in those with high pretreatment blood pressure levels or intracellular sodium concentrations. The patients in whom sympathetic reactivity was less blunted had the lowest response.

Acknowledgements. The authors gratefully acknowledge the technical help of Miss G. Lommelen, Y. Piccart, and Mr. K. Ipala and thank Mrs. Y. Toremans for secretarial help. Serum variables were determined in the St. Rafaël-Gasthuisberg Hospital Central Laboratory under the supervision of Dr. W. Lissens. Nitrendipine and matching placebo tablets and atenolol and matching placebo tablets were kindly supplied by Bayer and ICI, respectively. The research in this laboratory is partly supported by a grant from the N..F.W.O.

References

1. Hilton PJ (1986) Cellular sodium transport in essential hypertension. N Engl J Med 314: 222–229
2. Heagerty AM, Milner M, Bing RF, Thurston H, Swales JD (1982) Leucocyte membrane sodium transport in normotensive populations: dissociation of abnormalities of sodium efflux from raised blood pressure. Lancet 2: 894–896
3. Erne P, Bolli P, Bürgisser E, Bühler FR (1984) Correlation of platelet calcium with blood pressure. Effect of antihypertensive therapy. N Engl J Med 310: 1084–1088
4. Bruschi G, Bruschi ME, Caroppo M, Orlandini G, Spaggiari M, Cavatorta A (1985) Cytoplasmic free- (Ca^{2+}) is increased in the platelets of spontaneously hypertensive rats and essential hypertensive patients. Clin Sci 68: 179–184
5. Zidek W, Losse H, Vetter H (1982) Effect of nifedipine on blood pressure and on intracellular calcium in arterial hypertension. J Cardiovasc Pharmacol 4: S303–S305
6. Jones AW (1974) Altered ion transport in large and small arteries from spontaneously hypertensive rats and influence of calcium. Circ Res 34: S117–S122
7. Orlov SN, Postnov YV (1982) Ca^{2+} binding and membrane fluidity in essential and renal hypertension. Clin Sci 63: 218–224
8. Bolli P, Erne P, Hulthen UL, Ritz R, Kiowski W, Ji BH, Bühler FR (1984) Parallel reduction of calcium-influx-dependent vasoconstriction and platelet-free calcium concentration with calcium entry and β-adrenoceptor blockade. J Cardiovasc Pharmacol 6: S996–S1001
9. Haller H, Lenz T, Lüdersdorf M, Distler A, Philipp TH (1985) Changes in free intracellular calcium after nifedipine in patients with essential hypertension. (Abstract) J Hypertension 3: 410
10. Ambrosioni E, Costa FV, Montebugnoli L, Cavalliini C, Magnami B (1981) Effects of antihypertensive therapy on intralymphocytic sodium content. Drugs Exp Clin Res 7: 757
11. Heagerty AM, Bing RF, Thurston H, Swales JD (1983) Calcium antagonists in hypertension: relation to abnormal sodium transport. Br Med J 287: 1405–1407
12. Poston L, Gray HH, Crowther A, Dittrich HC, Hilton PJ, Webb-Peploe MM, MacGregor GA (1984) Cellular sodium concentration and vasoconstrictor state in hypertension. J Cardiovasc Pharmacol 6: S16–S20
13. M'Buyamba-Kabangu JR, Lijnen P, Groeseneken D, Staessen J, Lissens W, Goossens W, Fagard R, Amery A (1984) Racial differences in intracellular concentration and transmembrane fluxes of sodium and potassium in erythrocytes of normal male subjects. J Hypertens 2: 647–651
14. Weder AB, Torretti BA, Julius S (1984) Racial differences in erythrocyte cation transport. Hypertension 6: 115–123
15. Fyhrquist F, Puutula L (1978) Faster radioimmunoassay of angiotensin I at 37°C. Clin Chem 24: 115–118
16. Lijnen P, Amery A, Fagard R, Corvol P (1978) Direct radio-immunoassay of plasma aldosterone in normal subjects. Clin Chim Acta 84: 305–314
17. Lijnen P, Hespel P, Lommelen G, Laermans M, M'Buyamba-Kabangu JR, Amery A (1986) Intracellular sodium, potassium and magnesium concentration, ouabain-sensitive ^{86}rubidium-uptake and sodium efflux and Na^+, K^+ -contrasport activity in erythrocytes of normal male subjects studied in two occasions. Methods Find Exp Clin Pharmacol 8: 525–533
18. Walker BR, Shah RS, Ramanathan RB, Vanov SK, Helfant RH (1977) Guanabenz and methyldopa on hypertension and cardiac performance. Clin Pharmacol Ther 22: 868–874
19. Resnick LM, Laragh JH, Sealey JE, Alderman MH (1983) Divalent cations in essential hypertension. Relation between serum ionized calcium, magnesium and plasma renin activity. N Engl J Med 309: 888–891
20. M'Buyamba-Kabangu JR, Lepira B, Fagard R, Lijnen P, Ditu M, Tshiani KA, Amery A (1986) Relative potency of a beta-blocking and calcium entry blocking agent as antihypertensive drugs in black patients. Eur J Clin Pharmacol 29: 523–527

21. M'Buyamba-Kabangu JR, Fagard R, Lijnen P, Staessen J, Lissens W, Ditu M, Lepira B, Tshiani KA, Amery A (1987) Calcium entry blockade or β-blockade in long-term management of hypertension in blacks. Clin Pharmacol Ther 41: 45–54
22. Abson CP, Levy LA, Eyhcrabidi (1981) Once-daily atenolol in hypertensive Zimbabwean blacks. S Afr Med J 60: 47–48
23. Odia OJ, Cole TO (1986) Evaluation of a single daily dose of acebutolol 400 mg in the treatment of Nigerian hypertensives. Curr Ther Res 40: 680–684
24. Salako LA, Falase AO, Ragon A, Adio RA (1979) Beta-adrenoceptor blocking effects and pharmacokinetics of pindolol. A study in hypertensive Africans. Eur J Clin Pharmacol 15: 299–304
25. Seedat YK (1980) Trial of atenolol and chlorthalidone for hypertension in black South Africans. Br Med J 281: 1241–1243
26. Veterans Administration Cooperative Study Group on Antihypertensive Agents (1983) Efficacy of nadolol alone and combined with bendroflumethiazide and hydralazine for systemic hypertension. Am J Cardiol 52: 1230–1237
27. Isles CG, Johnson AOC, Milne FJ (1986) Slow release nifedipine and atenolol as initial treatment in blacks with malignant hypertension. Br J Clin Pharmacol 21: 377–383
28. Bühler FR (1983) Age and cardiovascular response adaptation. Determinants of an anti-hypertensive treatment concept primarily based on beta-blockers and calcium entry blockers. Hypertension 5 (Suppl III): 94–100
29. Müller FB, Bolli P, Erne P, Block LH, Kiowski W, Bühler FR (1984) Antihypertensive therapy with the long-acting calcium antagonist nitrendipine. J Cardiovasc Pharmacol 6: S1073–S1076
30. Bühler FR, Hulthen UL, Kiowski W, Bolli P (1982) Greater antihypertensive efficacy of the calcium channel inhibitor verapamil in older and low renin patients. Clin Sci 63: S439–S442
31. Tourkantonis A, Lasaridis A, Settas L (1984) Clinical experience with long-term nitren-dipine treatment in essential hypertension. J Cadiovasc Pharmacol 6: S1090–S1095
32. Ferrara LA, Fasano ML, Soro S (1985) Age-related antihypertensive effect of nitren-dipine, a new calcium entry blocking agent. Eur J Clin Pharmacol 28: 373–374
33. Blaustein MP (1980) How does sodium cause hypertension? A hypothesis. In: Zumkely H, Losse H (eds) Intracellular electrolytes and arterial hypertension. Thieme, Stuttgart, pp 151–157
34. Golenhofen K (1981) Differentiation of calcium activation processes in smooth muscle using selective antagonists. In: Bulbring E, Brading AF, Jones AW, Tomit T (eds) Smooth muscle: an assessment of current knowledge. Edward Arnold, London, pp 157–170
35. Hespel P, Lijnen P, Fiocchi R, Lissens W, Amery A (1986) Effect of calcium antagonism on intracellular concentrations and transmembrane fluxes of cations in erythrocytes of men at rest and during exercise. J Hypertens 4: 767–772

The Role of Renal Calcium Handling in the Hypotensive Response to Long-Term Nifedipine Administration in Essential Hypertensives

AKIHIKO NOZAWA, KENJIRO KIKUCHI, TOHRU HASEGAWA, HIROAKI KOMURA, SHINICHIRO SUZUKI, NAOTOSHI SATO, TOHRU OHTOMO, TAMAKI TAKADA, and OSAMU IIMURA[1]

Summary. This study was conducted in order to elucidate the significance of renal calcium handling in the hypotensive response to long-term nifedipine (Nif) (60 mg daily, t.i.d., for 4 weeks) therapy in 10 inpatients with mild to moderate essential hypertension (EHT).
  Single oral administration of Nif (20 mg) caused a rapid reduction of mean arterial pressure (MAP), and an enhancement of natriuresis as well as calciuria. Nif therapy for 1–4 weeks resulted in decreases of MAP and parathyroid hormone (PTH), while no significant change was observed in plasma ionized calcium (pCa^{2+}). Sustained increases in calciuria and a similar tendency in natriuresis were found 1 week after Nif therapy. Following 4 weeks of Nif therapy, pronounced calciuria continued, whereas natriuresis returned to the basal level. A significantly positive correlation between natriuresis and calciuria was recognized after single oral administration of Nif. This correlation, however, disapppeared following long-term Nif therapy. On the other hand, the calciuretic response negatively correlated with basal pCa^{2+} and the change in MAP following long-term Nif therapy.

Key words: Essential hypertension — Nifedipine — Natriuresis — Calciuria — Parathyroid hormone

Introduction

It has been proposed that an abnormality of calcium metabolism may play an important hypertensive role in essential hypertension. Epidemiologic studies suggest that dietary calcium deficiency and sodium overload may correlate with hypertension [1–3]. It has also been pointed out that renal calcium handling is closely related with sodium metabolism in the kidney [4]. It is less clear, however, how body calcium balance or renal calcium metabolism may contribute to the hypertensive mechanism. Recently, calcium antagonists have been widely used as potent antihypertensive agents in hypertensive patients. Therefore, the present study was performed to elucidate the significance of renal calcium handling in the antihypertensive response to long-term administration of the calcium antagonist, Nif, in patients with EHT.

[1] The 2nd Department of Internal Medicine, Sapporo Medical College, Sapporo, Japan

Materials and Methods

Ten mild-to-moderate EHT participated in this study. They were admitted to our hospital and received a fixed diet inlcuding 120 mEq of sodium, 75 mEq of potassium and 600 mg of calcium daily. Studies started in the early morning of the 14th day of hospitalization after overnight fasting. The patients were kept in the supine position, and renal clearance studies were performed. After emptying of the bladder, the clearance period started at 7 a.m. and lasted for 2 h. At 8 a.m. blood pressure was measured repeated by the ausculatory method immediately before blood sampling for the measurements of plasma creatinine, sodium, calcium, pCa^{2+} and intact component of PTH. Urine was collected at the endpoint of the clearance period for the measurements of creatinine, sodium, and calcium. Endogenous creatinine clearance (C_{cr}), urinary excretion of sodium ($U_{Na}V$) and calcium ($U_{Ca}V$), and fractional excretion of sodium (FE_{Na}) and of calcium (FE_{Ca}) were calculated from the values of measured plasma and urine concentration. Renal clearance was performed before and after first dose (20 mg) and long-term (60 mg daily, t.i.d., for 4 weeks) oral administration of a slow-released Nif tablet.

Creatinine was measured by the Jaffe method, and sodium and calcium concentration in the plasma and urine were measured by ion electrode method. PCa^{2+} and plasma PTH were measured by using calcium ion electrode (Radiometer, ICA-1) and radioimmunoassay, respectively.

Values were expressed as means ± standard error of mean. All statistical analyses were assessed by paired Student's t-test and simple correlation analysis.

Results

As shown in Table 1, a single administration of Nif resulted in a rapid reduction of MAP ($P < 001$), enhancement of calciuria ($U_{Ca}V$, $P < 0.005$; FE_{Ca}, $P < 0.05$) and natriuresis ($U_{Na}V$, $P < 0.001$; FE_{Na}, $P < 0.005$), and no significant changes in C_{cr}, pCa^{2+} and PTH. Nif therapy for 1–4 weeks resulted in a progressive reduction of MAP (1 week, $P < 0.005$; 4 weeks, $P < 0.001$) and a slight reduction in plasma PTH (1 week, $P < 0.1$). No significant change in pCa^{2+} was observed. A sustained increase in calciuria and a similar tendency in natriuresis were observed 1 week after Nif therapy. Following 4 weeks of Nif therapy, the increased calciuria continued, whereas natriuresis had returned to the basal level. A significant positive correlation between natriuresis and calciuria ($U_{Na}V$ vs $U_{Ca}V$, r = 0.917, $P < 0.0005$; FE_{Na} vs FE_{Ca}, r = 0.888, $P < 0.001$) after a single oral aministration of Nif was found. However, this correlation disappeared following long-term Nif therapy. On the other hand, as shown in Fig. 1, the calciuretic response to Nif negatively correlated with basal pCa^{2+} ($P < 0.05$) and positively with the fall in MAP ($P < 0.05$). The fall in MAP negatively correlated with basal pCa^{2+} (r = 0.678, $P < 0.05$) following long-term Nif therapy.

Table 1. Acute and chronic effects of nifedipine on mean parameters

	Single oral administration (n = 10)		Long-term administration (n = 9)		
	Basal	Result	Basal	1 Week	4 Weeks
MAP (mmHg)	115 ± 4	99 ± 4[c]	123 ± 2	105 ± 3[d]	99 ± 4[e]
C_{cr} (ml/min)	79.8 ± 5.0	89.8 ± 8.2	73.0 ± 5.4	83.5 ± 5.2	76.2 ± 5.7
$U_{Ca}V$ (μg/min)	87.0 ± 22.9	157.0 ± 33.5[c]	86.3 ± 18.8	158.1 ± 32.5[c]	178.1 ± 30.8[c]
FE_{Ca} (%)	1.07 ± 0.14	1.99 ± 0.42[b]	1.12 ± 0.17	1.83 ± 0.33[c]	2.03 ± 0.36[c]
$U_{Na}V$ (μEq/min)	124.3 ± 9.5	298.1 ± 34.0[e]	128.4 ± 5.6	174.8 ± 28.5	148.2 ± 30.7
FE_{Na} (%)	1.09 ± 0.14	2.50 ± 0.37[d]	1.20 ± 0.17	1.57 ± 0.29	1.46 ± 0.29
pCa^{2+} (mmol/l)	1.22 ± 0.01	1.22 ± 0.02	1.22 ± 0.01	1.20 ± 0.01	1.23 ± 0.02
PTH (pg/ml)	449.2 ± 49.8	426.8 ± 39.5	456.2 ± 42.3	403.3 ± 36.3[a]	404.0 ± 61.0

[a] $P < 0.1$; [b] $P < 0.05$; [c] $P < 0.02$; [d] $P < 0.005$; [e] $P < 0.001$

MAP, mean arterial pressure; C_{cr}, creatinine clearance; $U_{Ca}V$, urinary excretion of calcium; FE_{Ca}, fractional excretion of calcium; $U_{Na}V$, urinary excretion of sodium; FE_{Na}, fractional excretion of sodium; pCa^{2+}, plasma ionized calcium; PTH, parathyroid hormone

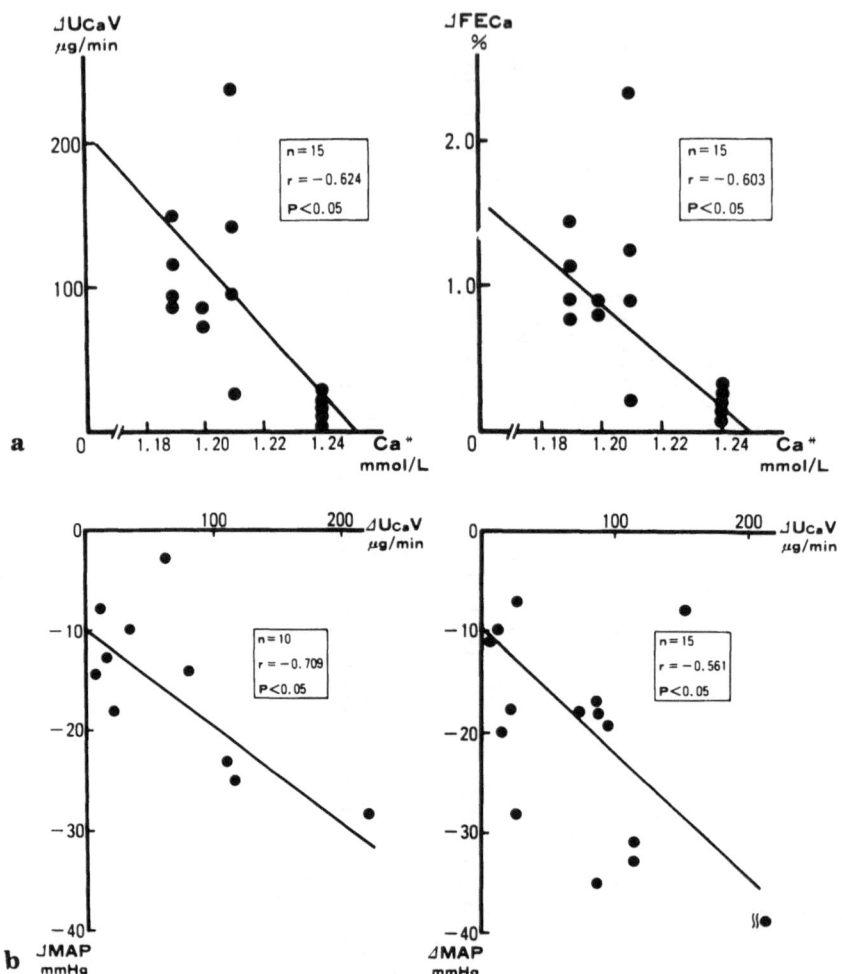

Fig. 1. a Correlation between plasma ionized calcium (pCa^2+) and change in urinary excretion of calcium ($\triangle U_{Ca}V$) or change in fractional excretion of calcium ($\triangle FE_{Ca}$) following long-term administration of nifedipine and **b** correlation between change in $\triangle U_{Ca}V$ and change in mean arterial pressure ($\triangle MAP$) following single (*left*) and long-term (*right*) administration of nifedipine in essential hypertensives

Discussion

Data from epidemiologic studies, clinical research [5] and basic investigations have suggested that abnormal calcium metabolism may be an important factor in the pathogenesis of human hypertension. Epidemiologic reports have indicated that dietary calcium deficiency may contribute to human hypertension and that an adequate calcium intake may reduce blood pressure in EHT. On the other hand, some reports have indicated that serum total calcium concentration is higher in hypertensive patients than in normotensive subjects [6]. In addition, acute elevation of extracellular calcium concentration in man by infusion of calcium salts has been reported to elevate blood pressure [7]. Thus, it is suggested that calcium may have a dual effect.

Recently, calcium channel blockers have been widely used in antihypertensive therapy. In the present study, we have investigated the significance of the body calcium balance and renal calcium handling in the antihypertensive effect of the calcium channel blocker, Nif.

Nif administration caused progressive reduction in blood pressure sustained calciuria and a transient natriuresis in EHT, while pCa^{2+} and C_{cr} did not change during therapy. Although the calciuretic response was positively correlated with the natriuretic response following a single oral administration of Nif, this relationship disappeared on long-term Nif therapy. Some reports have indicated that renal blood flow is significantly increased by Nif administration. Nif-induced calciuria may be related to renal hemodynamic changes in the acute phase of Nif therapy. On the other hand, long-term Nif administration was accompanied by sustained calciuria and reduction of plasma PTH. Similar results have been obtained after nitrendipine or verapamil [8, 9]. However the mechanism of reduction in plasma PTH following Nif therapy is not entirely clear. Furthermore, the calciuretic response to Nif negatively correlated with basal pCa^{2+} and positively to the change in MAP. As previously shown [10], following long-term Nif therapy the fall in MAP negatively correlated with pCa^{2+}.

References

1. MacCarron DA, Morris CD, Cole C (1982) Dietary calcium in human hypertension. Science 217: 267–270
2. Ackley S, Barret-Connor E, Suarez L (1983) Dairy products, calcium and blood pressure. Am J Clin Nutr 38: 457–461
3. MacCarron DA, Morris CD, Henry HJ, Stanton JL (1984) Blood pressure and nutrient intake in the United States. Science 224: 1392–1397
4. Augus ZS, Goldfarb S (1985) Renal regulation of calcium. The kidney. Raven Press, New York, pp 1323–1335
5. Siani A, Strazzullo P, Guglielmi S, Pacioni D, Giacco A, Lacone R, Mancini M (1988) Controlled trial of low calcium versus high calcium intake in mild hypertension. J Hypertens 6: 253–256
6. Kesteloot H, Geboers J (1982) Calcium and blood pressure. Lancet 1: 813—815
7. Valchakis ND, Frederics R, Velasquez M, Alexander N, Singer F, Maronde RF (1982) Sympathetic system function and vascular reactivity in hypercalcemic patients. Hypertension 4: 452–458
8. Ramp WK, Cooper CW, Ross III AJ, Wells Jr SA (1979) Effects of calcium and cyclic nucleotides on rat calcitonin and parathyroid hormone secretion. Mol Cell Endocrinol 14: 205–211
9. Cooper CW, Borosky SA, Farrell PE, Steinsland OS (1986) Effects of the calcium channel activator BAY-K-8644 on in vitro secretion of calcitonin and parathyroid hormone. Endocrinology 118:545–549
10. Resnick LM, Laragh JH (1985) Renin, calcium metabolism and the pathophysiologic basis of antihypertensive therapy. Am J Cardiol 56: H68-H74

Ventricular Function in Elderly Hypertensive Patients: A Radionuclide Assessment

Maurizio Petitto[1], Vincenzo Liguori[1], Salvatore Di Somma[1], Carmine Magnotta[1], Mario Ausiello[1], Maurizio Galderisi[1], Marcello Brignoli[1], and Oreste De Divitiis[2]

Summary. Radionuclide ventriculography (RNV) was used to study the influences of age and the duration of hypertension on left ventricular function in 3 groups of patients: 22 normotensive adults, 126 hypertensive adults, and 53 hypertensive elderly. The elderly hypertensive patients showed, in comparison with the normotensives, an increase of SVR, end-diastolic volume (EDV) and end-systolic volume (ESV), and reduced ejection fraction (EF) with comparable change in mean ejection rate (MER), cardiac output (CO), HR, stroke volume (SV), blood volume (BV), and systolic blood pressure (SBP)/ESV. In comparison with hypertensive adults, they had increased SVR with similarly increased BV, EF, ESV, and SBP/ESV and reduced CO, SV, EDV, and MER. Hemodynamic parameters had negative correlations with age and with duration of hypertension, while a positive correlation was recorded between SVR and age. Thus, advanced age provides an additional impairment to ventricular function to that already induced by hypertension by means of a further increase of SVR and reduced ventricular distensibility as the relation of BV to EDV shows.

Key words: Hypertension — Elderly — Ventricular function — Radionuclide ventriculography

Introduction

It is well known that in hypertensive patients both increased age and duration of hypertension induce greater vascular and cardiac damage with consequent increases in morbidity and mortality [1-3]. Our study aimed to evaluate the influences of age and the duration of hypertension on ventricular function. For this purpose we studied a group of elderly hypertensive (systolic and diastolic) pts with hypertension histories of at least four years for comparison with groups of normotensive and hypertensive adults.

Materials and Methods

The study consisted of 201 subjects free from heart failure studied by radionuclide ventriculography (blood pool, ^{99m}Tc) subdivided as follows:

---

[1] Cardioangiology Section, Second School of Medicine, Naples University, Napoli, Italy
[2] Department of Physiopathology, La Sapienza University, Rome, Italy

a) group A, 22 normotensive (diastolic blood pressure (DBP) < 90 mmHg), healthy
    adults (age < 60 years mean age 46 ± 9 years; 10 M, 12 F; blood pressure (BP)
    132 ± 11/78 ± 7 mmHg);
b) group B, 126 hypertensive (DBP > 90 mmHg), adults mean age 48 ± 8 years;
    (61 M, 65 F; BP 175 ± 12/105 ± 5 mmHg);
c) group C, 53 hyptertensive elderly (age ≥ 65 years mean age 69 ± 6 years);
    subjects (27 M, 26 F, BP 171 ± 13/103 ± 5 mmHg).

Patient characteristics are shown in Table 1. Groups A and B were comparable for
age; groups B and C for BP. The three groups were comparable for body surface
area.

Radionuclide venticulography was performed after at least 1 month free of treatment. First-pass technique was used to obtain cardiac output (CO), while ejection
fraction (EF) and mean ejection rate (MER) were assessed by blood pool. A single
administration of ^{99m}Tc serum albumin was injected i.v. at the dosage of 15 mCi,
after a supine rest of 30 min. Ohio-nuclear VP 450 φ-camera was used. Image
acquirement was performed on 32 frames with the patients in 45 degree left anterior
oblique (LAO) projection.

At the end of this assessment, HR, SBP, DBP, and mean arterial blood pressure
(MABP) were recorded by automatic screening devices (sphygmomanometer MOD
ADS 400). The statistical analysis was performed by unpaired t-test, comparing each
group of hypertensive patients with the control group and each other. For hypertensive groups, regression analyses of hemodynamic parameters with age, duration of
hypertension, and SVR were performed. In all 3 groups, regression equations
between BV on one hand, and SVR and EDV on the other, were also calculated.

Results

Means ± SD and the significance of differences of hemodynamic parameters in the
3 groups are shown in Table 2 and Fig. 1. Compared to the normotensive adults, the
hypertensive adults showed a significant increase in SVR, EDV, and ESV with comparable CO, HR, SV, and MER, but with reduced EF. In comparison with the
normotensive adults, the hypertensive elderly patients had significantly increased
SVR and ESV with comparable CO, SV, BV, EDV, SBP/ESV and significantly
reduced MER, and EF. In contrast to the hypertensive adults, the hypertensive
elderly subjects had an even greater increase in SVR with comparable BV, EF, ESV,
and SBP/ESV, but significantly reduced CO, SV, EDV, and MER.

The regression coefficients of the hemodynamic parameters with age, with dura-
tion of hypertension, and with SVR in the hypertensive groups are shown in Table 3.
The only significant positive correlation was between age and SVR. CO, SBP/ESV,
MER, stroke work index (SWI), SWI/EDV, cardiac index (CI), SV, and EF
demonstrated a negative correlation with age (Table 3). CO, CI, SV, SWI, and
SWI/EDV also had a negative correlation with the duration of hypertension. CO,
CI, SV, EF, EDV, SWI, and MER were negatively correlated with SVR (Table 3).
Furthermore, the hypertensive elderly patients showed, in comparison with the
hypertensive adults, higher incidence and severity of signs of vascular damage and

Table 1. Patient characteristics

	Normal subjects	Hypertensive patients	
	Adult	Adult	Elderly
n	22	126	53
Age (years)	46 ± 9	48 ± 8	68 ± 6
Hypertension duration (months)	—	33 ± 25	97 ± 53
M/F	10/12	61/65	26/27
SBP (mmHg)	132 ± 11	175 ± 12	171 ± 13
DBP (mmHg)	78 ± 7	105 ± 5	104 ± 5
Risk factors (n)			
Smoking	5 (22.7%)	65 (51.5%)	26 (49%)
Dyslipidosis	—	28 (22.2%)	19 (30%)
Diabetes	—	7 (5.5%)	9 (16.9%)
Obesity	—	21 (16.6%)	10 (18.8%)
ECG (n)			
Left ventricular hypertrophy	—	73 (57.9%)	40 (75.4%)
ST changes	—	23 (18.2%)	10 (18.8%)
$P_{RA} > 200$ ms	—	1 (0.07%)	2 (3.7%)
RBBB	—	6 (4.7%)	5 (9.4%)
LBBB	—	3 (2.3%)	4 (7.5%)
LAE	—	10 (7.9%)	4 (7.5%)
Fundus oculi (n)			
Stage I	—	95 (75.3%)	33 (62.6%)
Stage II	—	31 (24.6%)	20 (37.7%)
Proteinuria (n)	—	7 (5.5%)	6 (11.3%)
Creatinine > 15 mg/l	—	8 (6.3%)	8 (15%)

SBP, systolic blood pressure; DBP, diastolic blood pressure, ST, surface tension; P_{RA}, mean right atrial pressure; RBBB, right bundle branch block; LAE, left atrial enlargement

ECG alteration (proteinuria, fundus oculi, left ventricular hypertrophy etc). A negative correlation was found between SVR and BV. This relationship was significant for the normotensive (SVR = 2038 −0.157 BV; r = −0.42; P 0.05) and the hypertensive (SVR = 2413 −0.121 BV; r = −0.40; P 0.001) adults and not significant for the elderly patients (r = −0.25 ns). The relationship of EDV to BV was significant in the normotensive (EDV = 3.26 + 0.027 BV; r = 0.68; P 0.001) and the hypertensive (EDV = 92.25 + 0.011 BV; r = 0.29; P 0.001) adults and not significant for the elderly hypertensives (r = 0.22 ns).

Discussion

The elderly hypertensives although selected as free from signs or symptoms of heart failure, showed, at the radionuclide ventriculography, an impaired ventricular function in comparison with not only the normotensive subjects but also with the adults who had comparable degree of systolic and diastolic hypertension. Our results seem to demonstrate that this impairment is essentially due to two main causes: a) a deficit of left ventricular compliance, and b) the increase of SVR and afterload.

Table 2. Hemodynamic parameters and significance of differences between normal subjects (group A), and adult (group B) and elderly (group C) hypertensive patients

Parameter	Group A	Group B	Group C	A-B	A-C	B-C
SBP	132.27 ± 11.92	175.02 ± 12.26	171.50 ± 13.57	0.001	0.001	NS
DBP	78.86 ± 7.22	105.51 ± 5.24	104.01 ± 5.12	0.001	0.001	NS
MABP	97.13 ± 8.68	129.15 ± 8.37	125.78 ± 7.16	0.001	0.001	NS
HR	74.09 ± 7.39	72.53 ± 12.63	73.58 ± 8.70	NS	NS	NS
CO	5.87 ± 0.68	6.00 ± 0.85	5.55 ± 0.72	NS	NS	0.005
SV	79.43 ± 9.24	84.37 ± 16.61	75.98 ± 13.59	NS	NS	0.005
EDV	124.88 ± 22.19	143.90 ± 29.22	134.01 ± 17.16	0.005	NS	0.05
ESV	45.18 ± 16.62	59.61 ± 22.02	57.24 ± 13.44	0.005	0.005	NS
BV	4.41 ± 0.55	4.68 ± 0.78	4.66 ± 0.40	NS	NS	NS
SVR	1343.59 ± 222.65	1745.46 ± 278.35	1854.37 ± 320.23	0.001	0.001	0.05
EF	64.86 ± 7.53	58.73 ± 10.51	56.73 ± 8.60	0.02	0.001	NS
SWI/EDV	499.09 ± 92.98	565.10 ± 120.58	538.49 ± 94.72	0.02	NS	NS
MER	2.25 ± 0.34	2.06 ± 0.57	1.84 ± 0.45	NS	0.001	0.02
SBP/ESV	3.37 ± 1.39	3.37 ± 1.34	3.21 ± 1.15	NS	NS	NS

Values given are means ± SD.
SBP, systolic blood pressure; DBP, diastolic blood pressure; MABP, mean arterial blood pressure; CO, cardiac output; SV, stroke volume; EDV, end-diastolic volume; ESV, end-systolic volume; BV, blood volume; EF, ejection fraction; SWI, stroke work index; MER, mean ejection rate

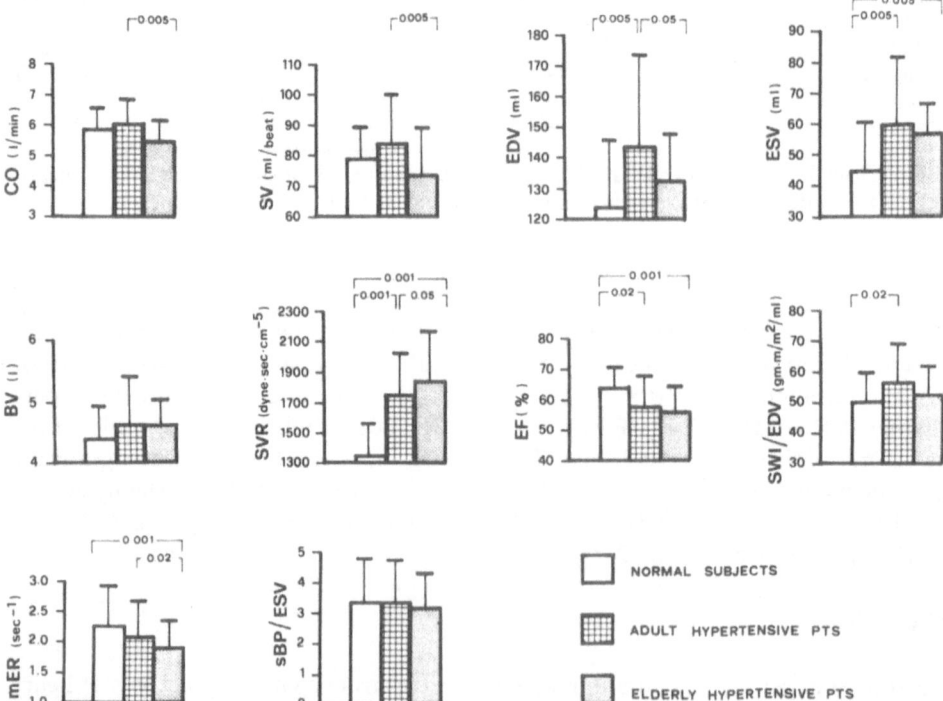

Fig. 1. Hemodynamic parameters (mean ± SD) in the 22 normotensive adults, the 126 hypertensive adults, and the 53 elderly subjects studied. *CO*, cardiac output; *SV*, stroke volume; *EDV*, end-diastolic volume; *ESV*, end-systolic volume; *BV*, blood volume; *EF*, ejection fraction; *SWI*, stroke work index; *mER*, mean ejection rate; *sBP*, systolic blood pressure

Table 3. Correlation coefficients (r) and probabilities (P) of hemodynamic parameters in terms of age, duration of hypertension, and SVR in hypertensive groups (adult and elderly, $n = 179$)

	Age		Duration		SVR	
	r	P	r	P	r	P
SBP	−0.11	NS	−0.07	NS	—	—
DBP	−0.10	NS	−0.04	NS	—	—
MBP	−0.11	NS	−0.07	NS	—	—
SBP/ESV	−0.15	(0.05)	−0.11	NS	−0.07	NS
MER	−0.18	(0.05)	−0.05	NS	−0.28	(0.001)
BV	0.05	NS	0.4	NS	−0.35	(0.001)
SVR	0.14	(0.05)	0.13	NS	—	—
HR	0.007	NS	0.04	NS	−0.03	NS
EDV	−0.08	NS	−0.08	NS	−0.26	(0.001)
ESV	0.02	NS	−0.004	NS	0.08	NS
EF	−0.16	(0.05)	−0.07	NS	−0.32	(0.001)
SWI	−0.22	(0.01)	−0.19	(0.01)	−0.27	(0.001)
SWI/EDV	−0.20	(0.01)	−0.19	(0.01)	0.005	NS
CO	−0.19	(0.01)	−0.17	(0.05)	−0.86	(0.001)
CI	−0.24	(0.001)	−0.20	(0.01)	−0.62	(0.001)
SV	−0.19	(0.01)	−0.16	(0.05)	−0.54	(0.001)

CI, cardiac index; see Table 2 for other abbreviations

In fact, the most relevant manifestation of dysfunction is represented by a reduced CO, due to the reduced SV (HR being comparable). This effect on the SV is mainly due to the behaviour of EDV. Elderly EDV was reduced in comparison with that of the hypertensive adults who had an increased EDV in respect to the normotensive subjects. This reduction of EDV in the elderly must be attributable to a deficit of distensibility of the left ventricle in diastole. In fact, it is in the presence of a unchanged BV and with a comparable HR, evident. The relationship of EDV to BV had an analogous behaviour in hypertensive adults, as in the normotensives, but the same relationship was not significant in the hypertensive elderly.

A deficit of ventricular compliance has been described in the elderly and in adult hypertensive patients as well [6]. This deficit most likely has different meanings and pathological bases in hypertensives [7] and in the elderly [8]; attributable in the former group to ventricular hypertrophy [6, 7] and in the latter, to the increased rigidity of the connective component of the ventricle. On the other hand, a deficit of contractility could not explain the deficit of function in the elderly. In fast, ESV did not show a significant difference for the elderly in comparison with hypertensive adults, and neither did the systolic ratio SBP/ESV, a reliable index of contractility [9].

That SVR was significantly higher in the elderly in comparison with the adult hypertensive patients, could provide an explaination for the reduction of MER as the relationship between these two parameters shows (Table 3). The relationship between SVR and BV shows that the hypertensive adults have an analogous behaviour to normotensive adults, SVR showing the normal trend to reduction with increasing BV even if at higher levels. This negative relation is lost in the elderly hypertensive, whose SVR, besides being higher, is not able to adjust itself to the BV. Thus, the increased afterload is further explaination for the impairment of ventricular function which the negative relations between SVR and the main indices of ventricular function (EF, CO, and SV) confirm (Table 3).

The significant negative correlation between SVR and EDV (Table 3) connects the two principal mechanisms of alterated ventricular function in elderly hypertensive patients. Furthermore, SVR correlates positively with age, while the parameters of ventricular function (CO, SV, MER, SWI, SWI/EDV) show a negative correlation to age and hypertension duration (Table 3). The increase of SVR and its lack of regulation capability could express greater vascular alteration. The higher incidence of signs of vascular damage we found in the elderly (Table 1) could be a manifestation of this alteration.

In conclusion, our results show the advanced age is an additional factor contributing to ventricular dysfunction in hypertensives through two principal mechanisms: (a) the reduced diastolic distensibility and (b) the increased afterload. Thus, ventricular dysfunction increases with age and duration of hypertension.

References

1. Gordon T (1964) Blood Pressure of adults by age and sex. Vital Health Stat [11]: 1-6
2. Ambrosio GB, Zamboni S, Vanuzzo D, Regato R (1980) La presenza di ipertensione nella comunita. G Ital Cardiol 10: 1280-1285
3. Dyear AR, Stamler J, Shekelle RB (1977) Hypertension in the elderly. Med Clin North Am 61: 513-529
4. Sowera JR (1985) Hypertension in elderly. Boehringer Ingelheim
5. Messerli FH, Ventura HO, Glade V (1983) Essential hypertension in the elderly: Hemodynamics, intravascular volume, plasma renin activity, and circulating catecholamine levels. Lancet 2: 983-985
6. Messerli FH, Devereaux RB (1983) Introduction to left ventricular hypertrophy. Good or evil? Am J Med 26: 1-3
7. Fouad FM, Slominski JM, Tarazi RC (1984) Left ventricular diastolic function in hypertension: relation to left ventricular mass and systolic function. J Am Coll Cardiol 3: 1500-1506
8. Lakatta EG (1987) Do hypertension and aging have a similar effect on the myocardium? Circulation 75 (Suppl I) 69-77
9. Sagawa K (1981) The end-systolic pressure-volume relation of the ventricle: definition, modifications and clinical use. Circulation 63: 1223-1227

Distensibility of Large Arteries in Elderly Hypertensive Patients After Chronic Treatment with Nicardipine SR

R. CARRETTA, M. BARDELLI, S. MUIESAN, F. VRAN, B. FABRIS, F. FISCHETTI, and L. CAMPANACCI[1]

Summary. The brachial arterial compliance and the carotid blood flow were determined in 16 hypertensives older than 60 years (60–85; 67 ± 6.5), after 15 days of *placebo* or 2 months of therapy with *nicardipine SR* (40 mg b.i.d.), administered randomly following a crossover design, in a single-blind protocol. The hemodynamic parameters were determined 8 h after the last pill of *nicardipine SR* was taken. The study was performed both before and 2 h after the administration of 40 mg of nicardipine. Mean arterial blood pressure was significantly reduced after 40 mg of nicardipine, both in the patients on *placebo* (130 ± 12 vs 112 ± 13 mmHg; $P < 0.001$) and in the patients receiving chronic treatment with *nicardipine SR* (118 ± 13 vs 108 ± 10 mmHg; $P < 0.01$).

The brachial arterial compliance and the carotid blood flow were increased after 40 mg of nicardipine both when the patients were on *placebo* (2.1 ± 0.9 vs 2.4 ± 0.8 cm^4 dyne$^{-1} \times 10^{-7}$, $P < 0.05$; and 9.2 ± 1.8 vs 11.0 ± 2.9 ml/s, $P < 0.002$, respectively) and when they were receiving chronic treatment with *nicardipine SR* (2.1 ± 1.4 vs 2.8 ± 1.7 cm^4 dyne$^{-1} \times 10^{-7}$, $P < 0.05$; and 8.9 ± 2.5 vs 9.9 ± 2 ml/s, $P < 0.05$, respectively).

These results show that the drug increases arterial distensibility and carotid blood flow.

Key words: Large arteries — Compliance — Flow — Nicardipine SR

Introduction

Distensibility of the large-arteries is of crucial importance in determining the value of systolic and diastolic blood pressures [1]. Although this concept has been well known for a long time, it has recently received renewed interest because of the development of ultrasound techniques which allow researchers to study the structural and functional characteristics of the large arteries in different diseases, namely, in essential hypertension. In this field of research, the effect of many antihypertensive drugs on large-arteries distensibility has been evaluated [2]. It has been reported recently that the acute and chronic treatment of arterial hypertension with nicardipine (calcium antagonist of the dihydropyridine group) enhances arterial compliance (an index of the distensibility of the wall of the large arteries) [2]. Therefore, we have evaluated the effects of acute and chronic treatment on arterial compliance with a slow-release formula of nicardipine, both before and 2 h after the administration of the drug to elderly hypertensive patients.

---

[1] Institute of Medical Pathology, Trieste University, Trieste, Italy

Materials and Methods

The study was performed in 16 hypertensive patients older than 60 years (range 60–85; mean age 67 ± 6.5). Each patient was randomly assigned to therapy with placebo or with nicardipine SR (40 mg b.i.d.). The placebo was given for 2 weeks, while the nicardipine, for 2 months. At the end of these periods, the order of administration of the drugs was reversed, following a crossover single-blind protocol. At the end of each period of treatment, a hemodynamic study was performed 8 h after the last pill of placebo or nicardipine SR was taken. The study was then repeated 2 h after the administration of 40 mg of nicardipine. The arterial compliance was determined by measuring the arterial diameter (D) with two-dimensional echography and the arterial pulse wave velocity (PWV) by piezoelectric microphones, following the formula:

$$C = \pi D^2/4\eta \ (PWV)^2$$

where η is the blood viscosity.

The carotid blood flow was calculated by measuring the arterial diameter (B-mode echography) and the mean blood velocity (MV) using a continous-wave Doppler, following the formula:

$$Q = \frac{\pi D^2}{4} \times MV$$

The mean blood velocity was determined by calculating the area under the envelope designed by the subsequent modes of the frequencies (measured every 5 ms). The data were expressed as mean $\pm$ SD. The statistical analysis of the data was performed with the Student's t-test.

Results

The systolic and diastolic blood pressures were significantly reduced after chronic treatment with nicardipine SR. The administration of 40 mg of nicardipine further reduced the systolic and diastolic blood pressures during both the placebo and the active treatment periods (Fig. 1) However, in 3 patients, after 40 mg of nicardipine, the reduction of the systolic blood pressure was lower than 15 mmHg and that of the diastolic was lower than 10 mmHg. These patients were considered nonresponders. The data concerning them were analysed separately.

The heart rate was slightly, although significantly, raised after chronic treatment with nicardipine SR, while the increment was more evident after the administration of 40 mg of nicardipine in the patients treated with placebo (Fig. 1).

The arterial compliance of the brachial artery was enhanced by the administration of 40 mg of nicardipine both in the patients treated with placebo and in those treated with nicardipine SR. In "at rest" conditions, 8 h after the last pill was taken, the arterial compliance did not differ from the placebo to the active treatment phase (Fig. 2).

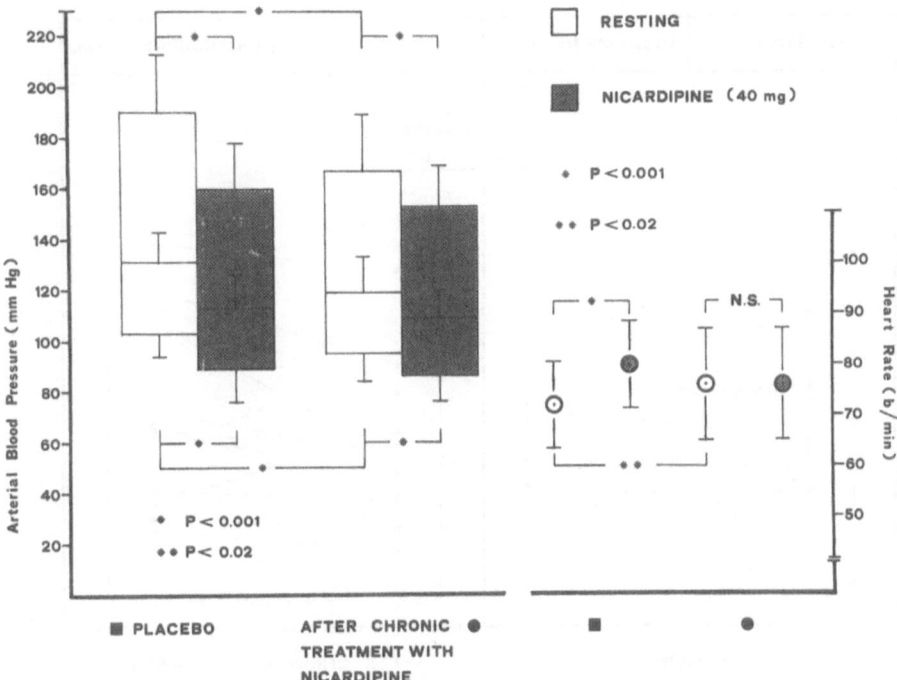

Fig. 1. Arterial blood pressure and heart rate in the different phases of the study

The diameter of the brachial artery was unchanged after 40 mg of nicardipine when the patients were on placebo (0.454 ± 0.068 vs 0.463 ±0.07 cm). Yet, when they were treated with the active drug, the 40 mg of nicardipine increased slightly, although significantly, the arterial diameter (0.435 ± 0.063 vs 0.449 ±0.066 cm).

The diameter of the brachial artery was unchanged after 40 mg of nicardipine when the patients were on placebo (0.454 ± 0.068 vs 0.463 ± 0.07 cm). Yet, when they were treated with the active drug, the 40 mg of nicardipine increased slightly, although significantly, the arterial diameter (0.435 ± 0.063 vs 0.449 ± 0.066 cm).

The diameter of the carotid artery did not change after 40 mg of nicardipine in either the placebo (0.761 ± 0.066 vs 0.770 ± 0.072 cm) or the active treatment (0.789 ± 0.130 vs 0.799 ± 0.128 cm) phase of the study.

Discussion

Arterial compliance is reduced in the essential hypertensive, partially as a consequence of the increase in diastolic blood pressure [1] and partially as a primary alteration contributing to the development of hypertension [3]. This is especially the case in systolic hypertension of the elderly. It has recently been reported that some antihypertensive drugs, particularly the calcium antagonists [2, 4, 5] and the angioteusin-converting enzyme (ACE) inhibitors [6], improved the arterial com-

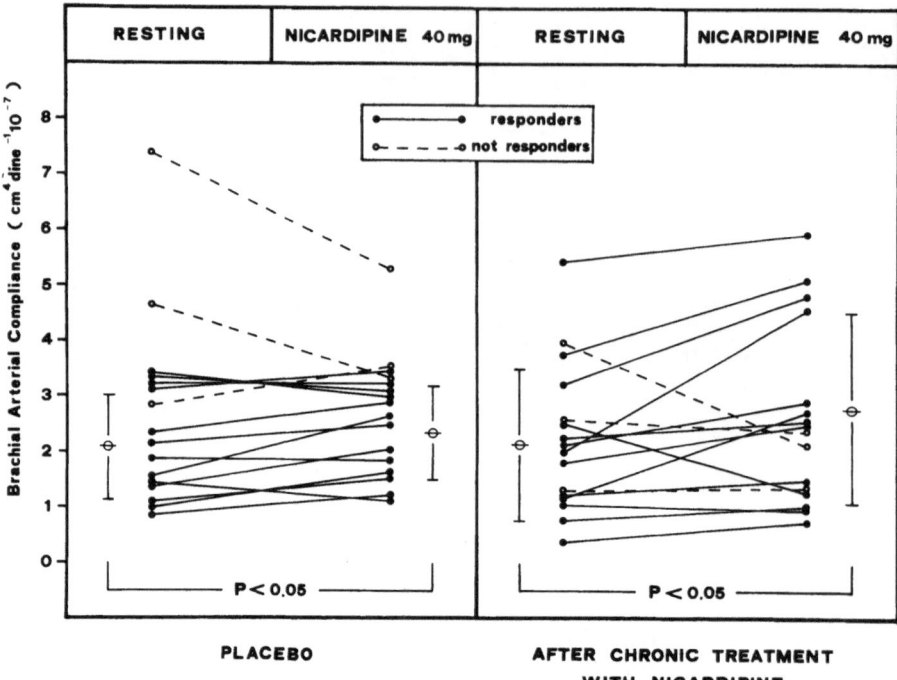

Fig. 2. Changes in the compliance of the brachial artery in the different phases of the study

pliance of adult hypertensive patients. In the present study, we have studied the effects of nicardipine, a calcium antagonist of the dihydropyridine group, in patients older than 60 years with the aim of assessing whether therapy with nicardipine could also modify arterial compliance in these patients.

The results of this study show that acute treatment with 40 mg of nicardipine enhances the forearm arterial compliance in elderly hypertensive patients, both when they were on placebo or receiving chronic treatment with nicardipine SR. This effect was due to a reduction of pulse wave velocity; although, in the patients receiving chronic treatment with nicardipine, a small increase in arterial diameter also contributed to this effect.

The reduction of pulse wave velocity, transmitted along the wall of the brachial artery, could be attributed to either structural and/or functional changes (since both are related to blood vessel distensibility) [1] or to transmural pressure [7]. It seems unlikely that only 2 months of therapy would be enough to change the structural characteristics of the arterial wall in elderly hypertensive patients. It would also explain why the increase in arterial compliance was not stable in these patients after therapy with nicardipine SR. On the other hand, the reduction of pulse wave velocity was probably not an indirect effect related to the reduction of blood pressure; since it was not evident in at rest conditions (8 h after the last pill was taken) in the patients receiving nicardipine SR as compared to the placebo phase; although the blood pres-

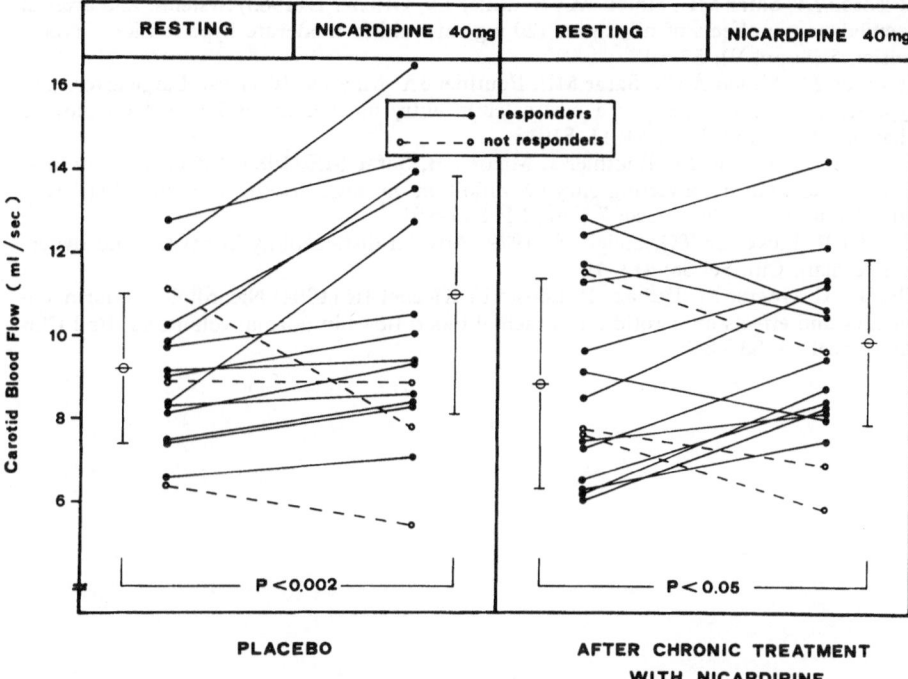

Fig. 3. Changes in the carotid blood flow in the different phases of the study

sure was, in that moment, still significantly reduced. Therefore, it seems likely that the enhancement of arterial compliance, observed after the administration of 40 mg of nicardipine, was a specific effect of the drug, although limited to that time.

A last consideration concerns the carotid blood flow. It is enhanced after acute administration of the drug in both the placebo- and in the nicardipine SR-treated patients, according to Thuillez et al. [8]. Since the carotid blood flow was increased, although there was significant blood pressure reduction, it appears that the administration of nicardipine does not incur the risk of cerebrovascular hypoperfusion.

In conclusion, the acute administration of 40 mg of nicardipine in elderly hypertensive patients improves arterial compliance and enhances the carotid blood flow, whether in patients taking placebo or nicardipine SR.

References

1. O'Rourke MF (1982) Arterial function in health and disease. Churchill Livingston
2. Levenson J, Simon A Ch, Bouthier J, Maarek B, Safar ME (1985) The effect of acute and chronic nicardipine therapy on forearm arterial haemodynamics in essential hypertension. Br J Clin Pharmacol 20: 1075–1135
3. Ventura MO, Messerli FM, Oigman W (1984) Impaired arterial compliance in borderline hypertension. Am Heart J 108: 132–137

4. Levenson JA, Safar ME, Simon AC, Bouthier JA, Griener L (1983) Systemic and arterial haemodynamic effects of nifedipine (20 mg) in mild-to-moderate hypertension. Hypertension 5 (Suppl V): 57-60
5. Levenson JA, Simon A Ch, Safar ME, Bouthier JA, Maarek BC (1984) Large arteries in hypertension: acute effects of a new calcium entry blocker nitrendipine. J Cardiovasc Pharmacol 6 (Suppl VII): S1011-S1015
6. Simon AC, Levenson JA, Bouthier J, Maarek B, Safar ME (1985) Effects of acute and chronic angiotensin-converting enzyme inhibition on large arteries in human hypertension. J Cardiovasc Pharmacol 7 (Suppl I) S45-S51
7. Gribbin B, Pickering TG, Sleight P (1979) Arterial distensibility in normal and hypertensive man. Clin Sci 56: 413-417
8. Thuillez C, Gueret M, Duhaze P, Lhoste F, Kiechel JR (1984) Nicardipine: pharmacokinetics and effects on carotid and brachial blood flows in normal volunteers. Br J Clin Pharmacol 18: 837-847

Effects of Nifedipine on Blood Pressure, Arterial Compliance and Left Ventricular Mass in Elderly Patients with Isolated Systolic Hypertension

Salvatore Novo[1], Emilio Nardi[2], Giovanni Noto[2], Giuseppe Licata[2], and Antonio Strano[3]

Summary. The aim of this study was to evaluate the effects of acute and chronic administration of slow-release nifedipine (SRN) on blood pressure (BP), aortic index (AI), average wall stress (AWS), left ventricular mass (LVM), and other hemodynamic parameters in elderly patients with isolated systolic hypertension (ISH) (systolic blood pressure [SBP] > 175 mmHg). We studied 10 patients (mean age 73.7 ± 5.6 years) in which after a washout period, in basal conditions, 3 h after the administration of SRN (20 mg), and 180 days after chronic therapy (40 mg daily), we evaluated the changes of BP, HR, AI, AWS, LVM, and other parameters obtained by means of echocardiography. After SRN we observed a significant decrease of SBP both in acute ($P < 0.005$ in supine and $P < 0.0125$ in upright position) and in chronic ($P < 0.0005$ in supine and $P < 0.005$ in upright position) therapies and a slight decrease of DBP, whereas HR did not show great changes. AI decreased significantly ($P < 0.01$ in acute and in chronic) as well as did systemic vascular resistance ($P < 0.025$ in acute and $P < 0.01$ in chronic). Moreover, we observed a significant diminution of AWS ($P < 0.01$) and LVM ($P < 0.01$) after 180 days of treatment. These results seem to show that SRN is useful in elderly patients with ISH, because it produces an improvement both of arterial compliance and of left ventricle function parameters.

Key words: Nifedipine — Hypertension — Elderly — Arterial compliance — Left ventricular mass

Introduction

Hypertension has been recognized as the single most potent, common, and remediable risk factor for cerebrovascular disease, congestive heart failure, and coronary disease, which are the major causes of cardiovascular morbidity and mortality in the elderly [1]. Moreover, it has been demonstrated that systolic hypertension is the most important risk factor for stroke, and that this risk is directly related to systolic blood pressure (SBP) values [2]. The prevalence of predominant or isolated systolic hypertension (ISH) is estimated to be 25% – 30% of men and women at the age of 80 years [3]. These data illuminate the problem and emphasize the need of finding a hemodynamic basis to obtain a reduction of SBP in the elderly.

---

[1] Institute of Chest Diseases, University of Catania, Catania, Italy
[2] Institute of Clinical Medicine, University of Palermo, Palermo, Italy
[3] Department of Internal Medicine, II University of Rome, Tor Vergata, Rome, Italy

The finding that in elderly subjects, systemic arterial compliance is reduced and inversely related to SBP elevation, suggests that a loss of distensibility of the aorta and large arteries is responsible for ISH [4, 5]. Therefore, the cause of the reduction of arterial compliance might be increased stiffness of the large arteries caused by functional or structural alterations of the arterial wall [4]. Judging from these observations, the most important agents for reduction of SBP are probably the vasodilating drugs that working on the large arteries, can produce an increase in arterial compliance. The selection of the most appropriate antihypertensive agent for elderly patients requires careful consideration, since the therapeutic window of most drugs is narrower in such subjects and serious adverse reactions may affect the expected benefits of treatment [6, 7]. Moreover, with greater age and longer histories of hypertension, baroflex sensitivity and beta adrenoceptor mediated function become blunted, plasma renin activity is often reduced, and vascular resistance is markedly elevated, as alpha adrenoceptor-medicated vasoconstruction prevails [8]. Thus, plasma renin activity relates indirectly to patient age. Drugs that interfere with beta adrenoceptor-mediated functions or with the renin-angiotensin system can be expected to be more effective in younger patients and in subjects with high renin levels [8]. Drugs that have a primarily vasodilator or volume-depletion effect and that thereby evoke reflex stimulation are more effective in older and low-renin patients [8].

On the basis of these considerations, calcium channel blockers seem to be particularly suitable for the treatment of ISH in the elderly, since these drugs generally do not cause postural hypotension, central nervous system responses, fluid retention, and other important adverse effects particularly undesirable in these patients. The calcium channel blocker, nifedipine, produces vasodilation-inhibiting vascular smooth muscle contractions. This action is used for hypertensive emergency therapy by means of sublingual administration and for chronic treatment for arterial hypertension, utilizing a slow-release preparation twice daily [9–11].

With these priciples in mind, we designed a study to investigate the effects of slow-release nifedipine tablets (SRN) on blood pressure (BP), arterial compliance, average wall stress (AWS), left ventricular mass (LVM) and other hemodynamic parameters in elderly patients with ISH.

Materials and Methods

We studied 10 elderly patients (6 males and 4 females) with an average age of 73.7 ± 5.6 years that were suffering from ISH (SBP > 175 mmHg) with normal values of diastolic blood pressure (DBP < 90 mmHg). Informed consent was obtained from all subjects. After a 1-week washout period, under basal conditions and 3 h after SRN (20 mg) administration, SBP, DBP, mean blood pressure (MBP), HR, and pressure rate product (PRP) in supine and in upright position were evaluated. In addition, the effects on the following hemodynamic parameters were also examined in supine position: end-diastolic (EDD) and end-systolic diameters of left ventricle (ESD), shortening fraction (SF), V_{cf}, stroke volume (SV), cardiac output (CO), ejection fraction (EF), aortic index (AI), and SVR. After 6 months of treatment with SRN (20 mg twice daily), all the subjects observed a 24-h washout period and repeated the same examinations before and after the administration of SRN. LVM and AWS were evaluated at the beginning and at the end of the study. BP values were determined according to recommendations of the American Heart Association [12]. Hemodynamic parameters were obtained by applying M-mode and two-dimensional echocardiography, using an instrument Irex III and a Cardio 80 Kontron computer for the elaboration of the data. The left ventricle dimensions were obtained when the ultrasonic beam was directed at the chamber between the mitral valve echoes and the papillary muscle echoes [13]. The diastolic diameter was taken at the peak of the R wave of ECG and from the trailing edge of the left side of the interventricular septum to the leading edge of the posterior endocardial echo [13]. The systolic diameter was taken at the peak downward motion of the interventricular septum [13]. SF was calculated by the following formula [14]: (EDD-ESD)/(EDD) $\times$ 100. VCF was obtained by (EDD-ESD)/LVET $\times$ EDD) ratio [14]. Ventricular volumes were obtained from two-dimensional images using Simpson's formula [15]. AI was obtained by pulse pressure (PP)/SV ratio [16]. SVR values were calculated by the following formula [17]: (MBP $\times$ 60 $\times$ 1332)/CO. AWS was derived in this way: SBP ($\frac{1}{2}$EDD + $\frac{1}{2}$ESD)/(average end-diastolic wall thickness + average end-systolic wall thickness). Measurements for the detection of LVM, made in accordance with Penn Convention, were used in the modified cubed formula [18]: [18]: 1.04 (EDD + left ventricle septal thickness + posterior wall thickness)^3 − (EDD)^3 − 13.6. Patients with abnormal left ventricle wall kinesis were excluded from the study in order to make echocardiographic measurements reproducible and reliable [19]. Student's t-test for paired data was used to calculate statistical significance.

Results

Changes in Blood Pressure, Heart Rate, and Pressure Rate Product

SRN produced a significant decrease of SBP both in acute and after 6 months of treatment in supine and upright position (Fig. 1, Table 1); the decrease of DBP was also significant but of minor evidence (Fig. 1, Table 1). HR showed a small but significant increase only after acute administration in supine position (Fig. 1, Table 1). PRP as well as MBP and PP decreased significantly after acute administration and after chronic therapy both in supine and in upright position (Fig. 1, Table 1). After 6 months of treatment, before the last drug administration, only SBP and PP were significantly reduced in comparison to basal conditions (Fig. 1, Table 1).

Changes of Hemodynamic Parameters, Average Wall Stress, and Left Ventricular Mass

After SRN administration, EDD and ESD decreased significantly both in acute and in chronic treatment (Table 1). SV and CO increased (Table 1), whereas SVR and AI decreased (Fig. 1, Table 1). These changes were evident after a single administration

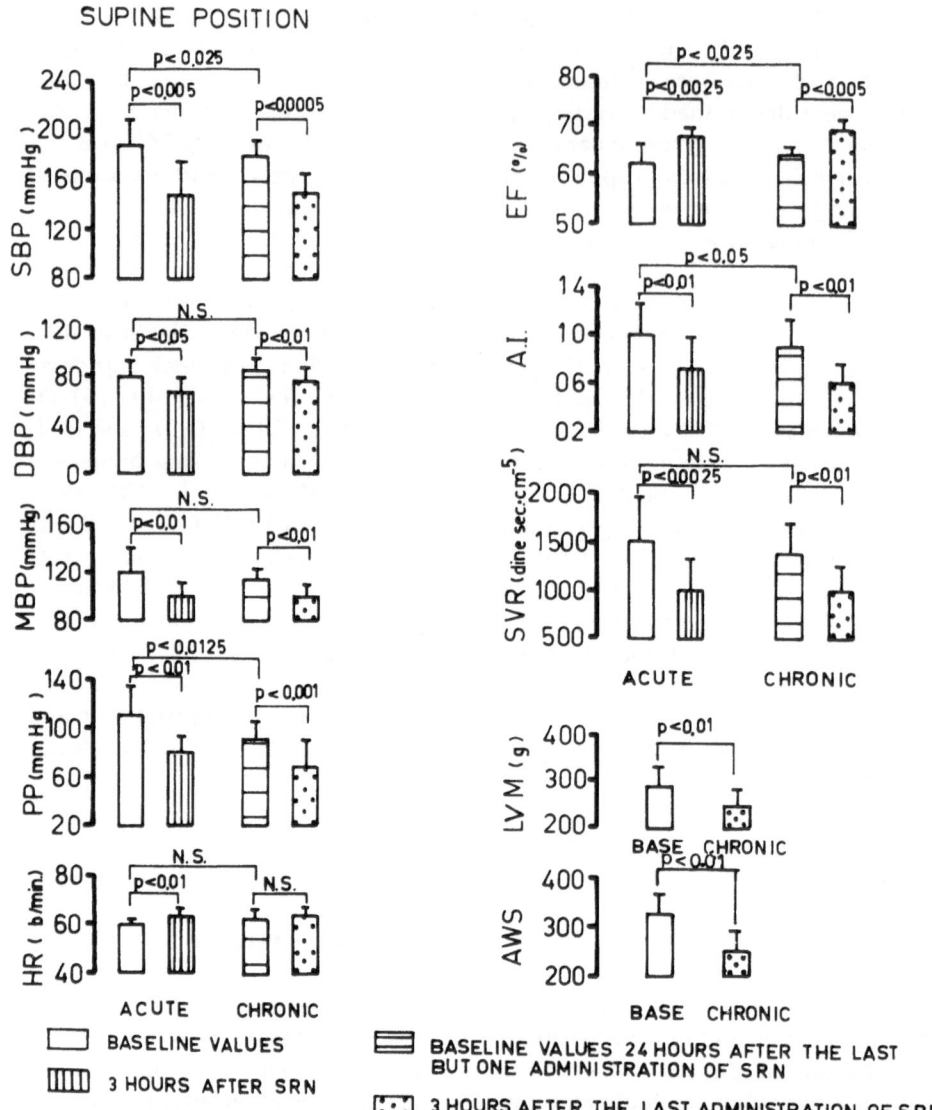

Fig. 1. Effects of acute (20 mg) and chronic (40 mg daily for 6 months) administration of slow-release nifedipine. *SBP*, systolic blood pressure; *DBP*, diastolic blood pressure; *MBP*, mean blood pressure; *PP*, pulse pressure; *EF*, ejection fraction; *AI*, aortic index; *LVM*, left ventricle mass; *AWS*, average wall stress

of SRN, as well as after the last drug administration after 6 months of treatment. We also observed a significant reduction of EDD and AI before the last SRN tablet provided for the study in comparison to basal conditions (Fig. 1, Table 1). Echocardiographic indexes of left ventricular function showed a significant improvement; in particular, we observed an increase of SF, EF, and VCF both after acute administration and after chronic therapy (Fig. 1, Table 1). Moreover, we also observed a

Table 1. Effects of acute (20 mg) and chronic (20 mg twice daily) administration of slow-release nifedipine (SRN).[a]

	Acute		Chronic		1→2 P<	1→3 P<	3→4 P<
	Baseline values	Three hours after SRN	Baseline values (24 H after SRN)	Three hours after SRN			
SBP supine (mmHg)	193.75 ± 20.43	152.5 ± 22.7	178.57 ± 10.2	147.14 ± 18.4	0.005	0.025	0.0005
SBP upright (mmHg)	179.8 ± 23.5	146.25 ± 20.37	167.14 ± 5.6	142.14 ± 14.9	0.0125	0.05	0.005
DBP supine (mmHg)	81.25 ± 14.36	71.25 ± 8.69	85.7 ± 5.3	77.85 ± 6.3	0.05	N.S.	0.01
DBP upright (mmHg)	85.0 ± 19.14	68.75 ± 8.53	87.85 ± 2.6	78.57 ± 6.9	0.01	N.S.	0.01
MBP supine (mmHg)	118.75 ± 19.5	98.25 ± 9.36	116.65 ± 5.6	100.9 ± 8.6	0.01	N.S.	0.01
MBP upright (mmHg)	116.6 ± 20.51	94.58 ± 12.47	113.28 ± 2.5	99.74 ± 5.3	0.01	N.S.	0.005
HR supine (beats/min)	59.0 ± 2.44	64.5 ± 3.0	62.7 ± 2.8	64.1 ± 3.1	N.S.	N.S.	N.S.
HR upright (beats/min)	68.75 ± 6.5	74.5 ± 4.4	72.1 ± 4.3	73.8 ± 4.2	0.01	N.S.	N.S.
PRP supine	11431 ± 2935	9836 ± 1930	10479 ± 1910	9431 ± 1986	0.01	N.S.	0.005
PRP upright	12361 ± 3710	10895 ± 2520	12050 ± 1872	10489 ± 1672	0.025	N.S.	0.005
PP supine (mmHg)	112.5 ± 22.9	81.25 ± 13.5	92.85 ± 9.9	69.28 ± 17.1	0.01	0.0125	0.001
PP upright (mmHg)	94.8 ± 18.7	77.5 ± 15.0	79.28 ± 5.3	63.57 ± 18.6	0.01	0.01	0.01
EDD (cm)	5.9 ± 0.48	5.7 ± 0.43	5.4 ± 0.6	5.2 ± 0.6	0.01	0.025	0.05
ESD (cm)	3.8 ± 0.33	3.5 ± 0.25	3.7 ± 0.24	3.4 ± 0.5	0.0005	N.S.	0.05
Stroke volume (ml)	107.9 ± 16.0	112.4 ± 19.4	105.6 ± 15.5	114.7 ± 16.3	0.0025	N.S.	0.0025
Cardiac output (l/min)	6.3 ± 1.17	7.2 ± 1.31	6.6 ± 1.12	7.3 ± 1.2	0.0025	N.S.	0.01
Ejection fraction	62.3 ± 2.20	68.2 ± 1.70	64.3 ± 2.1	69.5 ± 1.9	0.0025	0.025	0.005
Aortic index	1.04 ± 0.25	0.73 ± 0.18	0.87 ± 0.21	0.60 ± 0.17	0.01	0.05	0.01
SVR (dine.s.cm^{-5})	1504 ± 429	1094 ± 275	1412 ± 325	1097 ± 243	0.025	N.S.	0.01
Shortening fraction (%)	34.2 ± 1.4	38.6 ± 1.3	31.4 ± 4.5	34.6 ± 5.4	0.005	0.05	0.01
V_{cf} (circ/s)	1.02 ± 0.17	1.35 ± 0.05	1.14 ± 0.13	1.39 ± 0.9	0.0125	0.05	0.01

SBP, systolic blood pressure; DBP, diastolic blood pressure; MBP, mean arterial blood pressure; PRP, pressure rate product; PP, pulse pressure; EDD, end-diastolic diameter of left ventricle; ESD, end-systolic diameter of left ventricle
[a] In acute, the parameters were evaluated in basal conditions (after pharmacological washout) and 3 h after the drug administration; after 6 months of treatment the same parameters were evaluated 24 h after the last but one SRN administration and then again 3 h after the last drug tablet.

diminution of AWS (from 325.6 ± 47.8 to 248.9 ± 48.7) and of LVM (from 288.7 ± 40.7 to 246.3 ± 38.6) after 6 months of treatment (Fig. 1).

Discussion

Several studies have demonstrated the efficacy of nifedipine in the treatment of arterial hypertension [9–11]; the results of this study show the usefulness of this drug in elderly patients with ISH as well. We obtained a marked decreased of SBP (owing to the significant decrease of SVR), while the diminution of DBP was of minor evidence. A slight reflexive increase in HR (evident only after acute administration in supine position) was also noticed. The decrease of SBP could depend on the diminution of calcium overload present in large arteries of elderly patients [20], and this data is strengthened by the significant diminution of AI, expressive of the improvement in arterial compliance. This result is particularly appreciable in these patients, both because arterial calcinosis appears to be an inevitable consequence of aging [21], and because the intensity and extent of arterial calcium accumulation can be considerably enhanced by hypertension. So, it is possible that the finding of a particularly sensitive response to treatment with calcium antagonists in elderly subjects [21] may be explained by the elevated arteriolar calcium content being responsible, in part, for the increase in SVR. This would mean that nifedipine interferes with the fundamental pathogenetic process of arterial calcinosis and its consequences. On the other hand, it has been demonstrated that some calcium antagonists, such as verapamil, diltiazem, nifedipine, and other 1, 4-dihydropyridine derivates, proved to be able to protect the arterial walls against calcium overload and structural alterations in a variety of animal disease models [22].

In our study we also observed, after 6 months of treatment, a decrease both of AWS and of LVM. These results are very important,because it has been demonstrated that cardiac hypertrophy has a closer correlation with SBP then DBP which suggests that reduced arterial distensibility and compliance may stimulate cardiac hypertrophy through a disproportionate increase in SBP [23]. On the basis of these observations, it is possible to suppose that the improvement in arterial compliance and the diminution of AWS induced by SRN chronic administration, play an important role in the reversal of cardiac hypertrophy. In conclusion, the overall impression obtained from our study is that nifedipine is effective and may be considered a possible first-choice agent for the treatment of ISH in elderly patients; because the efficacy is coupled with an improvement in arterial compliance thus interfering with the possible pathogenetic mechanism responsible for both the increase in SBP and its harmful consequences.

References

1. Kannel WB, Gordon T (1978) Evaluation of cardiovascular risk in the elderly: The Framingham Study. Bull NY Acad Med 54: 573–591
2. Subcommittee on Risk Factors and Stroke of the Stroke Council (1987) Risk factors in stroke. AHA Focus Series. American Heart Association. Stroke 3 (1): 9–14

3. Kannel WB, Dauber TR, McGee DL (1980) Perspectives on systolic hypertension: The Framingham Study. Circulation 61: 1179–1182
4. Simon ACh. Safer ME, Levenson JA, London GM, Levy BI, Chau NPh (1979) An evaluation of large arteries compliance in man. AM J Physiol 237: 550–554
5. Safar ME, Laurent St, Asmar RE, Savafian A, London GM (1987) Systolic hypertension in patients with arteriosclerosis obliterans of the lower limbs. Angiology 4: 287–295
6. Ben-Ishay D, Leibel B, Stessman J (1986) Calcium channel blockers in the management of hypertension in the elderly. Am J Med 81 (Suppl VIA): A30-34
7. Anonymous (1985) Treatment of hypertension in the over-60s. Lancet 1: 1369–1370 (editorial)
8. Laragh JH, Bühler FR, Chobanian A, Hansson L, Zachariah PK (1987) Calcium antagonists in hypertension: update 1986. J Cardiovasc Pharmacology 9 (Suppl IV): 1–3
9. Zanchetti A (1987) Role of calcium antagonists in systemic hypertension. Am J Cardiol 59: 130–136
10. Strano A, Novo S, Modica R, Nardi E, Donia G (1986) Hemodynamic effects of acute administration of slow-release nifedipine in elderly patients with systolic hypertension. Am J Nephrol 6 (Suppl I): 91–94
11. MacGregor GA (1986) Hypertension. In: Krebs R (ed) Treatment of cardiovascular diseases by Adalat (nifedipine). Schattauer, Stuttgart New York, pp 231–258
12. Kirkendall WM, Burton AC, Epstein FH, Fresis ED (1967) Recomendations for human blood pressure determination by sphygmomanometer. Circulation 36: 980–987
13. Sahn DJ, DeMaria A, Kisslo J, Weyman A (1978) Recomendations regarding quantitation in M-mode echocardiography: results of a survey of echocardiographic measurements. Circulation 58: 1072–1083
14. Quinones MA, Pickering E, Alexander JK (1978) Percentage of shortening of the echocardiographic left ventricular dimension. Its use in determining ejection fraction and stroke volume. Chest 74: 59–65
15. Eaton LW, Maughan WL, Shoukas AA, Weiss JL (1979) Accuration volume determination in the isolated ejecting canine left ventricle by two-dimensional echocardiography. Circulation 60: 320–327
16. Tarazi RC, Magrini F, Dustan HP (1975) The role of aortic distensibility in hypertension. In: Miller P, Safar MD (eds) International symposium on hypertension. Boehringer Ingelheim, Monaco, pp 133–138
17. Novo S, Licata G, Pinto A, Davì G, Strano A (1983) Haemodynamic effects of an antihypertensive combination between labetalol and chlortalidone administered for 6 months. J Hypertens 1 (Suppl II): 353–360
18. Devereux RB, Reichek N (1977) Echocardiographic determination of left ventricular mass in man. Anatomic validation of the method. Circulation 55: 613–618
19. Martin MA, Fieller NRJ (1979) Echocardiography in cardiovascular drug assessment. Br Heart J 41: 536–543
20. Simon ACh, Levenson JA, Safar ME (1985) Hemodynamic mechanisms of and therapeutic approach to systolic hypertension. J Cardiovasc Pharmacol 7: 22–27
21. Fleckenstein A, Frey M, Fleckenstein-Grün G (1986) Antihypertensive and arterial anticalcinotic effects of calcium antagonists. Am J Cardiol 57: 1–10
22. Fleckenstein A (1988) Future prospects in calcium antagonist therapy: prevention of arteriosclerotic vascular damage. Abstract of Verapamil Satellite Symposium of the 25 Anniversary International Symposium on Calcium Antagonists in Hypertension, Basel, February 9-11, 1988. p 3
23. Bouthier JD, DeLuca N, Safar ME, Simon ACh (1985) Cardiac hypertrophy and arterial distensibility in essential hypertension. Am Heart J 109: 1345–1352

Long-Term (12-Month) Antihypertensive, Metabolic, and Renal Hemodynamic Effects of Nifedipine and Nisoldipine

CLARA WITTENBERG[1] and JOSEPH B. ROSENFELD[2]

Summary. The antihypertensive, metabolic, and renal effects of nifedipine (NF) 40–80 mg/day and nisoldipine (NS) 10–20 mg/day were monitored in 32 patients with mild and moderate hypertension for a 12-month period. Blood pressure was significantly reduced in both groups after 12, 24, and 52 weeks of therapy. Systolic blood pressure (SBP) was reduced from 165 ± 14 to 147 ± 21 mmHg $(P < 0.01)$ and diastolic (DBP) from 104 ± 6 to 88 ± 9 mmHg $(P < 0.001)$ at the end of the treatment with NF. In the NS group, SBP was reduced from 171 ± 13 to 148 ± 9 mmHg $(P < 0.01)$, and DBP was reduced from 104 ± 5 to 93 ± 12 mmHg $(P < 0.01)$. There were no significant changes in the heart rate during this period. Plasma renin activity (PRA) decreased from an initial value of 1.8 ± 2.5 ng%/ml per h to 1.22 ± 1.06 ng%/ml per h in the NF group and increased from 1.28 ± 1.53 ng%/ml per h to 1.5 ± 2.05 ng/ml per h in the NS group. Both changes were not significant. Plasma aldosterone did not change in the NF group (11.1 ± 4.0 ng% vs 11.0 ± 4.3) and significantly increased from 10.2 ± 4.3 ng% to 13.6 ± 4.3 $(P < 0.05)$ in the NS group. Urine aldosterone increased in both groups, but not significantly. No significant changes were observed with both drugs in the lipid profile. In both groups, oral glucose tolerance test was not significantly different after 12 months. Glomerular filtration rate (GFR, insulin clearance) increased from 88 ± 20 ml/min to 92 ± 18 ml/min and renal plasma flow (RPF-PAH clearance) decreased from 400 ± 98 ml/min to 366 ± 86 ml/min in the NF group. In the NS group, GFR increased from 93 ± 17 ml/min to 94 ± 20 ml/min and RPF from 357 ± 70 ml/min to 363 ± 95 ml/min. All these changes were non-significant. The changes in urinary excretion of sodium and potassium were also not significant. Both NF and NS proved to be effective antihypertensive agents having no undesirable metabolic or renal effects during 12 months of follow-up.

Key words: Nifedipine — Nisoldipine — Hypertension — Renal function — Metabolic effects

Introduction

Chronic essential hypertension is characterized by increased peripheral vascular resistance [1]. Drugs with a dilatatory effect on the arterial wall will therefore be indicated as a therapeutical modality [2]. It has been more than a decade since it was demonstrated that calcium entry blockers promote systemic vasodilation [3, 4]. Recent reports have described the antihypertensive effect of calcium entry blockers in patients with mild to moderate essential hypertension [5–11]. The effects of this

---

[1] Hypertension Clinic, Beilinson Medical Center, Tel Aviv, Israel
[2] University Sackler School of Medicine, Petah Tikva, Israel

class of drugs on plasma renin, aldosterone, lipoproteins, and carbohydrate meta-bolism have also been examined [12-19]; but only few studies have investigated the long-term effects of diltiazem [5] and nifedipine [6]. The aim of our study was to evaluate the long-term safety and efficacy of the new dihydropyridine derivative nisoldipine (NIS) and compare it to nifedipine (NIF) in relation to blood pressure, plasma renin activity (PRA), aldosterone concentration, and serum lipoprotein frac-tions in essential hypertension patients followed for 12 months.

Subjects and Methods

The study comprised 32 subjects (26 men and 6 women, mean age 53 ± 7 years). All subjects had grade I-II essential hypertension according to WHO criteria. All had supine diastolic blood pressure readings of 95 mmHg or more on at least 3 occasions during a 4-week placebo period. All patients were known to our hypertension clinic, those with secondary forms of hypertension as well as other cardiovascular or major illnesses having been excluded by routine clinical evaluation.

Placebo Run-in Period

Suitable patients entered a 4-week placebo washout during which they were seen at 2-week intervals (Fig. 1). Those with a supine diastolic blood pressure between 95 and 125 mmHg at the end of this period were randomly allocated to either NIF 20 mg b.i.d. or NIS 10 mg once daily (od).

Treatment Period

After 2 weeks of active treatment (step I), patients not reaching goal diastolic blood pressure of < 95 mmHg (non-responders) had their NIF dosage increased to 40 mg b.i.d. or NIS dosage increased to 20 mg od (Fig. 1). Those who had not reached goal diastolic blood pressure (non-responders) after 4 weeks of active treatment (step II) had oxprenolol retard (80-160 mg od) added to the calcium blockers (step III).

Follow-up went on for 52 weeks. Case files included demographic data as well as information concerning past, concomitant, and inter-current diseases. Adverse effects were asked for and recorded on a side effect questionnaire at each visit. Supine and standing blood pressures, heart rate, and weight were checked every 2nd week during the placebo run-in and first 8 weeks of active treatment. From then on, visits took place once a month for responders and every 2nd week for non-responders. Blood pressure was measured twice in 2 positions: after 5 min supine and after 2 min standing. The mean of the 2 consecutive readings was recorded. Measurements were performed with a standard sphygmomanometer in the morning between 8:30 and 10:00 before the morning tablet intake. Phase V of Korotkoff sound was recorded as diastolic blood pressure. Insulin [20], total cholesterol [21], triglycerides [22], HDL [23], ApoA and ApoB [24] were determined by standard methods usage in our laboratory. An analysis of variance and 2 subsequent t-tests were used to examine the significance of changes in blood pressure produced by treatment. All data are reported as mean values ± standard error of mean (SEM) [25, 26].

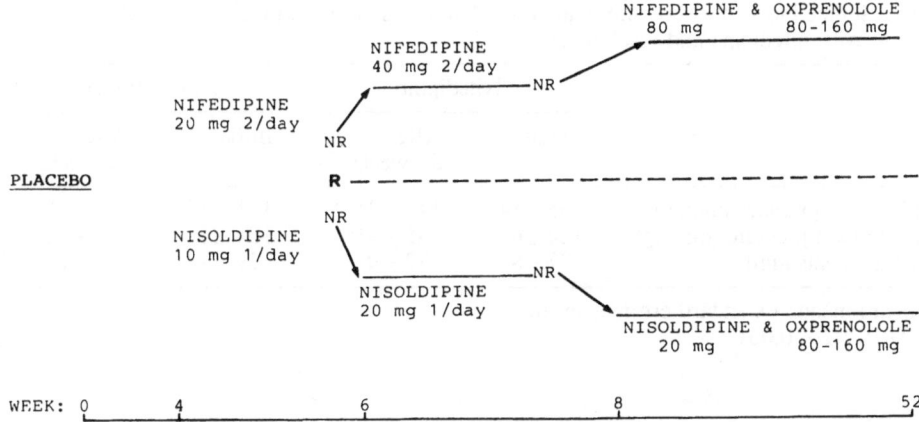

Fig. 1. Design of the study. *NR*, no response; *R*, response

Results

Blood Pressure and Heart Rate

Both supine systolic and diastolic blood pressure values were significantly reduced by NIF and NIS (Table 1). Systolic blood pressure (SBP) was reduced by 17 mmHg, and diastolic blood pressure (DBP), by 16 mmHg at the end of the treatment with NIF. In the NIS group, SBP was reduced by 23 mmHg and DBP by 11 mmHg. Mean heart rate in the supine position was not affected by NIS and was slightly and insignificantly reduced by NIF.

Metabolic Effects: Serum Lipid Changes

In the NIF group, no changes were seen in cholesterol, low density lipoprotein (LDL), and high density lipoprotein (HDL) at the end of 52 weeks (Table 2). Serum triglycerides decreased by 16%, ApoA lipoprotein decreased by 3.3%, and ApoB lipoprotein increased by 12%. At the end of 52 weeks of treatment with NIS, serum cholesterol decreased by 7%, LDL by 11.7%, and HDL by 13.3%. Serum trigly-cerides increased by 12.5%, ApoA lipoprotein decreased by 12% and ApoB lipo-protein increased by 18.5%.

Hormonal and Laboratory Parameters

PRA did not change significantly, being 1.8 ng/ml per h before and 1.22 ng/ml per h at the end of 52 weeks in the NIF group (Table 3). PRA rose from 1.28 ng/ml per h to 1.5 ng/ml per h in the NIS group. Plasma aldosterone did not change in the NIF group (11.1 ng% vs 11 ng%) and significantly increased from 10.2 ng% to 13.6% ng% ($P < 0.05$) in the NIS group. Urine aldosterone increased from 8.4 ng% to 10.8 ng% in the NIF group and from 8.8 ng% to 10.4 ng% in the NIS group.

Table 1. Supine blood pressure and heart rate of subjects before and after 52 weeks of treatment with nifedipine and nisoldipine

	Nifedipine		Nisoldipine	
	Initial	After 52 weeks	Initial	After 52 weeks
Systolic blood pressure (mmHg)	165 ± 14	147 ± 21**	171 ± 13	148 ± 9*
Diastolic blood pressure (mmHg)	104 ± 6	88 ± 9**	104 ± 5	93 ± 11*
Heart rate (beats/min)	77 ± 8	72 ± 9	79 ± 12	76 ± 6

Values are means ± standard error of mean.
$*P < 0.01$; $**P < 0.001$

Table 2. Serum lipids (mg/dl) before and after 52 weeks of treatment with nifedipine and nisoldipine

	Nifedipine		Nisoldipine	
	Pretreatment	After 52 weeks	Pretreatment	After 52 weeks
Serum cholesterol	229 ± 56	222 ± 51	225 ± 50	209 ± 30
HDL	48 ± 12	48 ± 12	45 ± 12	39 ± 8
LDL	144 ± 43	145 ± 37	154 ± 40	136 ± 35
VLDL	30 ± 15	24 ± 6	35 ± 12	33 ± 10
Serum triglycerides	146 ± 62	123 ± 31	152 ± 67	171 ± 66
ApoA lipoprotein	213 ± 26	206 ± 52	210 ± 39	185 ± 28
ApoB lipoprotein	108 ± 17	121 ± 48	108 ± 22	128 ± 50

Values are means ± standard error of mean.
HDL, high density lipoprotein; LDL, low density lipoprotein; VLDL, very low density lipoprotein

Renal Function and Electrolyte Excretion

At the end of the NIF and NIS treatments no significant changes were observed in the insulin clearance glomerular filtration rate (GFR)(Table 4). Renal plasma flow (RPF) as measured by the para-aminohippuric acid (PAH) clearance showed a 10% decrease at the end of 52 weeks in the NIF group, whereas the RPF insignificantly increased from 357 ml/min to 363 ml/min on NIS. At the end of 52 weeks of NIF and NIS, no significant changes in urinary excretion of Na and K were observed.

Side Effects

Moderate ankle swelling was experienced by 3 patients in the NIF group. Seven patients in the NIS group and five in the NIF group complained of headaches. Six in the NIS group and three in the NIF group complained of palpitations approximately 1-2 h after each dose. Six patients in the NIS group complained of mild fatigue. Most side effects disappeared after 2 months of treatment.

Table 3. Hormonal and laboratory parameters before and after 52 weeks of treatment with nifedipine and nisoldipine

	Nifedipine		Nisoldipine	
	Pretreatment	After 52 weeks	Pretreatment	After 52 weeks
Plasma renin activity (ng/ml per h)	1.8 ± 2.5	1.22 ± 1.06	1.28 ± 1.53	1.5 ± 2.05
Plasma aldosterone (ng%)	11.1 ± 4.9	11.0 ± 4.3	10.2 ± 4.3	13.6 ± 4.3*
Urine aldosterone (ng%)	8.4 ± 3.6	10.8 ± 3.9	8.8 ± 3.5	10.4 ± 6

*$P < 0.05$

Table 4. Renal function and electrolyte excretion before and after 52 weeks of treatment with nifedipine or nisoldipine

	Nifedipine		Nisoldipine	
	Initial	After 52 weeks	Initial	After 52 weeks
GFR (Insulin clearance) (ml/min)	88 ± 50	92 ± 18	93 ± 17	94 ± 20
RPF (PAH clearance) (ml/min)	400 ± 98	366 ± 36	357 ± 70	363 ± 95
Urinary sodium (mmol/24-h)	95 ± 46	91 ± 40	112 ± 42	115 ± 25
Urinary potassium (mmol/24-h)	41 ± 13	45 ± 13	42 ± 15	42 ± 12

GFR, glomerular filtration rate; RPF, renal plasma flow; PAH, para-aminohippuric acid

Discussion

Therapy with NIS resulted in a marked blood pressure reduction at the end of the 52 weeks of treatment. Contrary to the observation of Bühler et al. [27], claiming that mainly old and low-renin subjects respond to calcium entry antagonists, the young patients in our small group responded as well as the old ones. No orthostatic hypotension occurred, and the hypotensive effect was well maintained on monotherapy or with the addition of beta-blockers (5 patients in the NIF group and three in the NIS group).

The treatment was not equally tolerated. Those patients who complained of mild side effects stayed in the study, and their complaints disappeared within 1–2 weeks. Flush headache and palpitations, however, were experienced by a relatively large number and resulted in 3 dropouts.

A decrease in the heart rate in the supine position was recorded after the 52nd week with NIF and NIS treatment. This effect is similar to the one described with diltiazem and probably reflects a negative inotropic effect by direct action on the sinus node [28].

It should be pointed out that NIF and NIS did not have the same effect on PRA and aldosterone in plasma and urine. In the NIF group, PRA showed a decrease from 1.8 ng/ml per h to 1.22 ng/ml per h, whereas in the NIS group, there was a mild increase from 1.28 ng/ml per h to 1.5 ng/ml per h. In the NIF group, no changes in plasma aldosterone were observed, whereas in the NIS group there was an increase from 10.2 ng% to 13.6 ng%. Urinary aldosterone excretion increased at the end of both treatments. With the exception of plasma aldosterone in the NIS group, all other changes were not statistially significant.

At the end of 52 weeks of NIF, no significant changes were observed for total cholesterol, very low density lipoprotein (VLDL), LDL, and HDL; whereas in the NIS group a clear tendency to decrease was observed in these parameters. In the NIF group, triglycerides decreased by 16% and ApoA by 3.3%, while ApoB increased by 12%. NIS had an opposite effect on triglycerides: they increased by 12.5%. ApoA decreased by 12% and ApoB increased by 18.5% with NIS. Further studies are needed in order to clarify the effects of these 2 calcium entry blockers on different lipid functions in hypertensive patients.

Both NIF and NIS caused an increase of urinary aldosterone excretion at the end of 52 weeks; however, as these effects were accompanied by a decrease of PRA in the NIF group and an increase in the NIS group, it can be assumed that the increase of the urine aldosterone rate was not directly linked to PRA.

NIS proved to be as efficacious as NIF, as most of the observed changes in the lipid profile, renal function, PRA, and aldosterone were not significant at the end of 12 months of treatment. Both drugs can therefore be useful in the management of patients with hypertension, diabetes mellitus, and lipid disturbances.

References

1. Freis ED (1960) Hemodynamics in hypertension. Physiol Rev 40: 27–54
2. Koch-Weser J (1974) Vasodilating drugs in the treatment of hypertension. Arch Intern Med 133: 1017–1027
3. Bender F (1968) Die medikamentöse Behandlung von Herzrhythmus-störungen. Therapiewoche 18: 1803–1808
4. Brittinger WD, Schwarzbeck A, Wittenmeier KW (1970) Klinisch-experimentelle Untersuchungen über blutdrucksenkende Wirkung von Verapamil. Dtsch Med Wochenschr 95: 1871–1877
5. Chaffman M, Brogden RN (1985) Diltiazem: a review of its pharmacological properties and therapeutic efficacy. Drugs 29: 387–454
6. Sorkin EM, Clissold SP, Brogden RN (1985) Nifedipine: a review of its pharmacodynamic and pharmacokinetic properties, and therapeutic efficacy, in ischemic heart disease, hypertension and related cardiovascular disorders. Drugs 30: 182–274.
7. Lederballe-Pedersen O, Mikkelsen E, Christensen NJ, Kornerup HJ, Pedersen EB (1979) Effect of nifedipine on plasma renin, aldosterone and catecholamines in arterial hypertension. Eur J Clin Pharmacol 15: 235–240
8. Aoki K, Sato K, Kawaguchi Y, Yamamoto M (1982) Acute and long-term hypotensive effects and plasma concentrations of nifedipine in patients with essential hypertension. Eur J Clin Pharmacol 23: 197–201

9. Klein W, Brandt D, Vrecko K, Härringer M (1983) Role of calcium antagonists in the treatment of essential hypertension. Circ Res 52 (Suppl I): 174–181
10. Olivari MT, Bartorelli C, Polese A, Fiorentini C, Moruzzi P, Guazzi MD (1979). Treatment of hypertension with nifedipine, a calcium antagonist agent. Circulation 59: 1056–1062
11. Spivack C, Ockern S, Frishman W (1983) Calcium antagonists: clinical use in the treatment of systemic hypertension. Drugs 25: 154–177
12. Hiramatsu K, Yamagishi F, Kubota T, Yamada T (1982) Acute effects of the calcium antagonist, nifedipine, on blood pressure, pulse rate, and the renin-angiotensin-aldosterone system in patients with essential hypertension. Am Heart J 104: 1346–1350
13. Lewis GRJ, Steward DJ, Lewis BM, Bones PJ, Morley KD, Janus ED (1981) The antihypertensive effect of oral verapamil: acute and long-term administrations and its effects on the high-density lipoprotein values in plasma. In: Zanchetti A, Krikler DW (eds) Calcium antagonism in cardiovascular therapy. Excerpta Medica, Amsterdam, pp 270–277
14. Trost BN, Weidmann P (1984) Effects of nitrendipine and other calcium antagonists on glucose metabolism in man. J Cardiovasc Pharmacol 6: S986–S995
15. Wada S, Nakayama M, Masaki K (1982) Effects of diltiazem hydrochloride on serum lipids: comparison with beta-blockers. Clin Ther 5: 163–173
16. MacGregor GA, Rotellar C, Markandu ND, Smith SJ, Sagnella GA (1983) The acute response to nifedipine is related to pretreatment blood pressure. Postgrad Med J 59 (Suppl II): 91–94
17. Inouye IK, Massie BM, Benowitz N, Simpson P, Loge D (1984) Antihypertensive therapy with diltiazem and comparison with hydrochlorothiazide. Am J Cardiol 53: 1588–1592
18. Franz IW (1980) Differential antihypertensive effect of acebutolol and hydrochlorothiazide/amiloride hydrochloride combination on elevated exercise blood pressure in hypertensive patients. Am J Cardiol 46: 301–305
19. Oelkers W, Schöneshofer M, Blümel A (1974) Effects of progesterone and four synthetic progestagens on sodium balance and the renin-aldosterone system in man. J Clin Endocrinol Metab 39: 882–890
20. Hebing LG (1979) Determination of total serum insulin. Diabetologia 8: 260–266
21. Siedel J et al. (1981) Total cholesterol — enzymatic calorimetic method. J Clin Chem Clin Biochem 19: 838
22. Bergmeyer HU (1966) Methods of enzymatic analysis, 2nd edn. Verlag Chemie, Weinheim; Academic Press, New York London
23. Lopes-Virella MF et al. (1977) HDL-C. Clin Chem 23: 882
24. Dacol P, Kostner GM (1983) ApoA and ApoB determination. Clin Chem 29(6): 1045–1050
25. Hollander M, Wolfe DA (1973) Nonparametric statistical methods. Wiley, New York, p 503
26. Krauth J (1971) A locally most powerful tied rank test in a Wilcoxon situation. Ann Math Stat 42: 1949–1956
27. Bühler FR, Hulthen UL, Kiowski W, Bolli P (1983) Greater antihypertensive efficacy of the calcium channel inhibitor verapamil in older and low renin patents. Clin Sci 63: S439–S442
28. Kawai C, Konishi T, Matsuyama E (1981) Comparative effects of three calcium antagonists, diltiazem, verapamil and nifedipine, on the sinoatrial and atrioventricular nodes: experimental and clinical studies. Circulation 63: 1035–1042

Long-Term Hemodynamic and Metabolic Effects of Nitrendipine Vs Hydrochlorothiazide in Hypertensive Patients over 70 Years of Age*

Rene W.M.M. Jansen[1], Henk J.J. Van Lier,[2] and Willibrord H.L. Hoefnagels[1]

Summary. Diuretics and calcium antagonists both have been advocated for the treatment of hypertension in the elderly. In a double-blind, placebo-controlled, and parallel study, the hemodynamic, metabolic, and side effects of the new dihydropyridine derivative, nitrendipine, (20 mg once daily) were compared with those of hydrochlorothiazide (50 mg once daily). Blood pressure (BP) was significantly reduced ($P < 0.01$) by both nitrendipine ($13/10 \pm 4/3$ mmHg; $n = 15$) and hydrochlorothiazide ($25/11 \pm 4/2$ mmHg; $n = 16$; mean $\pm$ standard error of mean [SEM]). However, the reduction in systolic BP was greater after hydrochlorothiazide than after nitrendipine ($P = 0.02$). Both treatments had no effect on heart rate (HR) and body weight. Plasma potassium decreased (0.6 mmol/l) after hydrochlorothiazide and increased (0.2 mmol/l) after nitrendipine. Plasma glucose, uric acid, and plasma renin activity (PRA) increased only after hydrochlorothiazide. Both treatments had no effects on plasma cholesterol and triglycerides. No significant correlations were found in the nitrendipine group between mean BP reduction and basal PRA or age. Edema and flushing were the main adverse reactions during nitrendipine. We concluded that nitrendipine effectively lowered BP in patients 70 years or older, without the potentially harmful metabolic side effects of hydrochlorothiazide.

Key words: Elderly — Hypertension — Treatment — Nitrendipine — Hydrochlorothiazide

Introduction

The risk of cardiovascular disease increases in old age. Recently it has been demonstrated that antihypertensive treatment in the elderly results in reduced cardiovascular mortality and morbidity [1]. Diuretics and calcium antagonists both have been advocated for the treatment of hypertension in the elderly [2]. Since essential hypertension is hemodynamically characterized by an increased vascular resistance [3], the decrease in peripheral resistance as a primary mechanism of antihypertensive action is a favorable hemodynamic effect. Moreover, calcium

[1] Division of General Internal Medicine, Department of Medicine, University Hospital Nijmegen, Nijmegen, The Netherlands
[2] Department of Statistical Consultation, University of Nijmegen , Nijmegen, The Netherlands
* This study was supported financially by a grant from Bayer Nederland B.V.

antagonists may also facilitate diuresis and natriuresis [4, 5]. The main limitation of calcium antagonists is the short duration of their hypotensive action. Nitrendipine is a new, long-acting calcium antagonist belonging to the dihydropyridine group and can be administered in a once-daily dose [6]. Therefore, we performed a comparative study of the blood pressure lowering effects of long-term treatment with nitrendipine and hydrochlorothiazide in hypertensive patients 70 years or older.

Patients and Methods

In this study 31 hypertensive patients (aged 70–84 years) were included. Fifteen patients were treated with nitrendipine (mean age 72 ± 2 years, mean $\pm$ SD) and 16 patients with hydrochlorothiazide (mean age 75 ± 4 years). Patients with the following diseases were excluded from the study: angina pectoris, congestive heart failure, myocardial infarction or cerebrovascular accident if less than one year before the study, insulin dependent diabetes millitus, gout, accelerated or malignant hypertension, and/or a plasma creatinine concentration more than 150 μmol/l. The study was approved by the local ethical committee and all patients gave written informed consent. Patients were enrolled in the study if they had, after a washout period of 10 weeks, a supine diastolic blood pressure between 95 and 120 mmHg or a systolic BP of 180 mmHg or more as measured on 3 consecutive visits. BP was measured using a standard sphygmomanometer. BP and HR values are presented as the means of 2 measurements taken after 20 min of rest. Standing BP and HR were measured after 2 min in the standing position. The study was designed as a double-blind, parallel study of 12-week duration. After a washout period of 10 weeks, all patients received single-blind placebo therapy for 4 weeks. Patients were treated in a randomized order with 20 mg of nitrendipine in 1 daily dose or with 50 mg of hydrochlorothiazide in 1 daily dose. Patients visited the outpatient clinic every 4 weeks after an overnight fast and 24 h after medication. They were questioned for side effects using non-leading questions. At each visit BP, HR, and body weight were recorded. At the end of the placebo period and after 12 weeks of treatment, blood samples were collected for determination of plasma electrolytes, creatinine, glucose, calcium, uric acid, cholesterol, triglycerides, PRA, plasma aldosterone, plasma norepinephrine [7], and plasma drug levels. Compliance was established by pill counting and measurements of plasma drug levels. Plasma hydrochlorothiazide levels were assayed by a HPLC method [8]. Plasma nitrendipine levels were analyzed using capillary column gas chromatography with electron capture detector [9] with the limit of detection being 0.2 ng/ml.

Statistical comparisons between paired observations were made with Student's t-test when appropriate; otherwise, Wilcoxon's signed rank test was used. The Mann-Whitney test was used to compare the group on continuous parameters. Differences in proportions were tested with the Fisher exact test. To study the independent effects of age and basal PRA on BP responses, a multiple regression analysis was used. All values given in tables and text are expressed as mean $\pm$ SEM, unless otherwise indicated.

Results

Both treatments caused a significant fall of BP after 12 weeks of therapy (Table 1). Comparison of the BP reductions revealed that the fall of supine systolic BP was significantly greater after hydrochlorothiazide than after nitrendipine treatment ($P = 0.02$). Fourteen patients on hydrochlorothiazide (88%) and 11 patients on nitrendipine (73%) reached a supine diastolic BP lower than 95 mmHg or a diastolic BP reduction greater than 10 mmHg. None of the patients had orthostatic hypotension during the placebo period. After 4 weeks of treatment, a fall in systolic BP of more than 20 mmHg with compliants of dizziness was found in 2 patients, one in each group. No orthostatic hypotension was found at 8 and 12 weeks. Neither treatment had any effect on HR in the supine and upright positions, nor did body weight change during either active treatment. The biochemical effects (Table 2) show a significant decrease of plasma potassium and a significant increase of plasma glucose and plasma uric acid during treatment with hydrochlorothiazide. In contrast, these biochemical parameters remained unchanged during nitrendipine, except for a slight, but significant, increase of plasma potassium. Neither treatment had effect on cholesterol (total cholesterol, low-and high-density lipoprotein cholesterol) or triglycerides. PRA, aldosterone, and norepinephrine did not change during nitrendipine, whereas PRA increased significantly during hydrochlorothiazide treatment. Both drugs had significantly different effects on PRA ($P < 0.001$) and plasma norepinephrine ($P < 0.05$). The reduction of mean arterial pressure in response to hydrochlorothiazide, but not to nitrendipine treatment, was significant correlated to basal PRA (r = -0.54, $P = 0.03$). No significant correlations were found between the reduction of mean arterial pressure during either treatment and age. No major

Table 1. Mean values of blood pressure (BP) and heart rate before and after treatment with nitrendipine or hydrochlorothiazide

		Baseline	Placebo	12 Weeks of treatment
Nitrendipine				
Systolic BP	Supine	190 ± 6	$177 \pm 5^{++}$	$164 \pm 5**$
(mmHg)	Standing	185 ± 6	178 ± 7	$166 \pm 6*$
Diastolic BP	Supine	105 ± 1	102 ± 1	$92 \pm 1***$
(mmHg)	Standing	108 ± 1	105 ± 2	$97 \pm 3*$
Heart rate	Supine	78 ± 3	74 ± 3	75 ± 3
(beats/min)	Standing	83 ± 4	85 ± 4	81 ± 4
Hydrochlorothiazide				
Systolic BP	Supine	186 ± 4	$177 \pm 6^{+}$	$153 \pm 5***$
(mmHg)	Standing	183 ± 3	175 ± 5	$150 \pm 5***$
Diastolic BP	Supine	103 ± 1	$98 \pm 2^{++}$	$87 \pm 2***$
(mmHg)	Standing	108 ± 2	105 ± 3	$94 \pm 3***$
Heart rate	Supine	73 ± 2	$68 \pm 2^{+}$	70 ± 2
(beats/min)	Standing	81 ± 3	80 ± 2	82 ± 3

* treatment versus placebo: *$P<0.05$; **$P<0.01$; ***$P<0.001$
+ placebo versus baseline: +$P<0.05$; ++$P<0.01$

Table 2. Biochemical values before and after 12 weeks of therapy

	Hydrochlorothiazide		Nitrendipine		Significance between treatments
	Before	After	Before	After	
Plasma sodium (mmol/l)	142 ± 1	140 ± 1*	143 ± 1	142 ± 1*	NS
Plasma potassium (mmol/l)	3.7 ± 0.1	3.1 ± 0.1***	3.5 ± 0.1	3.7 ± 0.1**	P < 0.001
Creatinine (μmol/l)	82 ± 4	82 ± 5	78 ± 3	79 ± 4	NS
Glucose (mmol/l)	4.9 ± 0.1	5.2 ± 0.2*	5.5 ± 0.6	5.4 ± 0.5	P < 0.05
Total calcium (mmol/l)	2.29 ± 0.03	2.31 ± 0.03	2.38 ± 0.04	2.33 ± 0.04	NS
Uric acid (mmol/l)	0.30 ± 0.02	0.36 ± 0.03**	0.30 ± 0.02	0.32 ± 0.02	P < 0.05
Total cholesterol (mmol/l)	5.8 ± 0.2	5.7 ± 0.2	6.0 ± 0.3	5.8 ± 0.3	NS
HDL-cholesterol (mmol/l)	1.1 ± 0.1	1.1 ± 0.1	1.2 ± 0.1	1.2 ± 0.1	NS
LDL-cholesterol (mmol/l)	4.0 ± 0.2	3.9 ± 0.2	4.2 ± 0.3	3.9 ± 0.2	NS
Triglycerides (mmol/l)	1.4 ± 0.1	1.5 ± 0.1	1.4 ± 0.2	1.5 ± 0.2	NS
PRA (nmol/1 per h)	0.67 ± 0.16	1.26 ± 0.28***	0.62 ± 0.10	0.56 ± 0.08	P < 0.001
Aldosterone (nmol/l)	0.24 ± 0.04	0.28 ± 0.13	0.16 ± 0.20	0.20 ± 0.06	NS
Plasma NE (nmol/l)	1.95 ± 0.17	2.33 ± 0.31	2.06 ± 0.22	1.78 ± 0.20	P < 0.05

$*P < 0.05$; $**P < 0.01$; $***P < 0.001$ (post-pretreatment values)

HDL and LDL, high-and low-density lipoprotein, respectively; PRA, plasma renin activity; NE, norepinephrine

side effects were found in either study group. Peripheral edema and flushing were the main adverse reactions during nitrendipine treatment, but these tended to decrease during the course of the study. The compliance rates, i.e., the percentages of patients who had used more than 95% of their medication, were 77% in the hydrochlorothiazide group and 88% in the nitrendipine group. Plasma hydrochlorothiazide levels ranged from 0.035 to 0.128 μg/ml (mean 0.072 $\pm$ 0.006 μg/ml), and plasma nitrendipine, from 0.2 to 13.7 ng/ml (mean 3.0 $\pm$ 1.0 ng/ml). One patient on nitrendipine had plasma values is of nitrendipine below the detection limit.

Discussion

This study showed that monotherapy with 20 mg nitrendipine once daily effectively lowered BP without increasing HR in patients of 70 years or older. Hydrochlorothiazide (50 mg once daily) also effectively lowered BP and the decrease in systolic BP was significantly greater than after nitrendipine. It must be emphasized that BP measurements in this study were made 24 h post-dose. At present, there is still some doubt whether nitrendipine given once daily is as effective as given twice daily [10–12]. Cozensi et al. [10] found that nitrendipine once daily was not sufficient to maintain the hypotensive effect over the full 24 h. Therefore, it remains an open question whether, in elderly patients, nitrendipine, given in a perhaps more appropriate b.i.d. schedule, lowers BP as effectively as hydrochlorothiazide. The compliance rate as established by pill counting and plasma drug concentrations, were equally good in both groups and, therefore, cannot account for the observed differences in systolic BP response. The plasma concentrations of nitrendipine, measured 24 h post-dose, were comparable to those found by Kendall et al, [13], who studied the influence of age on the pharmacokinetics of nitrendipine in elderly patients with mild hypertension. In none of the patients did the therapy cause intolerable side effects. The 4 patients on nitrendipine who experienced edema and flushing considered these side effects merely inconvenient. Nitrendipine treatment was not accompanied by the number of potentially harmful biochemical effects observed during hydrochlorothiazide treatment. So, a decrease of plasma potassium and an increase of plasma uric acid and plasma glucose, as observed during hydrochlorothiazide treatment, were not found in the nitrendipine group. Nitrendipine treatment in patients of this age group appeared to have no influence on plasma cholesterol and triglycerides. These findings are in agreement with other studies [14–16], but in contrast to the study by Francischetti et al. [17], who found, after 12-months of treatment with nitrendipine, a decrease of high-density lipoprotein cholesterol in patients under 65 years of age. The effects of nitrendipine on PRA in patients 70 years or older have not yet been studied extensively. We found that PRA remained unchanged, in contrast to the significant rise found after hydrochlorothiazide treatment. Most studies in younger patients report a slight increase of PRA after short-term treatment with nitrendipine [4, 18]. This was also found in elderly hypertensive patients by Conen et al. [19]. The mean age in their study, however, was only 59 years. Unlike other studies [2, 18, 20], we did not find a correlation between basal PRA or age and the antihypertensive effect of nitrendipine. Recently, the absence of an age-dependent BP response with nitrendipine was also reported by Mehta et al. [21].

In conclusion, we found that nitrendipine effectively lowered BP in elderly patients without the potentially harmful metabolic side effects of hydrochlorothiazide.

Acknowledgments. The authors wish to express their gratitude to Dr. J. van Ree and colleagues for help in the selection of patients, to J. Willemsen who performed the plasma norepinephrine determinations, and the Y. Tan for determination of plasma hydrochlorothiazide levels. We thank Bayer Nederland B.V. for generously supplying nitrendipine and hydrochlorothiazide and for determination of plasma nitrendipine levels.

References

1. Amery A, Birkenhäger W, Brixko P, Bulpitt C, Clement D, Deruyttere M, De Schaepdryver A, Dollery C, Fagard R, Forette F, Forte J, Hamdy R, Henry JF, Joossens JV, Leonetti G, Lund-Johansen P, O'Malley K, Petrie J, Strasser T, Tuomilehto J, Williams B (1985) Mortality and morbidity results from the European working party on high blood pressure in the elderly trial. Lancet 1: 1349–1354
2. Bühler FR, Bolli P, Kiowski W, Erne P, Hulthén UL, Block LH (1984) Renin profiling to select antihypertensive baseline drugs: Renin inhibitors for high-renin and calcium entry blockers for low-renin patients. Am J Med 77: 36-42
3. Messerli FH, Ventura HO, Glade LB, Sungaard-Ruse K, Dunn FG, Frohlich ED (1983) Essential hypertension in the elderly: Haemodynamics, intravascular volume, plasma renin activity and circulating catecholamine levels. Lancet 2: 983–986
4. Luft FC, Aronoff GR, Sloan RS, Fineberg NS, Weinberger MH (1985) Calcium channel blockade with nitrendipine: Effects on sodium homeostasis, the renin-angiotensin system and the sympathetic nervous system in humans. Hypertension 7: 438–442
5. Leonetti G, Cuspidi C, Smapieri L, Terzoli L, Zanchetti A (1982) Comparison of cardiovascular, renal, and humoral effects of acute administration of two calcium channel blockers in normotensive and hypertensive subjects. J Cardiovasc Pharmacol 4: S319-S324
6. Müller FB, Bolli P, Erne P, Block LH, Kiowski W, Bühler FR (1984) Antihypertensive therapy with the long-acting calcium antagonist nitrendipine. J Cardiovasc Pharmacol 6: S1073-S1076
7. Hoffmann JJML, Willemsen JJ, Lenders JWM, Benraad ThJ (1986) Reduced imprecision on the radioenzymatic assay of plasma catecholamines by improving the stability of the internal standards. Clin Chim Acta 156: 221–226
8. Koopmans PP, Tan Y, van Ginneken CAM, Gribnau FWJ (1984) High performance liquid chromatographic determination of hydrochlorothiazide in plasma and urine. J Chromatogr 307: 445–450
9. Rämsch KD, Graefe KH, Scherling D, Sommer J, Ziegler R (1986) Pharmacokinetics and metabolism of calcium-blocking agents nifedipine, nitrendipine, and nimodipine. Am J Nephrol 6 (Suppl I): 73–80
10. Cosenzi A, Franca G, Piemontesi AM, Bellini G (1986) Once-a-day nitrendipine vs chlorthalidone in mild-to-moderate essential hypertension. Curr Ther Res 40: 99–106
11. Corsing C, Varchmin G, Stoepel K (1987) Once-daily nitrendipine: Therapy in longterm patients with essential hypertension (mild or moderate), efficacy and tolerance. J Cardiovasc Pharmacol 9 (Suppl IV): S136-S139
12. Groth H, Stimpel M, Edmonds D, Mosca R, Vetter W (1985) Nitrendipine in essential hypertension: Dose-finding and effects on renin-angiotensin system, J Hypertens 3: 419
13. Kendall MJ, Lobo J, Jack DB, Main ANH (1987) The influence of age on the pharmacokinetics of nitrendipine. J Cardiovasc Pharmacol 9 (Suppl IV): S96-S100

14. Lopez LM, Aguila E, Baz R, Mehta JL (1983) Absence of potentially adverse effects of hydralazine and nitrendipine on serum lipids. Clin Res 31: 844
15. Ferrara LA, Soro S, Fasano ML (1985) Effects of nitrendipine in glucose and lipid serum concentrations. Curr Ther Res 37: 614–618
16. Johnson BF, Romero L, Marwaha R (1986) Hemodynamic and metabolic effects of the calcium channel blocking agent nitrendipine. Clin Pharmacol Ther 39: 389–394
17. Francischetti EA, Oigman W, de A Fagundes VG, Sanjuliani AG, Cunha MC (1987) Long-term therapy with nitrendipine: Evalution of its antihypertensive and metabolic effects. J Cardiovasc Pharmacol 9 (Suppl IV) S107-S112
18. Pedrinelli R, Fouad FM, Tarazi RC, Bravo EL, Textor SC (1986) Nitrendipine, a calcium-entry blocker: Renal and humoral effects in human arterial hypertension. Arch Intern Med 146: 62–65
19. Conen D, Gerber A, Orfei R, Müller J (1987) Long-term therapy with nitrendipine: Effect on cerebral blood flow in elderly hypertensive patients. J Cardiovarc Pharmacol 9 (Suppl IV): S300-S302
20. Kiowski W, Bühler FR, Fadayomi MO, Erne P, Müller FB, Hulthén U., Bolli P (1985) Age, race, blood pressure and renin: Predictors for antihypertensive treatment with calcium antagonists. Am J Cardiol 56: H81-H85
21. Mehta J, Lopez LM, Deedwania PC, Fagan TC, Sternlieb CM, Vlachakis ND, Birkett JP, Schwartz LA (1987) Similar efficacy of nitrendipine in young ar 1 elderly hypertensive patients. Am J Cardiol 60: 1096–1100

Complications and the Choice of Antihypertensive Drugs in the Elderly

Mitsuaki Nakamaru, Toshio Ogihara, Hiroshi Mikami, Fuminori Masugi, Jitsuo Higaki, Atsuhiro Otsuka, Takeshi Hata, and Yuichi Kumahara

Summary. The presence of cardiovascular, respiratory, and metabolic complications which should be considered in the selection of antihypertensive drugs and the possible incidence of side effects was investigated in 1100 hypertensive patients over the age of 60 years. The prevalence of both cardiovascular and respiratory complications increased with age from 59% at 60 years to 80% at 80 years and from 13% at 60 years to 28% at 80 years respectively. On the other hand, the prevalence of metabolic complications decreased with age from 58% at 60 years to 38% at 80 years. The incidence of side effects in monotherapy was 12% for diuretics, 10% for beta-blockers, 2% for calcium antagonists, and 2% for converting enzyme inhibitors. In view of the presence of complications and side effects, the percentage of patients who should avoid specific antihypertensive drugs for first-line therapy was judged by physicians as 60% for diuretics, 27% for beta-blockers, 9% for converting enzyme inhibitors, and 6% for calcium antagonists. These judgements were mainly made because of diabetes mellitus (25%), hyperuricemia (18%), hyperlipidemia (16%), hypokalemia (11%), or renal insufficiency (10%) in the case of a diuretic, and chronic obstructive pulmonary disease (11%), heart failure (7%), or bradycardia (4%) in the case of a beta-blocker. There were considerably less patients who had contraindications to the use of calcium antagonists or converting enzyme inhibitors. We conclude that both calcium antagonists and converting enzyme inhibitors are drugs of choice for first-line therapy of hypertension in the elderly.

Key words: Hypertension — Complications — Antihypertensive drugs — Elderly hypertensives

Introduction

Drug therapy in the elderly is, in general, difficult. Absorption may be altered and delayed, and metabolism may be decreased by impaired renal and hepatic functions. Thus, altered pharmacokinetics makes the elderly more susceptible to drug side effects. Compliance is often poor in elderly patients. Elderly hypertensive patients also have many other illnesses, especially: cerebrovascular disease, heart disease, pulmonary disease, and diabetes mellitus. Special consideration should be given in the choice of an antihypertensive drug because of these coexisting diseases. In the present study, we surveyed the prevalence of dementia and cardiovascular, respiratory, and metabolic complications in 1100 elderly hypertensive patients. The fre-

[1] Department of Medicine and Geriatrics, Osaka University Medical School, Osaka, Japan

quency of antihypertensive drugs used and incidence of adverse side effects were also investigated. We evaluated the percentage of patients judged by physicians as unfit for a specific antihypertensive drug as first-line therapy because of the presence of complications and or side effects.

Materials and Methods

The present report was based on a chart review which we conducted August–December 1986. The study included 1100 hypertensive patients (480 males and 620 females) over 60 years of age (mean age 71 years) who had a systolic blood pressure of 160 mmHg or more, or a diastolic blood pressure of 90 mmHg or more, irrespective of antihypertensive drug therapy. Both hospitalized patients and outpatients were included in this study. The prevalence of dementia and cardiovascular, pulmonary, and metabolic complication which should be considered in the selection of antihypertensive drugs was surveyed. Cardiovascular complications included cerebrovascular disease, renal insufficiency, ischemic heart disease, heart failure, arrhythmias, and occulusive arterial disease. Pulmonary complications such as chronic obstructive pulmonary disease (COPD) were investigated. Metabolic complications included diabetes mellitus, hyperuricemia, hyperlipidemia, and electrolyte disturbances. The diagnoses of these complications were performed by personal physicians and further assessed by a committee consisting of ourselves. Diagnoses were based on the history of illness, clinical findings, laboratory data, and specific techniques such as computerized tomography of the brain for cerebrovascular disease, electrocardiogram or echocardiography for heart disease, and chest X-ray or spirogram for pulmonary disease. The diagnosis of diabetes mellitus was performed by a level of fasting blood glucose and 75 g oral glucose tolerance test in a untreated patient. Any patient already being treated by an oral hypoglycemic agent or insulin was diagnosed as having diabetes mellitus. Criterion for hyperlipidemia was a serum cholesterol level above 240 mg/dl in an untreated patient. Criterion for hyperuricemia was a serum uric acid level above 7 mg/dl in an untreated male subject and above 6 mg/dl in an untreated female subject. Criteria for hyperkalemia and hypokalemia were a serum potassium level above 5.2 mEq/1 and below 3.5 mEq/1, respectively. The frequency of antihypertension drugs used and side effects were also investigated. We requested personal physicians to select which antihypertension drugs should be avoided as first-line therapy because of the presence of complications and side effects. The results were also reevaluated by the committee consisting of ourselves.

Results

Figure 1 shows the prevalence of dementia and cardiovascular, respiratory, and metabolic complications. Dementia was observed in approximately 50% of hypertensive patients over 80 years of age, if borderline dementia was included. The prevalence of cardiovascular complications increased with age from 59% in patients

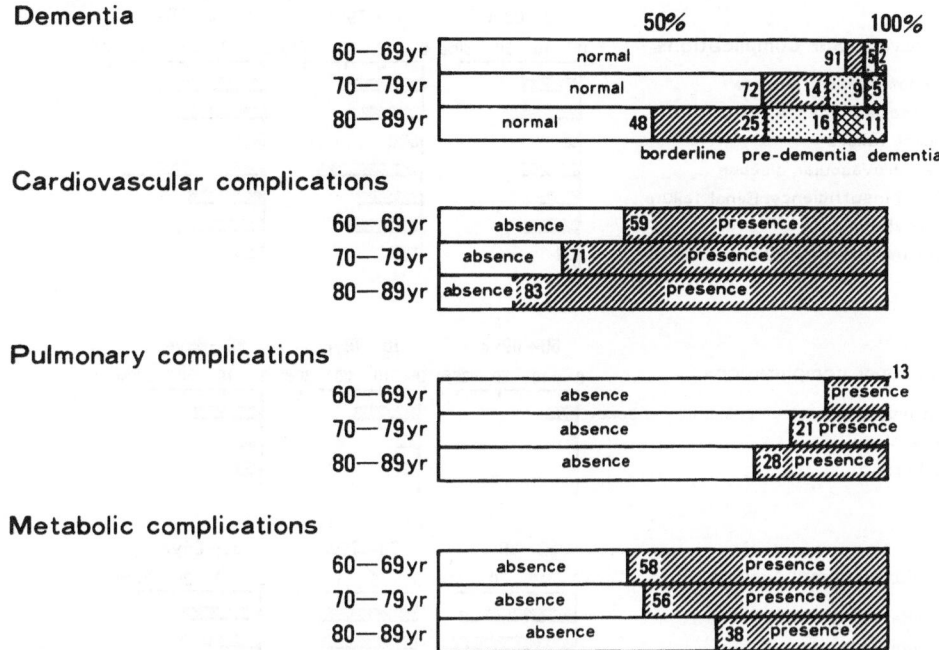

Fig. 1. The prevalence of dementia and cardiovascular, respiratory, and metabolic complications in elderly hypertensive patients

in their 60s to 80% in patients in their 80s. Their specific complications are listed in Fig. 2. Complications included ischemic heart disease, myocardial change revealed in electrocardiogram, cerebrovascular disease, renal insufficiency or renal failure, and arrhythmias. The prevalence of respiratory complications also increased with age from 13% in patients in their 60s to 28% in patients in their 80s. The most frequent complication was COPD as shown in Fig. 2. Metabolic complications including diabetes mellitus, hyperlipidemia, and hyperuricemia were observed in 58% of patients in their 60s and decreased with age.

The types of therapy were also surveyed in this study. Twenty percent of patients were treated by non-drug therapy and 80% received drug therapy (60% for monotherapy and 20% for combined therapy). The frequency of drugs used in monotherapy was 65% for calcium antagonists, 15% for diuretics, 6% for beta-blockers, and 5% for converting enzyme inhibitors. In combined therapy, calcium antagonists were also the most frequent drugs prescribed (36%), followed by diuretics (22%), converting enzyme inhibitors (18%), and beta-blockers (13%). The incidence of adverse side effects in elderly hypertensive patients treated by monotherapy was 12% for diuretics, 10% for beta-blockers, 2% for calcium antagonists, and 2% for converting enzyme inhibitors.

Judged by physicians, the percentage of patients who should avoid a specific antihypertensive drug as first-line therapy because of the presence of complications and side effects was 60% for diuretics, 27% for beta-blockers, 9% for converting enzyme

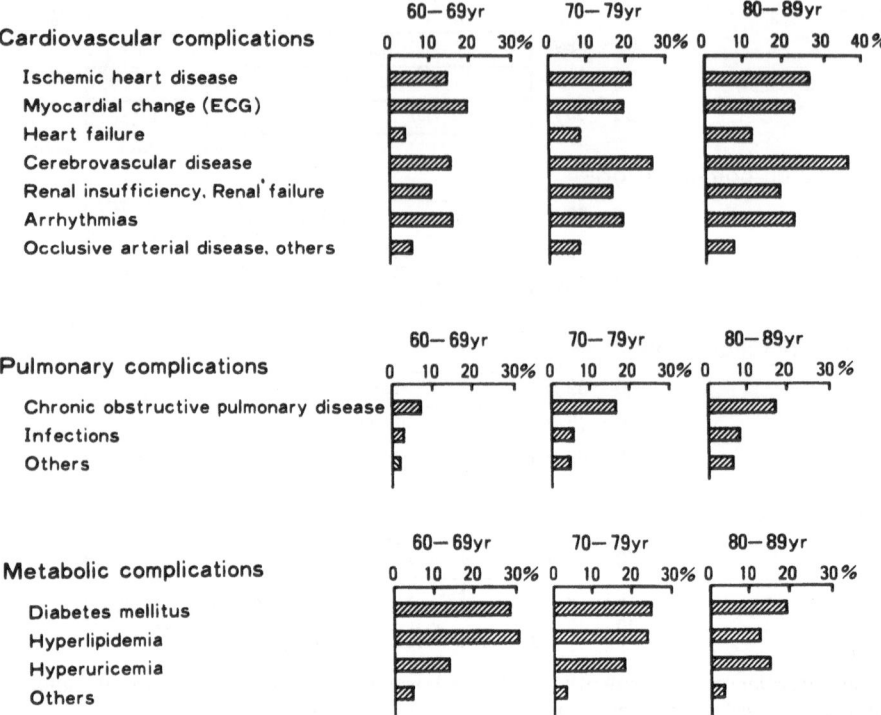

Fig. 2. Items of cardiovascular, respiratory, and metabolic complications in elderly hypertensive patients

inhibitors, and 6% for calcium antagonists. These judgements were mainly based on diabetes mellitus or hyperglycemia (25%), hyperuricemia (18%), hyperlipidemia (16%), hypokalemia (11%), or renal insufficiency (10%) for diuretics and COPD (11%), heart failure (7%), or bradycardia (4%) for beta-blockers. The reasons against use of a converting enzyme inhibitor were hyperkalemia (7%) or renal insufficiency (3%). There were markedly less patients who were judged unsuited to the use of a calcium antagonist.

Discussion

Recent clinical data indicate that hypertension in the elderly is a risk factor for cardiovascular complications and that treatment is safe and effective in reducing morbidity and mortality. In "The European Working Party on High Blood Pressure in the Elderly Trial," cardiovascular mortality was reduced in patients with diuretic therapy, owing to a reduction in cardiac deaths [1]. These findings are consistent with results of other major trials [2-4] and clearly show the benefit of therapy in elderly hypertensives. Concerning side effects, "The Hypertension Detection and

Follow-up Program" suggested that the elderly patients had considerably fewer side effects than the younger age group [3].

In the therapy of hypertension, the stepped-care approach is a widely accepted guideline [5]. Thiazide diuretics and beta-adrenoceptor blockers are used for steps 1 and 2, and vasodilators and adrenergic neuron blockers are suggested as steps 3 and 4. Diuretics are the most frequently used and the least expensive antihypertensive drugs and have demonstrated a reduction in morbidity and mortality in every major trial in which they have been used as a first-line therapy. However, they may induce well-known side effects such as hypokalemia, hyperglycemia, hyperuricemia, and hypercholesterolemia. Beta-blockers are not as effective as diuretics for mono-therapy in elderly patients [6]. Their use is usually contraindicated in patients with pulmonary disease or heart failure. They also cause hypertriglycemia and decreased high-density lipoprotein [7]. Adrenergic neuron blockers should not be used in elderly patients because they are susceptible to postural hypotension.

Medications used may have deleterious effects that negate the positive effects, especially in the elderly. Therefore, special attention should be payed when selecting therapy. In the present study, we investigated the prevalence of cardiovascular, respiratory, and metabolic complications which should be considered in the selection of antihypertensive drugs. Cardiovascular complications such as ischemic heart disease, heart failure, arrhythmias, cerebrovascular disease, renal disease, or occlusive arterial disease were observed in more than 60% of elderly hypertensive patients. Of these disorders, the use of beta-blockers is contraindicated in patients with heart failure, bradycardia, and occlusive arterial disease, and thiazide diuretics are usually ineffective in the presence of renal insufficiency and might even induce a further decrease in glomerular filtration rate. COPD was the most frequent respiratory complication in the elderly and its prevalence increased with age. The use of beta-blockers should be avoided in elderly patients with COPD. The prevalence of metabolic complications including diabetes mellitus, hyperlipidemia, or hyperuricemia decreased with age from 60% at 60 years to 40% at 80 years. It is possible that only a few of the hypertensive patients in their 80s with these complications may survive. The elderly may be more susceptible to the metabolic side effects of diuretics. Thus, their use may not be preferable in elderly patients with metabolic complications. As diuretics decrease extracellular fluid volume at the expense of potassium loss, the arrhythmic potential of hypokalemia may limit their use.

Ideally, therapy for the elderly should provide few side effects and have a simple regimen to enhance compliance. This study shows that the incidence of side effects observed in patients treated with diuretics or beta-blockers is more than that seen in patients treated with calcium antagonists or converting enzyme inhibitors. The presence or absence of dementia is examined in this study. Approximately 50% of patients over the age of 80 years have some sort of cognitive dysfunction if borderline dementia is included. This finding indicates that cerebral blood flow should not be decreased by antihypertensive therapy, and that physicians must keep in mind compliance in treatment hypertensive patients with dementia.

In view of the presence of complications and side effects, we evaluated the percentage of patients judged by physicians as being unsuited to the use of specific antihypertensive drug for first-line therapy. Diuretics were the most frequently avoided drug for first-line therapy of hypertension in the elderly. The main reasons cited were metabolic complications and renal insufficiency. Beta-blockers were also frequently avoided in many cases because of the presence of COPD, heart failure, bradycardia, or insulin-dependent diabetes mellitus. In contrast with diuretics or beta-blockers, both calcium antagonists and converting enzyme inhibitors were less frequently avoided for first-line therapy. In fact, calcium antagonists such as nifedipine, nicardipine, and diltiazem were the most frequently prescribed drugs for both monotherapy and combined therapy in this study. They are effective as monotherapy in elderly hypertension [8] but are more expensive compared to diuretics and have to be given 2 or 3 times daily. Development of long-lasting calcium antagonists is now in progress. Converting enzyme inhibitors, e.g., captopril or enalapril, seem to be effective for mild to moderate hypertension in the elderly [9, 10] and do not cause many unwanted side effects.

In conclusion, both calcuim antagonists and converting enzyme inhibitors appear to be preferable drugs for first-line therapy of hypertension in the elderly. To date, however, it is not clear whether these new drugs reduce cardiovascular mortality and morbidity, and have a more favorable effect on the quality of life. Prospective, controlled trials are necessary to ascertain their benefits.

References

1. Amery A, Birkenhäger W, Brixko A, Bulpitt C, Clement D, Fagard R, De Schaepdryver A, Dollery C, Deruyttere M, Forette F, Forte J, Hamdy R, Henry JF, Joossens JV, Leonetti G, Lund-Johansen P, O'Malley K, Petrie J, Strasser T, Tuomilehto J (1985) Mortality and morbidity results from the European working party on high blood pressure in the elderly trial. Lancet 1: 1349–1354
2. Veterans Administration Co-operative Study on Antihypertensive Agents (1972) Effects of treatment on morbidity in hypertension III. Influence of age. diastolic pressure and prior cardiovascular disease. Circulation 45: 991–1004
3. Hypertension Detection and Follow-up Program (1985) Detection and treatment of hypertension in older individuals. Am J Epidemiol 121 :371–376
4. Coope J, Warrender TS (1986) Randomised trial of treatment of hypertension in elderly patients in primary care. Br Med J 293: 1145–1151
5. The Joint National Committee on Detection, Evaluation, and Treatment of High Blood Pressure (1984) The 1984 report of the Joint National Committee on Detection, Evaluation, and Treatment of High Blood Pressure. Arch Intern Med 144: 1045–1057
6. Bühler FR, Burkhart F, Lütold BE, Küng M, Marbet G, Pfisterer M (1975) Antihypertensive beta blocking action as related to renin and age: a pharmacologic tool to identify mechanisms in essential hypertension. Am J Cardiol 36: 653–669
7. Weinberger MH (1985) Antihypertensive therapy and lipids: evidence, mechanisms, and implications. Arch Intern Med 145: 1102–1105
8. Bühler FR, Bolli P, Kiowski W, Erne P, Hulthen UL, Block LH (1984) Renin profiling to select antihypertensive baseline drugs: renin inhibitors for high-renin and calcium entry blockers for low-renin patients. Am J Med 77: 36–42
9. Jenkins AC, Knill JR, Dreslinski GR (1985) Captopril in the treatment of the elderly hypertensive patient. Arch Intern Med 145: 2029–2031
10. Woo J, Woo KS, Vallance-Owen J (1986) Captopril versus hydrochlorothiazide/triamterene in mild-to-moderate hypertension in the elderly. Lancet 2: 924

Quality of Life in the Treatment of Hypertension in the Elderly

Hiroshi Mikami, Toshio Ogihara, Mitsuaki Nakamaru, Fuminori Masugi, Jitsuo Higaki, Atsuhiro Otsuka, Takeshi Hata, and Yuichi Kumahara[1]

Summary. We evaluated the effects of 4 antihypertensive drugs on the quality of life (QOL) in patients over 60 years of age. Mild to moderate hypertensive patients ($n = 230$; systolic blood pressure (BP) > 160 mmHg and/or diastolic BP > 95 mmHg) without serious complications were enrolled in the study and randomly assigned to 4 different antihypertensive drugs: captopril, nicardipine, pindolol, and trichlormethiazide. At 0, 3, 6, and 12 months, clinical examinations were performed. QOL was assessed using a questionnaire, and cognitive function was evaluated by dementia screening scale. The percentage of withdrawals because of adverse effects by 12 months was significantly high in the pindolol group (24%). Hypotensive effects of the drugs were comparable, and there were no significant changes in cognitive function within each treatment group. In the nicardipine, captopril, and trichlormethiazide groups, significant improvements in QOL were noted at 6 months but became less significant at 12 months. In the pindolol group, QOL was rather worsened at 6 months, but at 12 months it was comparable with those of the other groups. Thus, the present study demonstrated that there are considerably different effects on QOL among the antihypertensive drugs in the treatment of elderly patients.

Key words: Quality of life — Antihypertensive treatment — Elderly hypertensives

Introduction

Recently, considerable effort has been focused on the evaluation of the effects of treatments on the QOL of hypertensive patients. With the rapidly increasing elderly population, evaluation of changes in the QOL of elderly hypertensives in response to treatment has become a matter of great clinical as well as social significance. In younger generations, different effects on the QOL have been demonstrated among widely used antihypertensive drugs [1], but, to our knowledge, there has been no report of this subject being studied in elderly people. The purpose of the present study was accordingly to evaluate the effects of treatment with 4 different antihypertensive drugs, which have been commonly used in Japan, during a 12-month period on the QOL of elderly hypertensive patients.

---

[1] Department of Medicine and Geriatrics, Osaka University Medical School, Osaka, Japan

Subjects and Methods

Two hundred and thirty elderly hypertensive patients (systolic BP > 160 mmHg and/or diastolic BP > 95 mmHg) of either sex over 60 years of age without serious complications were enrolled in the present study. After an observation period of at least 4 weeks, treatment of a 12-month period was initiated. Patients were randomly allocated to one of 4 antihypertensive drugs and given the initial doses as follows: Captopril ($n = 58$; 25–75 mg/day), nicardipine ($n = 59$; 40–80 mg/day), pindolol ($n = 56$; 10–20 mg/day), and trichlormethiazide ($n = 57$; 1–4 mg/day). For the first 3 months, the treatment was monotherapy as a rule. Trichlormethiazide (2–4 mg/day) was added to captropril, and captopril (25–75 mg/day) was added to the other drugs when BP control was not satisfactory.

At baseline and at the 3rd, 6th, and 12th month of treatment, the following examinations were performed: BP determination, hematological and biochemical tests, chest x-ray, electrocardigram, estimation of QOL, and cognitive function. BP was measured in sitting position and the baseline BP was an average of 2 BP values taken at the beginning and 2 weeks prior to the treatments. The hematological and biochemical tests included complete blood count, transaminases, alkaline phosphatase, blood urea nitrogen, serum creatinine, uric acid, serum electrolytes, serum lipids, creatinine phosphokinase, plasma glucose, and urinalysis. There were no statistically significant differences among the 4 groups in the number of patients, ages, systolic and diastolic BPs, heart rates, and cardiopulmonary ratios as determined on chest x-ray, hematological, and biochemical data. Estimation of QOL was performed by an interview using a questionnaire developed for this study [2]. The questionnaire consisted of 38 questions to evaluate the following 10 items: general well-being, will to work, physical symptoms, sleep scale, emotional status, cognitive function, sexual function, life satisfaction, self-control, and vigor. Each question was answered by one of 3 grades: 2 points ("good," "well," "yes," etc.); 1 point ("moderate"); or 0 points ("bad," "poor," "no," etc.). In each patient, the sum of points was divided by the number of questions within each item to represent the score of the item (full score = 2.0). The cognitive function was also evaluated by Hasegawa's dementia screening scale [3].

Statistical Analysis

Values are expressed as means ± SD. Chi-squared test was performed to assess the significant differences of the baseline data and withdrawal rates, etc. among the 4 treatment groups. Within each treatment group, one-way analysis of variance was performed to evaluate the effect of the treatment on the variables, and significant tests were followed by Dunnett's test to assess the significance of differences of the means at the 3 points of the treatment period from the baseline value. One-way analysis of variance was performed to evaluate the effect of the different treatments on the variables at each point of the treatment, and significant tests were followed by Dunnett's test to assess the significance of differences of the means of each variable among the 4 treatment groups. In the QOL estimation, the changes in scores of each item from the baseline value were calculated, and the significance of differences was tested by Student's t-test against zero. A P value of less than 0.05 was considered significant.

Results

During the 12-month treatment period, high withdrawal rates were observed in the pindolol and trichlormethiazide groups, most of which were due to adverse effects of the drugs (Table 1). In the pindolol group, the withdrawal rate amounted to 23.9% (11 of 56 patients). One patient was withdrawn because of insufficient BP reduction, and the remaining 10 patients were withdrawn due to the following reasons: development of asthma or dyspnea, increase in cardiopulmonary ratio, fatigue, gastrointestinal adverse effects (anorexia, nausea, epigastric pain, etc.), Raynaud's phenomenon, muscle cramp, and/or worsening of diabetes. In the trichlormethiazide group, seven out of 57 patients (15.2%) were withdrawn: 2 patients developed cerebrovascular accidents, and the other reasons given were nausea, muscle weakness, atrial fibrillation, photosensitivity, and development of diabetes mellitus. In the nicardipine group, only three of the 59 patients were withdrawn from the study. The reasons given were severe tinnitus, asthmatic dyspnea, and flushing of the face associated with headache. In the captopril group, one of the 58 patients was withdrawn because of an elevation of serum potassium level (5.2 to 5.8 mEq/1), and 4 patients were withdrawn due to insufficient BP control. In addition to these withdrawals, 35 patients were excluded from the study because of loss to follow-up (Table 1). Three patients died of concurrent diseases which were not related to the antihypertensive treatment, while other reasons were transference to other hospitals, default without notice, and loss to follow-up after discharge. Since these were not directly related to the treatment with the drugs, they were considered separately from the withdrawals due to adverse effects and insufficient BP reduction. For the remaining 169 patients, QOL and clinical evaluation was performed at the 12-month point (Table 1).

During the 12-month treatment period, all 4 antihypertensive drugs had significant and comparable hypotensive effects starting from the 1st month of treatment. The group BP levels at 12 months were $143 \pm 16/79 \pm 12$ mmHg for captopril, $140 \pm 16/75 \pm 12$ mmHg for nicardipine, $142 \pm 15/79 \pm 10$ mmHg for pindolol, and $143 \pm 12/80 \pm 11$ mmHg for trichlormethiazide ($P < 0.001$ from each control).

Table 1. Withdrawals during the 12-month period and the remaining patients at the 12-month point in the 4 treatment groups for quality of life assessment

	Captopril	Nicardipine	Pindolol	Trichlormethiazide
No. of enrolled patients	58	59	56	57
No. of withdrawals	5	3	11	7
Withdrawal rates	9.8%	5.8%	23.9%	15.2%
Reasons for withdrawals				
Insufficient BP reduction	4	3	1	0
Adverse effects	1	2	10	7
Loss to follow-up	7 (0)	7 (0)	10 (2)	11 (1)
(Death from concurrent diseases unrelated to treatment)				
No. of patients for quality of life evaluation of 12 months	46	49	35	39

The heart rate was significantly decreased only in the pindolol group (71 ± 2 beats/min). There was a significant reduction in the cardiopulmonary ratio only in the captopril group (from $52.9 \pm 6.0\%$ to $51.6 \pm 5.2\%$ at 6 months and $50.9 \pm 4.8\%$ at 12 months; both $P < 0.01$). In the trichlormethiazide group, the serum uric acid level was consistently higher than baseline and the serum potassium level was significantly low at 6 and 12 months, and there were transient increases in the levels of blood urea nitrogen and creatinine phosphokinase at 6 months. In the pindolol group, the serum level of creatinine phosphokinase was consistently higher than baseline, and the serum lipids were transiently lowered at 6 months. In the nicardipine group, at 3 months, there was a transient increase in pulse rate, and at 6 months, serum potassium level was low transiently. In the captopril group, there was no significantly changed biochemical variables.

There were changes in the QOL scores of the patients in response to the antihypertensive treatment in the cases of all 4 drugs, but degrees of the changes were different among the drugs. At 6 months (Fig. 1), the captopril group showed significant improvements in scores for general well-being, will to work, and sleep scale. In the nicardipine group, scores for general well-being, will to work, sleep scale, and emotional status were improved. In the trichlormethiazide group, improvements were noted in general well-being and physical symptoms. However, the pindolol treatment rather worsened scores of physical conditions. There were significant differences in the changes in the scores of general well-being, will to work, and sleep scale between the pindolol and nicardipine groups ($P < 0.05$). The pindolol group also had significantly less improvement in will to work, physical symptoms, and sleep scale as compared with the remaining 2 groups. However, these differences disappeared at the 12-month stage, and all the groups had similar improvements from baseline in the scale for general well-being. Furthermore, the captopril and nicardipine groups maintained significant improvements in sleep scale. The latter group, however, showed significant worsening of sexual function. In fact, the scores for sexual function scale had a tendency to decrease in all 4 groups. In all groups, there were no significant changes in life satisfaction, self-control or vigor throughout the study. The cognitive function was not greatly affected by these antihypertensive drugs within each treatment group, but there were some differences when comparison was made among the 4 groups. At 6 months, the pindolol group had a significant decrease in the scores for the dementia screening scale as compared with the captopril and trichlormethiazide groups. At 12 months, the trichlormethiazide group had significant improvements in comparison with the nicardipine group.

Discussion

It has been a matter of considerable controversy whether antihypertensive treatment in the elderly is beneficial or not. Recently, many epidemiological and clinical studies have shown significant beneficial effects of antihypertensive treatment in the elderly who are less than 85 years of age through the prevention of complications and prolongation of life expectancy [4]. With the rapidly increasing elderly population,

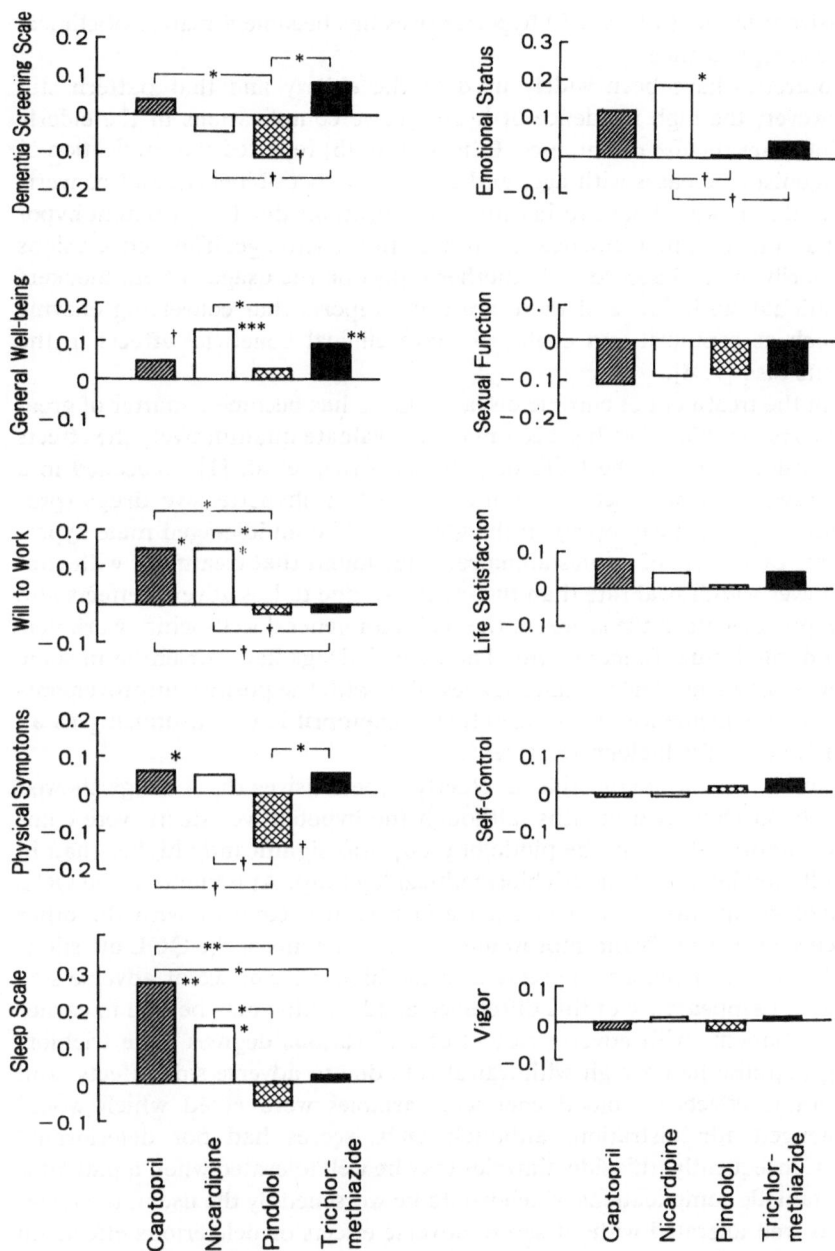

Fig. 1. Changes in scores of dementia screening scale and quality of life questionnaire from baseline to 6th month in 4 treatment groups. A positive change in score denotes improvement.
†$0.05 < P < 0.1$; *$P < 0.05$; **$P < 0.01$; ***$P < 0.001$

antihypertensive treatment for elderly hypertensives has become a matter of clinical as well as social significance.

Thiazide diuretics have been widely used in the elderly and that pattern still remains. However, the high incidence of hypertensive complications in the elderly often contraindicates the use of diuretics. Bühler et al. [5] reported that indication of calcium antagonists increases with age, and conversely, beta-blockers and converting enzyme inhibitors would have rather limited indications due to less potent hypotensive effect and increasing incidence of adverse effects with age. Their conclusions are not necessarily in good accord with another report on the usage of beta-blockers in an international study [6], and there are some reports that converting enzyme inhibitors, such as captopril and enalapril, have clinical beneficial effects in the elderly patients also [7, 8].

Recently, in the treatment of chronic diseases, QOL has become a matter of great interest, and considerable effort has been made to evaluate quantitatively the effects of antihypertensive drugs on the QOL of patients. Croog et al. [1] succeeded in a quantitative assessment of effects of commonly used antihypertensive drugs (propranolo, methyldopa, and captopril) on the QOL of white middle-aged male hypertensive patients by the use of a questionnaire. They found that treatment with captopril had a lower withdrawal rate than the other two due to less adverse effects and significant improvements in the scores of the scales for general well-being, work performance, and intellectual function, etc. The other 2 drugs had worsening in some items of QOL assessment. Their results suggest that with the positive improvements in QOL and its low incidence of adverse effects, captopril is very promising as an antihypertensive drug for lifelong treatment.

In the present study, we found that in elderly hypertensives the 4 drugs showed different effects on QOL at 6 months, although the hypotensive effects were comparable. The withdrawal rate in the pindolol group was significantly higher than in the others, followed by that of the trichlormethiazide group. At 6 months, the QOL of the pindolol group was rather worsened and was in a contrast with the other groups, which showed significant improvements in some items of the QOL questionnaire. This difference appears to be related to the higher incidence of adverse side effects, and the disappearance of this difference at 12 months may be due to earlier withdrawals of patients with adverse side effects of various degrees. The trichlormethiazide group also had a high withdrawal rate due to adverse side effects; and some unfavorable effects on blood chemical variables were noted which would prevent prolonged administration, although QOL scores had not deteriorated accordingly. Consequently, thiazide diuretics may be well tolerated when a patient is free from metablolic complications which would be worsened by the use of the drug. Captopril was well tolerated without severe adverse effects or deleterious effects on clinical variables despite there being a higher incidence of withdrawal due to insufficient BP reduction. This may be explained by the age-related decrease in the activity of the renin-angiotensin system [9] resulting in a reduced hypotensive response to angiotensin-converting enzyme inibitors. However, milder BP reduction is more often preferable for the aged, as is the significant cardiopulmonary ratio reduction in the absence of reflex tachycardia. These factors appear to have contributed interrelatedly to the improvement and maintenance of QOL in this group. Nicardipine also had favorable effects on QOL without serious deterioration of blood chemical variables. However, the cause of the relative worsening of cognitive function at 12 months as well as the significant worsening of sexual function is difficult to explain, because this drug is known to increase brain blood flow. The scores for sexual function were decreased in all 4 groups, but these kinds of questions put to elderly people are liable to encounter considerable tacit resistance due to their reluctance to answer such questions frankly. Consequently, the possibility remains that the results do not reflect the real status.

In summary, the 4 antihypertensive drugs exerted different effects on the QOL of the elderly hypertensives during the 12 month period. Captopril and nicardipine appear to be the drugs of choice for their favorable effects on QOL without serious adverse effects or deleterious effects on clinical parameters, while trichlormethiazide has only limited use in the elderly mainly because of its unfavorable effects on blood chemical variables. Pindolol has a considerably greater limitation in the treatment of hypertension in the elderly mainly due to its high incidence of adverse physical side effects without significant improvement in QOL. In conclusion, although quantitative evaluation of QOL in the elderly is associated with many difficulties, its significance will inevitably increase in the search for better drugs for the treatment of hypertension in the elderly.

References

1. Croog SH, Levine S, Testa MA, Brown B, Bulpitt CJ, Jenkins DJ, Klerman GL, Williams GH (1986) The effect of antihypertensive therapy on the quality of life. N Engl J Med 314: 1657–1664
2. Ogihara T, Mikami H, Nakamaru M, Masugi F, Otsuka A, Higaki J, Katahira K, Saito H, Kohara K, Rakugi H, Hata T, Kumahara Y (1988) Antihypertensive treatment with a converting enzyme inhibitor, captopril, and its effect on quality of life in the elderly. Geriat Med 26: 291–299 (in Japanese)
3. Hasegawa K (1984) Dementia screening scale. In: Israel L, Kozarevic D, Sartorius N (eds) Source book of geriatric assessment. Karger, Basel, pp 105–106
4. Davidson RA, Caranasos GJ (1987) Should the elderly hypertensive be treated? Arch Intern Med 147: 1933–1937
5. Bühler FR (1983) Age and cardiovascular response adaptation. Determinants of an antihypertensive treatment concept primarily based on beta-blockers and calcium entry blockers. Hypertension 5 (Suppl III): 94–100
6. Wikstrand J, Westergen G, Berglund G, Bracchetti D, Van Couter A, Feldstein CA, Ming KS, Kuramoto K, Landahl S, Meaney E, Pedersen EB, Rahn KH, Shaw J, Smith A, Waal-Manning H (1986) Antihypertensive treatment with metoprolol or hydrochlorothiazide in patients aged 60 to 75 years. JAMA 255: 1304–1310
7. Jenkins AC, Knill JR, Dreslinski GR (1985) Captopril in the treatment of the elderly hypertensive patients. Arch Intern Med 145: 2029–2031
8. Corea L, Bentiboglio M, Verdecchia P, Providenza M (1984) Converting enzyme inhibition vs diuretic therapy as first therapeutic approach to the elderly hypertensive patient. Current Ther Res 36: 347–351
9. Nakamaru M, Ogihara T, Higaki J, Hata T, Maruyama A, Mikami H, Naka T, Iwanaga K, Kumahara Y, Murakami K (1981) Effect of age on active and inactive plasma renin in normal subjects and in patients with essential hypertension. J Am Geriatr Soc 29: 379–382

Nisoldipine: A Replacement Therapy for Nifedipine and Other Vasodilators in the Treatment of Moderate to Severe Hypertension

A. Shamiss, E. Grossman, M. Bursztyn, and T. Rosenthal[1]

Summary. The efficacy of nisoldipine tablets was assessed in 51 patients with severe and moderate hypertension. Nisoldipine replaced nifedipine in 33 patients (group A), with and without beta-blockers. Nisoldipine replaced other vasodilators in 18 patients (group B), with beta-blockers and diuretics. The 2 groups were followed for 6 months. Blood pressure (mmHg) was reduced in group A from $176 \pm 21/101 \pm 22$ to $158 \pm 17/92 \pm 5$ ($P < 0.05$), and in group B from $169 \pm 26/99 \pm 11$ to $143 \pm 12/88 \pm 10$ ($P < 0.01$). None of the patients had aggravation of angina, cerebrovascular disease, or renal failure despite the significant blood pressure reduction. Five patients dropped out because of headaches and ankle edema: two from group A, and three from group B. Nisoldipine appears to offer an effective and safe substitute treatment for severe and moderate hypertensives resistant to, or intolerant of, nifedipine or other vasdilators.

Key words: Replacement triple therapy — Nisoldipine — Nifedipine — Arteriolar vasodilators

Introduction

Nisoldipine is a new derivative of dihydropyridine with chemical characteristics resembling those of nifedipine. Laboratory experiments have shown that nisoldipine is 10-100 times more effective than nifedipine and has both a longer duration of action and a highly selective vascular effect [1]. The present study was designed to examine the efficacy and safety of nisoldipine as a replacement therapy for nifedipine and other vasodilators in patients with severe hypertension who showed resistance or intolerance to their previous vasodilator treatment.

Material and Methods

Patients with moderate to severe hypertension were recruited from the Hypertension Unit of the Sheba Medical Center, Tel Hashomer. Group A consisted of 33 patients, 19 males and 14 females, ranging in age from 21 to 73 years (mean $\pm$ SD, 49 ± 11).

[1] Department of Medicine D, Hypertension Unit, Tel Aviv University Medical School, The Chaim Sheba Medical Center, Tel Hashomer, Israel

Group B consisted of 18 patients, 11 males and 7 females, ranging in age from 37 to 77 years (mean ± SD, 57 ± 12). Group A patients were being treated with nifedipine (40–120 mg/day) with (18 patients) or without (15 patients) beta-blockers, and group B patients were being treated with other vasodilators: hydralazine (10 patients), prazosin (5 patients), and enalapril (3 patients). Criteria for admission to the study included high blood pressure (< 160/95 mmHg) uncontrolled by the previous treatment or unbearable side effects. End organ damage in the patients was as follows: fundal changes in Keith-Wagener-Barker classification, 18 patients in grade II and 3 patients in grade III; left ventricular hypertrophy, 14 patients; renal failure (creatinine 1.5–2.3 mg/dl), 10 patients; and post-myocardial infarction and post-cerebrovascular accident, 1 patient each. Patients had the following concomitant diseases: diabetes mellitus, 7 patients; hydralazine-induced antinuclear factor (ANF), 2 patients; renal artery stenosis, 2 patients; and 1 patient each with systemic lupus erythematosus, nephrotic syndrome (diabetes mellitus), and nephrotic syndrome (focal glomerulosclerosis).

The study was conducted over an 8-month period. Patients were seen weekly in the outpatient clinic for the first 2 months, following which, nisoldipine (10 mg b.i.d.) was substituted for nifedipine or other vasodilators in groups A and B, respectively. The patients were then checked once a week for another 2 months. At each visit, blood pressure and pulse were measured in supine and standing positions both before and 2 h after medication was taken. Blood pressure measurements were taken by the physician each time, using the same standard mercury sphygmomanometer. Diastolic values were taken at the disappearance of 5th-phase Korotkoff sounds, and the average of 3 recordings was considered the representative pressure for each patient. If blood pressure was not controlled following 2 visits, the nisoldipine dosage was doubled. At each visit, body weight was measured and patients were asked and checked for the presence of side effects. Following 2 months of treatment, patients were examined every 2 weeks for another 4 months. Blood samples for urea, creatinine, glucose, blood count, electrolytes, uric acid, antinuclear factor, and urinalysis were taken at the beginning of the study and once a month thereafter. Plasma renin activity and aldosterone levels were measured at the beginning and end of the study for group A patients. Samples for the former were taken at 8:00 a.m. and analyzed using the New England Nuclear Kit according to the method of Haber et al. [2].

Aldosterone levels were measured by a modification of the Buhler method using specific antibodies prepared by the Weizmann Institute [3]. Results were expressed as mean ± standard error of mean (SEM). Student's t-test was used for comparison of results before and after nisoldipine substitution, and difference were considered significant if $P < 0.05$.

Results

Changes in body weight were insignificant, and no significant biochemical changes occurred in any of the patients during the study period (Table 1). Five patients (two in group A, and three in group B) dropped out because of headaches [3] and ankle

Table 1. Laboratory data of patients before and during replacement of nifedipine (group A) and other vasodilators (group B) by nisoldipine

Laboratory parameters	During nifedipine treatment	During other vasodilator treatment	End of study	
			Group A	Group B
Creatinine (mg/dl)	1.18 ± 0.07	1.08 ± 0.15	1.24 ± 0.6	1.08 ± 0.08
Glucose (mg/dl)	104 ± 7.5	95 ± 10	108 ± 5.4	96 ± 9
Sodium (mEq/L)	140 ± 1.2	143 ± 1.7	139 ± 1.2	139 ± 2.1
Potassium (mEq/L)	4.4 ± 0.09	4.1 ± 0.4	4.32 ± 0.08	4.2 ± 0.3
Cholesterol (mg/dl)	215 ± 5.2	211 ± 25	206 ± 6.5	215 ± 23
Triglycerides (mg/dl)	212 ± 31	203 ± 34	218 ± 38	201 ± 32
Plasma renin activity (ng/ml per h)	1.89 ± 0.51	—	1.48 ± 0.34	—
Aldosterone (ng/dl)	19.3 ± 2.1	—	20.1 ± 1.58	—
Sodium excretion (mEq/day)	159 ± 12	—	175 ± 20	—
Weight (kg)	82.8 ± 3.2	77 ± 13	82.6 ± 3.1	76 ± 13

edema [2]. Four patients who suffered from headache and three who developed polyuria tolerated the drug and continued the study to its end. Twenty out of the 33 patients in group A achieved the desired reduction in blood pressure with the initial dose of 10 mg b.i.d. Seven additional patients required an increased dose (20 mg b.i.d.) for improved blood pressure control. Sixteen out of the 18 patients in group B who entered the study because of uncontrolled blood pressure achieved the desired reduction in blood pressure: 13 patients with a dose of 10 mg b.i.d., and 3 patients with a maximal dose of 20 mg b.i.d. The course of the reduction in blood pressure in the 2 groups is shown in Fig. 1, and 2, respectively. Blood pressure was reduced from $176 \pm 21/101 \pm 22$ mmHg to $158 \pm 17/92 \pm 5$ mmHg ($P < 0.05$) in group A, and $169 \pm 26/99 \pm 11$ mmHg to $143 \pm 12/88 \pm 10$ mmHg ($P < 0.01$) in group B.

Discussion

The results of the study indicate that nisoldipine is an effective hypotensive agent and may replace other vasodilators like nifedipine [4], hydralazine, prazosin, and apresoline in the treatment of moderate to severe hypertensive patients who are resistant to or intolerant of these drugs. The benefit of nisoldipine over nifedipine was clearly shown in the 24-h blood pressure monitoring when significantly improved

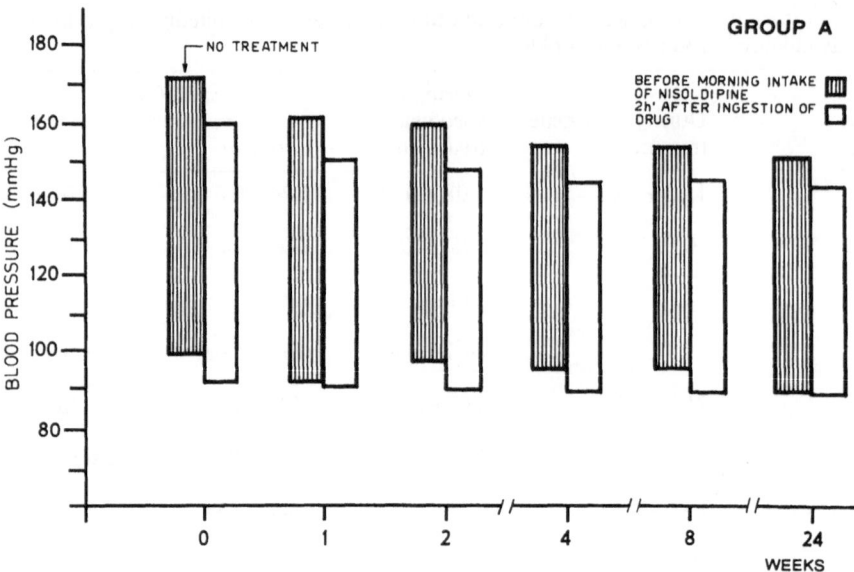

Fig. 1. Blood pressure of patients treated with nisoldipine, previously treated with nifedipine

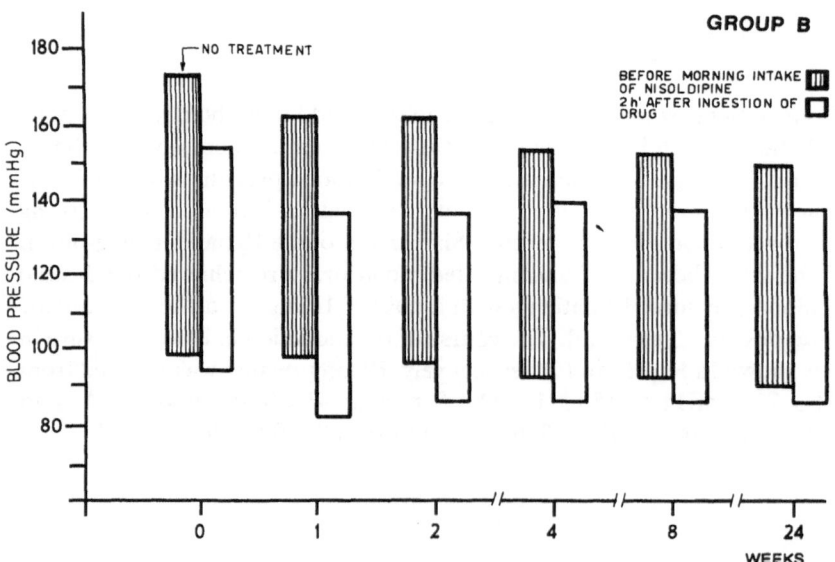

Fig. 2. Blood pressure of patients treated with nisoldipine, previously treated with different vasodilators

control was sustained even after 12 h in many patients, indicating the prolonged hypotensive effect of the drug.

With regard to other vasodilators, most of the patients in group B were resistant to previous treatment, and all of them exhibited the desired reduction in blood pressure with a maximal dose of 20 mg b.i.d. Few patients were referred to the replacement therapy because of adverse effects of their vasodilator drug. In 2 patients with drug-induced lupus, the antinuclear factor disappeared on the replacement therapy by the end of the study. The incidence of severe side effects, such as headaches, flushing, and palpitations, was low, and only 5 patients withdrew from the study because of them: two in group A, and three in group B. Although most of the patients in the present work were treated concomitantly with beta-blockers, it is noteworthy that the decrease in blood pressure with nisoldipine in the 2 groups was not accompanied by significant tachycardia, a finding in agreement with Knorr [5]. With regard to biochemial parameters, our data show no significant changes during the study period.

In conclusion, besides its greater hypotensive effect, nisoldipine appears to offer additional benefits over other vasodilators in patients with moderate to severe hypertension, namely, longer duration of action, and lower incidence of side-effects.

References

1. Kazda S, Garthoff B, Ransch KD, Schluter G (1983) Nisoldipine: New drugs annual. In: Criabine A (ed) Cardiovascular drugs. Raven Press, New York, pp 243
2. Haber E, Koerner T, Page LB, Kliman B, Purnode A (1969) Application of radio-immunoassay for angiotensin 1 to the physiologic measurements of plasma renin activity, in normal human subjects. J Clin Endocrinol Metab 29: 1349-1355
3. Buhler FR, Sealey E, Laragh JH (1974) Radioimmunoassay of plasma aldosterone. In: Laragh JH (ed) Hypertension Manual. Yorke Medical Books, New York, pp 655
4. Grossman E, Rosenthal T (1988) Nisoldipine: A replacement therapy for nifedipine in the treatment of severe hypertension. Clin Cardiol 11: 325-328
5. Knorr A (1982) Antihypertensive effect of nisoldipine, a new calcium antagonist. Br J Pharmacol 76 (Suppl I): 254

Panel Discussion

Chairmen: A. Zanchetti (Milan)
              T. Omae (Osaka)

Discussants: A. Amery (Leuven)
              W. H. Birkenhäger (Rotterdam)
              K. Kuramoto (Tokyo)
              C. Bulpitt (London)
              C. Dollery (London)
              P. Lund-Johansen (Bergen)

Concept of Antihypertensive Treatment in the Elderly

Kuramoto (Tokyo): The level of blood pressure to be treated in the elderly depends on the daily activity and target organ complications of each individual subject. Generally speaking, when systolic blood pressure exceeds 170 mmHg or diastolic blood pressure exceeds 90 mmHg consistently for a certain period of time, I would recommend treating the patient. This dividing line is based on a prospective study we performed in elderly hypertensives. The relationship between the pretreatment blood pressure level and cardiovascular end points was analyzed in the placebo group of the study: cardiovascular end points were significantly higher when systolic blood pressure exceeded 170 mmHg or when diastolic blood pressure exceeded 90 mmHg. The mean age of the patients in this study was 76.5 years. Therefore, we treated patients 60–69 years old when their blood pressure exceeded 160/90, because they are still active in social life. The average life expectancy in Japan is about 75 years for males and 80 years for females. In patients aged 70–79, I start treatment when blood pressure exceeds 170/90. Over 80 years of age, I usually do not start antihypertensive treatment unless there are dangerous complications or symptoms related to hypertension, but I continue to treat hypertensive patients aged 80 years or more if they are already under treatment.

Zanchetti (Milan): I think the question about which blood pressure level should be treated is always a particularly difficult question to answer. Although we have some guidelines derived from the larger controlled trials, these mostly refer to younger or middle-aged patients; as far as the elderly are concerned, it is a particularly difficult question to answer. Our opinions may differ, so I would like to ask Professor Lund-Johansen if he has some other comments.

Lund-Johansen (Bergen): Yes, I think the levels mentioned by Dr. Kuramoto are a bit lower than those generally recommended in the Scandinavian countries. One reason why I think the levels have been set higher is the argument that hypertension is so common in the elderly. If you should follow the rules just suggested by Dr. Kuramoto, a large percent of the elderly population would have to be on antihypertensive treatment.

Kuramoto: This is one viewpoint, but, as I said, the level mentioned should be a consistent level of blood pressure, meaning a blood pressure level which has been maintained for a certain period of time.

Zanchetti: I think a particularly disturbing problem is that most of the treatment trials have taken diastolic blood pressure as a guideline, while in the elderly, the change is predominantly systolic. This gives great difficulties. I do not know whether Professor Dollery, who participated in the MRC trial (which again took diastolic blood pressure as a guideline), can add something or tell us his opinion.

Dollery (London): I think it is important to distinguish between evidence and opinion. As Antoon Amery showed in his review, there's a rather limited amount of evidence from randomized, controlled trials in the elderly, and essentially that concerns all people who have both systolic and diastolic pressure elevations. Taking the EWPHE data and other data into account, when there is both systolic and diastolic elevation, I would say — at least up to the age of 80 and provided people have not got other severe illnesses that clearly make treatment not worthwhile — advancing cancer, dementia, or something of that kind — I would set the diastolic level for treatment a bit higher than Dr. Kuramoto, probably around 100 mmHg; and the systolic pressure level at 175 or 180 mmHg in elderly people. But as you say, isolated systolic hypertension is a very common situation, and on that, until we have the outcome data from the SHEP study — of which we saw a poster today — and from the study that Professor Amery is just starting, we really do not know. There is some evidence that isolated systolic hypertension is associated with increased morbidity and mortality, but whether that suggests an association or a causal association — and the two are very different things — I do not know. At the present moment I am fairly cautious about treating systolic hypertension only. It is fairly common to see elderly persons with a pressure of around 200/85-90, and if you let them rest and you see them once or twice, perhaps the blood pressure comes down to about 180/80 . . . . What do you do then? It is not difficult to lower the systolic pressure a bit, but if you lower the diastolic pressure very much then you are going to impair perfusion to vital areas. At the present moment I feel rather conservative about that kind of patient, and I usually do not treat them, or if I do, it is with very mild treatment.

Zanchetti: Well, we have to face some difference of opinion, because I quite agree it is a matter of opinion, rather than of evidence so far. At the beginning of this symposium we had a nice presentation by Dr. Ueda showing that even pure systolic hypertension is a risk. Then it seems we should tell the doctors it is risk, but this risk should not be decreased simply because we do not have the evidence yet. It is not so simple to say, "Do not do anything until you have the evidence." We should distinguish between evidence and opinion, but then action is a different thing from a trial.

Dollery: The problem I have is that I have seen quite a lot of elderly people whose lives have been made fairly miserable by inappropriately aggressive antihypertensive therapy. So, I think this is an age group where you have to weigh things rather carefully.

Zanchetti: Should it be a matter of trial and error — careful trying and careful correction? Professor Amery, one of the slides you showed indicated there was about the same advantage in treating elderly patients with systolic blood pressure between 160 and 180 mmHg and those with higher systolic blood pressure. Do you share the opinion that systolic blood pressure should be very high before starting treatment, or do you favor the opinion that whenever it is higher than 160, provided diastolic is 90 or 95 or over, the patient should be treated, carefully of course?

Amery (Leuven): We all agree that systolic blood pressure is a major risk factor. This is no to be discussed, and that was already emphasized by several people today. Still, we do not know if by decreasing it we shall also decrease the risk; that is the whole problem. Treatment will certainly provoke some side effects, and are the side effects that we provoke worth being provoked? If you look at the data of the EWPHE I have presented, all these patients had increased systolic and diastolic blood pressures, even after 3 months of placebo treatment. So, on the basis of these data, I would not say that we can advise treatment in isolated systolic hypertension. In isolated systolic hypertension, I would look more at the patient than at the pressure and try to see if there is any reason, apart from the pressure, to treat the patient — I mean, other symptoms, other signs, other complications. If there are no other complications, no other signs or symptoms, I would be very hesitant until we have the results of intervention trials. This opinion is based on the scanty evidence provided by the two trials which have been published. In the trial by Coop et al. on treatment of hypertension in the elderly, as far as isolated systolic hypertension was concerned, no indication was found of a better outcome of treatment. If there was any difference, it was in the reverse direction. On the other hand, there is the evidence of the pilot trial of SHEP. There have been oral reports at meetings, but no published data, suggesting that treatment could be of some advantage. So, the situation is balanced, and in this situation I would be hesitant. If the diastolic blood pressure is above 95 at repeated measurements, I would treat the patients, but otherwise I would wait and observe the patients carefully.

Zanchetti: I think we should move now to another point. Which weight should be given to the presence or absence of cardiovascular complications, and which complications, in deciding whether to start treatment and how to perform treatment.

Birkenhäger (Rotterdam): This is just to underscore what has been said this afternoon about the ranking order of causes of death in several countries.

As you can see in Table 1, all circulatory diseases are running far beyond other conditions, for instance, neoplasma, as has also been shown by Dr. Ueda in his impressive series. If you look at the specific causes of death (or for that matter, chronic morbidity) in hypertension, it is quite evident that ischemic heart disease remains rather constant throughout the entire age range. In Japan, we have this well-known low-incidence of ischemic heart disease, but if we then move to stroke, we see that Japan's score is very high indeed. Stroke mortality shows a clear pro-

Table 1. Mortality rate per 100,000 for hypertension, stroke, and ischemic heart disease in developed countries during 1980 (after World Health Statistics Annual 1982 and 1984)

	55-64 years		65-74 years		> 75 years	
	Male	Female	Male	Female	Male	Female
Hypertension						
United States	27.0	16.6	56.6	46.6	158.0	177.6
England and Wales	17.7	8.3	47.5	30.3	101.6	99.1
Australia	14.8	9.5	46.4	29.2	124.9	159.7
Japan	9.4	5.8	47.7	35.7	313.3	332.5
Stroke						
United States	74.6	56.8	258.0	188.6	1114.6	1115.9
England and Wales	114.1	82.2	434.5	334.7	1517.1	1662.9
Australia	120.4	79.6	411.7	284.1	1568.1	1803.0
Japan	204.2	117.9	770.5	476.4	2788.5	2300.6
Ischemic heart disease						
United States	579.9	188.5	1349.0	602.6	3605.0	2651.4
England and Wales	712.6	203.4	1590.2	661.5	3300.6	2099.6
Australia	592.6	186.3	1506.3	637.1	3446.5	2365.8
Japan	92.1	31.1	270.5	143.7	801.6	600.6

gression with age as far as the incidences are concerned, with the exception of Australia, which is very particular. (I think it is time for me to move to Australia, that is, if it would be agreeable to Austin Doyle, which I doubt.) We have seen that many of these kinds of complications have now been proven to be preventable by adequate treatment of hypertension.

The second table serves to solve one of the dilemmas in comparing the outcome of the different trials. I guess every one of you has realized that the incidence rates of cardiovascular complications: mainly ischemic heart disease, congestive heart failure, and stroke, have been presented in very different ways. We have witnessed at the main meeting that it was difficult to compare the incidence rates in the different trials. I would like to emphasize that converting event rates to 1 000 patient-observation years would greatly facilitate the comparison of trial results.

Table 2 shows that the general population experiences a cardiovascular event rate of 10 per 1 000 observation years (study 1). If we then look at some data from Framingham (study 2), we see that separated young low-pressure male subjects have an incidence of 6 per 1 000 observation years, while this is tripled in old people with low pressure. This rate of 20 per 1 000 observation years is the same as in young people with high pressure. In old people with high pressure we observe an impressive increase (50 cardiovascular events per 1 000 patient years). This provides a firm basis for interpreting the results of the intervention trials. When focusing on the placebo groups, we see that the MRC trial (study 4) has engaged subjects who were hardly more at risk than the general population from study 1. So, in fact, there was not much to gain in this particular trial by active treatment. As it happened, the benefits were indeed marginal: a reduction from 12 to 10 events per 1 000 observation years, but then that was the best which could have been expected. It is obviously not fair to extrapolate these results to the general hypertensive population. Let us

Table 2. Cardiovascular risk: incidence per 1 000 observation years

Study (No. and type)	Sex	Included	(treated)	Source
1. General population	M/F	10		WHS Ann.
2. Young, low pressure	M	6		FRAM.
Old, low pressure	M	20		FRAM.
Young, high pressure	M	20		FRAM.
Old, high pressure	M	50		FRAM.
3. Adults, mild hypertension	M/F	24	(17)	ANBPS
(60 + years)	M/F	35	(23)	ANBPS
4. Adults, mild hypertension	M	12	(10)	MRC
5. 60 + years, moderate hypertension	M/F	64	(32)	EWPHE

now take the Australian trial (study 3). Here we see a more realistic rate of events in the placebo group, which is similar to the Framingham data in young hypertensives. Apparently, the returns of treatment now become more substantial. The benefits become even more obvious in the older subgroup in the Australian trial, with 35 events per 1 000 being reduced to 23 by active treatment. Of course the climax of this table is to be observed at the bottom (study 5), which has been discussed by Professor Amery. It is quite clear that at this level of cardiovascular risk you can really achieve a substantial improvement by treatment, even though the residual event rate remains increased.

I think it is highly probable that we will obtain further improvement in the next decade. Some few key issues in treatment have already been discussed. I like to stress that we should titrate the treatment according to the pressure with the subject up in order to prevent cerebral ischemia as a hazard of treatment. This has already been pointed out by Professor Bulpitt several years ago and seems to be supported by the findings from Professor Omae's department, presented at this meeting, regarding cerebral blood flow. Secondly, we should take the J-shape phenomenon with regard to coronary perfusion at extremely low diastolic pressures more seriously than we have done so far. Cruickshank's findings appear to have been supported by other trials. The third point is that the potential advantages of newer antihypertensive product should be put to the test. Professor Amery has mentioned a coming trial in Europe, and I assume that Japan has both the population and the resources to conduct similar trials. Before that, we cannot say anything sensible about the true potential of the newer classes of antihypertensive drugs.

Amery: I would like to comment on the J-shaped curve in the elderly. This J-shaped curve has been discussed on many occasions, but some further interest has been raised by the recent paper of Cruickshank in the *Lancet*. Now, it is clear there should be a J-shaped curve somewhere if you go too low with pressure. However, if you take the data published by Cruickshank in the *Lancet*, and if you realize that what he gives is mean and standard errors, it is very clear the difference between the 3 groups is statistically not significant — that is one point. Furthermore. I do not think it has been proven by that paper that the J-shaped curve was caused by the treatment. I think this is a point which is still open for discussion. We do not know really what is the egg and what is the chicken. In other words, is it because the pressure is brought very low that the patients die sooner, or is it the opposite — because they are in bad shape they get low blood pressure and then they die sooner? I would like to see that first analyzed, compared with untreated patients, to see if this was anything to do with treatment or not.

Birkenhäger: First of all, I think that the query about the chicken and the egg is correct, but the same thing did not apply to systolic pressure, which would then weaken your argument, I think. Moreover, there are several other findings, for instance, from the Göteborg Primary Prevention Trial, also demonstrating an upward move in risk in those who had diastolic in-treatment pressures below 85. There are several other data in publication which I am not allowed to cite. If you consider isolated systolic hypertension, this issue becomes even more urgent of course, because the SHEP trial has shown that you can get reductions towards 55 mmHg diastolic. I think it makes sense to keep in mind the physiology, since the myocardium is perfused during the diastole.

Zanchetti: I think that once again we should distinguish between evidence, hints, and opinions. As far as the J-shaped curve is concerned, we have hints, and we have a good explanation for this — this is why these hints seem to be particularly persuading, but certainly we need stronger evidence. Certainly there must be a point of inflection, a blood pressure level below which the risk turns to an increase. Whether it is 85 or 80 mmHg or lower, certainly needs clearer evidence. I think we should now proceed to discuss another point, the problem — which is certainly very important — of the effects of treatment on the quality of life of the elderly hypertensive.

Bulpitt (London): I think the biggest problem of hypertension in the elderly is in the very elderly. We can more or less assume that in a man who is fit and in his early 60s the results relevant to middle-aged men will still apply, but when you get to the very elderly, things are very difficult. Dr. Kuramoto has told you that a woman in Japan has an expectation of life of 80 years and a man, 75. Now I can tell you that we cannot reach those levels in Europe or the USA, but still we have this difference of 5 years — a woman lives 5 years longer than a man in most developed industrialized countries, on average. In America, Sidney Katz did some studies on activities of daily living to work out how active these women were in the extra 5 years of life. He found they were not very active — they were disabled and impoverished, because they did not draw the pensions that their husband drew; they were confined to the house; and they were confined often to the wheelchair with arthritis. He actually concluded that it was not worth living an extra 5 years as a woman. So I think it is very important that we worry about this quality of life aspect. Most experts in geriatric medicine treat their patients to keep them well and active in the community; they actually treat on the basis of quality of life. They are also struck by the finding (as you have seen in many studies and a recently finished study) that the elderly with high levels of blood pressure do rather well. They live quite a long period of time. This, I imagine, is because their cardiovascular system is suffcently good to enable them to live for some time. However, I think the geriatricians have gone too far in the negative aspects of it, because they forget that prevention may still have a place in the elderly. As you saw from Dr. Birkenhäger's comments, a lot of the elderly, especially in Japan, are still dying of strokes. However you look at that — certainly from the quality of life angle — it is not a nice way to go (with a stroke). The patients will often say they do not take any notice of your advice, because they want to go quickly and die quickly and not linger in the hospital. Unfortunately, I am afraid a stroke is just the sort of condition where they will end up in the worst situation. Professor Birkenhäger pointed out that it is the elderly that get high stroke rates, and we certainly know what Professor Amery showed that at least under the age of 80 you can prevent strokes in about 40%. In the elderly, reduction of a lot of strokes — and 40% is a lot — has a considerable impact. In the EWPHE trial, for example, every 90 patients you treat for 1 year you save one stroke, whereas according to MRC trial, it is 840 middle-aged men and women that you have to treat for 1 year to save a stroke. So, there is a lot of potential for doing a lot of good in the elderly. These are all theories, though; there is very little evidence, especially in the very elderly, as to benefits. Therefore, there are going to be big attempts to measure the quality of life of treated elderly hypertensives to make sure that the people are still ambulant and well and in the community. A poster was shown today by Dr. Mikami and his colleagues where they compared an ACE inhibitor, a calcium channel blocker, a diuretic, and a beta-blocker on the quality of life of a group of elderly in Japan. They found that the ACE inhibitor and the calcium channel blocker were the best in preserving the quality of life. This may be the sort of pattern we are going to find, although it is very difficult to be certain at this moment. It is true that drugs like methyldopa may cause postural hypotension, and it is very important to monitor blood pressure on the standing pressure in the elderly. Having said that, in the European working party trial where methyldopa was an additional drug, we did not get so much trouble as you might expect. I think it is because the tablets were started as a small dose of 250 mg at night. Some of the elderly patients thought this was one of the better sleeping tablets that they had come across. So, I do not really want to predict what would be good for the quality of life in the elderly, especially the very elderly. I think we just have to wait for these trials to tell us the answers. Fortunately with SHEP, with the Systeur (the trial that is going to be started by the European working party), I know that quality of life measures are planned and that we will have an estimate of the psychological and physical well-being, the social well-being, and all the things that are very important in deciding whether an elderly person's life is worth living or not.

Zanchetti: What is the opinion of the members of the panel about the types of drugs that should be used in treating the elderly, and how one class or the other could be chosen?

Dollery: It seems to me, looking at the evidence of the European working party trial, that the diuretics are the drug to beat, because the diuretics are of low cost, they are simple for the patients to take, and there is evidence of long-term efficacy. All of the other drugs we are talking about, which may have marginal advantages in terms of side-effect profile — although again, low doses of diuretics have a relatively favorable side-effect profile — these other drugs have to show that they can beat the diuretics. When I am treating elderly patients with moderate hypertension, I start with a diuretic (usually either Dyazide or Moduretic 25, which is one of the arms of the treatment we are using in the MRC elderly hypertension trial) unless there are some specific contraindications to using them in a particular patient. For example, I would not use them in somebody who had maturity onset diabetes or a history of gout.

Zanchetti: Would you use the same large doses of thiazides as were used in the MRC trial?

Dollery: No, I think I indicated I have retreated a bit from there. When I said Moduretic 25, that is the half-strength Moduretic.

Lund-Johansen: Well, I think the easiest type of problem is when we have patients with other diseases, and this appears very frequently in the elderly. So, we have special cases where there would be a special indication for one class of drug and contra-indications to others. We can take, as an example, the patient with hypertension and coronary heart disease. If this patient is able to tolerate a beta-blocker, I think this would be the drug of first choice in most countries. If there are contraindications to beta-blockers, a calcium antagonist would be the first choice. Often we have to use the combination of a beta-blocker and a calcium antagonist. If we have patients with hypertension and peripheral vascular disease, obviously the beta-blockers would be contraindicated and we would prefer a drug not reducing peripheral blood flow. I could continue with these special types of patients, and I think we all remember these patients when we make the first choice of drugs. Nevertheless, what I have seen quite often is that people tend to forget the contraindications when they change. So I think that is one important message: if the first drug does not work and you have to change, do not forget the original contraindications and problems of your patient. Apart from that, I think we can decide what drug to use on the basis of the pharmacological properties of the drug, including their hemodynamic effects, and, as I have shown, they are widely different from one compound to another. I agree with all other speakers that we should take the blood pressure in the standing position in the elderly and that we should not make life miserable for any elderly hypertensive patient. In most cases, however, it is a matter of trial and error.

Zanchetti: I think Professor Weidmann suggested that if a patient has diabetes (even type 2 diabetes, which is present very often in the elderly patient), then a calcium antagonist might be the drug of first choice.

Weidmann (Bern): I would fully agree with Professor Dollery, in fact. The point I made is that the calcium antagonists and the converting enzyme inhibitors, too, from their side-effect profile, seem very acceptable, perhaps more acceptable than diuretics. Of course if we take the one major fact of the long-term prognosis, I would fully agree that the only hard data we really have is that diuretics do reduce morbid events. The comment I made was that antihypertensive treatment of diabetics seems to me to be somewhat easier with calcium antagonists and converting enzyme inhibitors than with diuretics, but I do not think we do have the proof of the superiority of any one of these classes at this time.

Zanchetti: What do you think, Colin, about the pathophysiological evidence that the elderly generally have a reduced blood volume? Is this something which makes the advantage of diuretics somewhat unexpected?

Dollery: Certainly it is a reasonable argument, but I have to become very cautious about predicting outcome based on theoretical considerations. We were talking about that earlier concerning coronary artery disease and myocardial infarction in hypertension, where I am still puzzled that we have not done better. So, I think one has to be cautious. I think the real message is we do need trials with these other drugs. I am very anxious to see large-scale comparative trials launched which will preferably take as a benchmark a standard drug like a diuretic and then compare ACE inhibitors and calcium antagonists, because we need to know. If they are better, we need to know; if they are worse, we need to know. If they are the same, we need to know; because if they are the same, then we can simply observe the contraindications and choose which seems to be best on the symptom profile. We don't know, and it is a big extrapolation to say that they will be the same. I think my bet is that they will not be exactly the same.

Weidmann: Since we heard so many interesting comments about the J-curve on the potential risk of excessive reduction in blood pressure, I think one point in the elderly which I would consider is the postprandial fall in blood pressure. I would like to ask the panelists whether any of you have data on the effects of drugs on postprandial blood pressure. Should we study more in that area?

Bulpitt: It has been said that something like 20% of the very elderly would have huge postprandial falls in systolic blood pressure and an even larger proportion would have a fall of at least 20 mmHg on standing up. So, recently one of my senior house officers, Dr. McCray, repeated these studies on my inpatients. Now they were inpatients, but they were fit to stand up; and he did the measurements after breakfast. He found nobody (out of about 30 people) who had fall of systolic pressure of 40 mmHg and only two had a fall of 20. I asked him to repeat the measurements after lunch; and then he did find a larger fall, but still he found nobody with a systolic fall of 40 and only one or two more with a fall of 20. Whether it was before lunch or after lunch, the diastolic pressure still went up when the patients stood up. It was the systolic that came down, and the difference was 13 mmHg after lunch and 9 mmHg before lunch. So, postprandial measurement does make a difference, but in no way is the difference of the size that some previous studies have led us to believe.

Zanchetti: We have a final point to discuss, and this is the problem of age. Personally, as a doctor, I refrain from the general concept that there is a retirement age from the possibilities of treatment: I think our patients should be treated at any age. Here again, the matter is to make the balance between possible advantages and possible disadvantages.

Amery: I have shown a slide where we looked at the event rate expressed per 1 000 patient years as asked by Professor Birkenhäger, in function of age in treated and untreated patients. As you may remember, there was an interaction between treatment effect and age, suggesting that the treatment effect was decreasing with age. In fact, above age 80 in these patients, there was no real evidence that we did decrease the event rate. Again, I do not know if it was because of the age that we did not decrease the event rate or if, in this particular group, there was something else which we could not identify in our study. Nevertheless, I would hesitate to advocate antihypertensive therapy in a hypertensive patient above age 80 without any other disease and without any complaints just because he has somewhat higher pressure. I would look first at the patient, and then at his pressure.

Birkenhäger: That does not mean that you should not continue treatment in somebody who has been successfully treated before and came into the age range beyond 80. This slide you showed applied only to those above 80 upon entering treatment, right?

Amery: That is of course correct.

Zanchetti: You do not imply that patients successfully treated for 20 or more years should stop treatment on their 80th birthday?

Birkenhäger: I said it, because you used the term "retirement from treatment."

Zanchetti: I quite agree. I was simply joking. Are there other comments on this problem of age? Is there any comment about the debated point at what age you should consider a patient as an elderly patient?

Omae (Osaka): The most difficult problem in the treatment of aged people is that biological aging does not parallel calendar aging. It very much varies from person to person. That is why epidemiological data or data obtained by studies of groups do not necessarily apply to individual persons. This also applies to cardiovascular diseases, too. It is my experience, for instance, that in a few very aged individuals there is very slight or apparently no cerebral atherosclerosis. Therefore, I think as Dr. Kuramoto pointed out, that treatment should be directed to individuals. So, if a hypertensive subject has a young cardiovascular system, even at the age of 80, I think he or she should be treated. However, if we lower blood pressure too much, this might be very harmful in some patients. In my opinion there are three possibilities in the elderly hypertensive. Some patients can get a beneficial effect from antihypertensive treatment; in some patients there are no beneficial nor detrimental effects; some other patients get harmful effects from antihypertensive treatment, especially those with very severe atherosclerosis or insufficient perfusion to various organs.

Bulpitt: I think we were helped in this respect in the EWPHE trial by having selected patients who biologically were not too old; because, as we all realize, the more the aorta gets stiff and noncompliant, the more the systolic blood pressure goes up and the diastolic goes down. One entry criteria for the EWPHE trial was having a high diastolic; so, I think the patients entered in the EWPHE trial perhaps selected themselves as people whose cardiovascular system was not as old as it might have been. Maybe that is one reason why the trials based on diastolic blood pressure have done so well.

Omae: There are data presented by Yokouchi et al. at the Japanese Society of Hypertension several years ago. At an old people's home, for those over the age of 80, there was no relationship between the blood pressure and life expectancy or mortality. This agrees with the data of the EWPHE trial. Eighty years, therefore, is the age limit for treatment when groups are considered; but in clinical terms, some of the individuals with very old ages can be treated with benefit.

Amery: Professor Bulpitt, I would like to know what you really meant when you said that the higher the diastolic blood pressure the younger the vascular tree.

Bulpitt: Yes, I think there is a real concept that we have not got to grips with, that of burnt-out diastolic hypertension. There are people who at the age of 60-65 may have diastolic values of 95-100 mmHg, and, therefore, have sustained diastolic hypertension. As they get older, the pulse pressure widens, the aorta gets more stiff, diastolic pressure comes down, and they end up by having isolated systolic hypertension. They no longer have diastolic hypertension. If they still had diastolic hypertension, maybe their cardiovascular tree would be a little younger, Of course, this is the theory, and evidence is scanty.

Lund-Johansen: Well, since I have some 20-year follow-up data on this, I can say that this is exactly what happened in my patients, who were treated for 20 years with conventional treatment. Diastolic blood pressure was well controlled; but somewhat to my surprise, when I looked at the intra-arterial recordings at rest and during exercise, these patients had, exactly as you said, been changed over to having isolated systolic hypertension when they were between 60 and 69.

Zanchetti: I think that after Professor Amery very well summarized the evidence from his own trial and the other trials, we can conclude that the elderly hypertensive can be treated with benefits that often are greater than the disadvantages. How the elderly hypertensive should be treated is still an open question. The drugs which were used in the EWPHE trial gave benefits greater than disadvantages, but they were anyway drugs that were chosen in the 1970s, because there were widely used at that time. Now we have new classes of drugs, and we have learned today that one of these classes, the calcium antagonists, has very interesting properties that seem particularly useful in the elderly. However, as has been pointed out by several speakers, we need to have trials showing these drugs have long-term benefits. It is in some way refreshing to know that the new Systeur (the new trial on hypertension in the elderly that Professor Amery is planning and to which our group is happy to participate) is considering a calcium antagonist as the drug of first choice for the treatment arm of the trial.

Author Index

Alli, C. 117
Amery, A. 17, 157
Applegate, W.B. 135
Asmer, R.G. 143
Ausiello, M. 177
Avanzini, F. 117

Bardelli, M. 183
Bettelli, G. 117
Borhani, N.O. 135
Brignoli, M. 177
Bursztyn, M. 227

Campanacci, L. 183
Carretta, R. 183
Chikamori, T. 123
Colombo, F. 117
Corso, R. 117
Curb, J.D. 135
Cutler, J.A. 135

Davis, B.R. 135
De Divitiis, O. 177
Devoto, M.A. 117
Di Somma, S. 177
Distante, A. 127
Di Tullio, M. 117
Dollery, C.T. 33

Fabris, B. 183
Fagard, R. 17, 157
Ferrari, P. 85
Fischetti, F. 183
Fujishima, M. 3
Furberg, C.D. 135

Garderisi, M. 177

Grossman, E. 227

Hasegawa, T. 171
Hasuo, Y. 3
Hata, T. 213, 219
Hawkins, C.M. 135
Higaki, J. 213, 219
Hoefnagels, W.H.L. 205

Iimura, O. 171
Inoue, I. 151
Ishida, H. 123

Jansen, R.W.M.M. 205

Kajiyama, G. 151
Kawamoto, A. 123
Kido, K. 151
Kikuchi, K. 171
Komura, H. 171
Kumahara, Y. 213, 219
Kuriyama, Y. 69
Kuzume, O. 123

L'abbate, A. 127
Lakatos, E. 135
Lattanzi, F. 127
Laurent, St. 143
Leonetti, G. 103
Lepira, B. 157
Licata, G. 189
Liguori, V. 177
Lijnen, P. 157
Lukarini, A.R. 127
Lund-Johansen, P. 53

Magnotta, C. 177
Marchioli, R. 117
Mariotti, G. 117
Masugi, F. 213, 219
Matsubayashi, K. 123
Matsumoto, K. 151
Matsuura H. 151
M'Buyamba-Kabangu,
  J.R. 157
McFate Smith, W. 135
Mikami, H. 213, 219
Muiesan, S. 183

Nakamaru, M. 213, 219
Nardi, E. 189
Newman, C.M. 33
Noto, G. 189
Novo, S. 189
Nozawa, A. 171

Ogihara, T. 213, 219
Ogura, H. 123
Ohtomo, T. 171
Omae, T. 3, 69
Omvik, P. 53
Orsini, E. 127
Oshima, T. 151
Otsuki, T. 151
Otsuka, A. 213, 219
Ozawa, T. 123

Page, L.B. 135
Perry, H.M., Jr. 135
Petitto, M. 177
Picano, E. 127
Probstfield J.L. 135

Radice, M.   117
Rosenfeld, J.B.   197
Rosenthal, T.   227

Safar, M.E.   143
Safavian, A.M.   143
Salvetti, A.   127
Sato, N.   171
Sawada, T.   69
Severi, S.   127
Shamiss, A.   227
Shimada, K.   123
Shingu, T.   151

Soubies, Ph.L.   143
Staessen, J.   17
Strano, A.   189
Suzuki, S.   171

Takada, T.   171
Taioli, E.   117
Tognoni, G.   117
Trost, B.N.   85

Ueda, K.   3

Van Hoof, R.   17
Van Lier, H.J.J.   205
Villella, M.   117
Vran, F.   183

Weidmann, P.   85
Wittenberg, C.   197

Zanchetti, A.   103
Zussino, A.   117

Key Word Index

Aging   123
Angiotensin-converting enzyme
   inhibitors   85
Antihypertensive drugs   69, 213
Antihypertensive medication   33
Antihypertensive therapy   17, 143
Antihypertensive treatment   85, 219
Arterial compliance   143, 189
Arteriolar Vasodilators   227
Atenolol   157
Autonomic nervous system   123

Blacks   157
Blood pressure   117, 123

Calcium antagonists   53, 103
Calcium channel blockers   85
Calciuria   171
CBF autoregulation   69
Cerebral circulation   69
Combination treatment   103
Complications   213
Compliance   183
Control of bood pressure   117
Coronary artery disease (CAD)   127

Diltiazem   53
Dipyridamole   127
Drug treatment   135

Echocardiography   127
Elderly   17, 33, 117, 177, 189, 205
Elderly hypertension   3, 123
Elderly hypertensives   213, 219
Epidemiology   17
Erythrocyte sodium   157

Essential hypertension   143, 151, 171
Exercise   53

Flow   183

Glucose metabolism   85

Hemodynamics   53, 123
Hemodynamic TIA   69
Hisayama study   3
Hydrochlorothiazide   205
Hypertension   17, 53, 69, 103, 117, 127,
   157, 177, 189, 197, 205, 213
Hypertension accompanying diabetes
   mellitus   85
Hypotensive response   33

Intracellular calcium   151

Large arteries   183
Left ventricular mass   189
Lipids   85
Lymphocytes   151

Metabolic effects   197
Mortality   17
Myocardial infarction   3

Natriuresis   171
Nicardipine SR   183
Nifedipine   53, 151, 171, 189, 197, 227
Nisoldipine   53, 197, 227
Nitrendipine   157, 205

Parathyroid hormone 171
Pathogenesis 85
Pharmacokinetics 33
Plasma renin activity 151
Prevention 135
Pulse wave velocity 143

Quality of life 135, 219

Radionuclide ventriculography 177
Renal function 197
Replacement triple therapy 227

Stroke 3, 135
Survival curves 3
Systolic hypertension 135

Tiapamil 53
Total mortality 135
Treatment 205
Treatment status 117

Ventricular function 177
Verapamil 53